DRUGS
OF CHOICE
current perspectives on drug use

DRUGS
OF CHOICE
current perspectives on drug use
SECOND EDITION

RICHARD G. SCHLAADT

University of Oregon

PETER T. SHANNON

Lane County Mental Health Department

PRENTICE-HALL, Englewood Cliffs, New Jersey 07632

Library of Congress Cataloging-in-Publication Data

SCHLAADT, RICHARD G., (date)
   Drugs of choice.

   Includes bibliographies and index.
   1. Drugs. 2. Psychotropic drugs. 3. Drug
utilization—United States. 4. Substance abuse—
United States. I. Shannon, Peter T. II. Title.
RM301.S43 1986   362.2'9   85-17001
ISBN 0-13-220740-0

Cover design: Joe Curcio
Manufacturing buyer: Barbara Kittle

Printed in the United States of America

10   9   8   7   6   5   4   3   2   1

ISBN 0-13-220740-0 01

PRENTICE-HALL INTERNATIONAL, INC., *London*
PRENTICE-HALL OF AUSTRALIA PTY. LIMITED, *Sydney*
EDITORA PRENTICE-HALL DO BRASIL, LTDA., *Rio de Janeiro*
PRENTICE-HALL CANADA INC., *Toronto*
PRENTICE-HALL HISPANOAMERICANA, S.A., *Mexico*
PRENTICE-HALL OF INDIA PRIVATE LIMITED, *New Delhi*
PRENTICE-HALL OF JAPAN, INC., *Tokyo*
PRENTICE-HALL OF SOUTHEAST ASIA PTE. LTD., *Singapore*
WHITEHALL BOOKS LIMITED, *Wellington, New Zealand*

CONTENTS

PREFACE   xvii

1

INTRODUCTION   1

THE GRAY AREA   1
  Individual Differences   2
  Quality Control   2
  Set   3
  Setting   4
  Legality   4

PERSPECTIVE ON DRUGS   4
    Caffeine   5
    Alcohol   5
    Nicotine   5
    Stimulants and Sedatives   6
    Marijuana   7
    Hallucinogens   7
    Opiates   7
    Volatile Substances   8
DRUG TECHNOLOGY   8
    Over-the-Counter Drugs   10
    Commercial Drugs   11
    Recreational Drugs   11
    Herbal Preparations   12
    Illegal Drugs   12
SUMMARY   13
NOTES   13

WHY PEOPLE USE DRUGS

15

INTRODUCTION   15
PSYCHOLOGICAL FACTORS   16
    Recreation/Social Facilitation   16
    Social Facilitation   16
    Sensation Seeking   16
    Religious/Spiritual Factors   18
    Altered States   18
    Rebellion and Alienation   19
SOCIOLOGICAL FACTORS: PEER PRESSURE AND GROUP ENTRY   20
DEPENDENCY STATES:PSYCHOLOGICAL PERSPECTIVES   20
    Existential/Psychoanalytic View   20
    The Adlerian Theory of Ego Compensation   22
DEPENDENCY STATES:SOCIOLOGICAL PERSPECTIVES   22
DEPENDENCY STATES:BIOLOGICAL MECHANISMS   23
    Philosophical Concerns   23
    Biochemical Theory   23
    Enkephalins and Endorphins   24
SUMMARY   26
NOTES   26

THE DRUG SCENE

28

INTRODUCTION   28
THE YOUTH DRUG SCENE   29
   Background   29
   Drugs on Campus   32
   Drugs in the Military   33
   Drugs and Athletics   35
THE ADULT DRUG SCENE   39
   Alcohol   39
   Tranquilizers and Sedative-Hypnotics   39
   Nicotine   40
   Caffeine   40
   Aspirin   40
   Amphetamines   41
   Marijuana   41
   Opiates   41
   The Workplace   41
THE SENIOR CITIZEN DRUG SCENE   43
   Types of Drug Use   44
SUMMARY   47
NOTES   47

PHARMACOLOGY
basic concepts of drug activity

50

SPECIFIC PHARMACOLOGY   50
CONSUMER SAFETY   51
   The Chemical (Drug) Being Considered   51
   The Receptor Mechanisms Affected   51
   The Dosage and Method of Administration   52
   The Kinds of Drug Interactions That Will Likely Take Place   55
   The Potential for Allergic Reactions   55
   The Potential for Tolerance and the Potential for Physical Dependence   55
THE NERVOUS SYSTEM AS AN ELECTRICAL SYSTEM   59
ANATOMY AND PHYSIOLOGY   61
   Central Nervous System   61
   Peripheral Nervous System   65
SUMMARY   71
NOTES   71

5

STIMULANTS

73

AMPHETAMINES 73
    Introduction 73
    Dexedrine 76
    Methamphetamine 76
METHYLPHENIDATE (RITALIN) 78
    Physical and Psychological Effects 79
    Hyperkinesis 79
    Educating the Hyperkinetic Child 80
COCAINE 81
    Introduction 81
    History 82
    Physiological and Pharmacological Effects 83
    Psychological and Sociological Effects 86
    Medical Use 86
CAFFEINE (XANTHINES) 87
    Introduction 87
    History 89
    Physical Effects 91
    Caffeinism 91
    Decaffeinated Coffee 94
MDA (METHYLENEDIOXYAMPHETAMINE) 94
LOOK-ALIKE DRUGS 95
SUMMARY 95
NOTES 96

6

TOBACCO
america's number one
preventable hazard

99

HISTORY 99
CHEMISTRY 100
THE 1979 SURGEON GENERAL'S REPORT 101
PHYSIOLOGICAL EFFECTS 102
    Gases 103
CHRONIC DISEASE 103
    Cardiovascular System 104
    Strokes (Apoplexy) 106
    Respiratory Diseases 106
    Lung and Other Cancers 107

SIDE EFFECTS   107
    Metabolism   107
    Appetite Reduction   108
    Fetal Nutrition and Pregnancy   109
    Exercise and Physical Performance   110
    Sexual Activity   110
    Other Health Factors   111
    Nicotine and Coffee Intake   111
    Vitamins   111
PSYCHOLOGICAL EFFECTS   112
    The Smoking Habit   112
    Reasons for Smoking and Not Smoking   112
    Types of Smokers   113
ALTERNATIVES TO SMOKING AND CONSEQUENT PROBLEMS   114
KICKING THE HABIT   115
    Methods   115
    Benefits of Quitting   115
    Changing to Other Forms of Tobacco Consumption   116
TOBACCO AND THE NONSMOKER   121
    Effects of Tobacco Smoke on Nonsmokers   121
    Nonsmokers' Rights   122
DIVERSIFICATION   123
SUMMARY   126
NOTES   126

7

DEPRESSANTS AND THE BODY

130

INTRODUCTION   130
SEDATIVE-HYPNOTICS   130
    Classification   130
    Physical Effects   131
    Barbiturates   131
    Methaqualone   133
MINOR TRANQUILIZERS   134
    Classification   134
    History   134
    Physical Effects   135
    Valium (Diazepam)   135
    Librium (Chlordiazepoxide)   138
MAJOR TRANQUILIZERS (ANTIPSYCHOTICS)   139
    Classification   139
    Current Use   139
    Physical Effects   140
DELIRIANTS (VOLATILE SUBSTANCES)   140

Classification 140
History 141
Physical Effects 141
Psychological Effects 142
SUMMARY 142
NOTES 143

ALCOHOL
america's number one
drug problem

145

INTRODUCTION 145
CONSUMPTION OF ALCOHOL IN THE UNITED STATES 146
    Youth 146
    Adults 147
    The Elderly 147
HISTORY 147
WHY DO PEOPLE DRINK? 148
    Advertising 148
    Peer Acceptance, Search for Adulthood, and Rebellion 149
    Changing Sex Roles 150
    Gender and Culture 150
    Sex 150
PHYSIOLOGICAL EFFECTS 151
    Circulatory System and Blood 151
    Nervous System 153
    Liver 154
    Digestive System 155
    Kidneys 155
    Body Temperature 156
    Fetal Alcohol Syndrome 156
    Cancer 156
    Testosterone Level 157
EFFECTS OF DRINKING ON THE INDIVIDUAL AND SOCIETY 157
    Economic Costs 157
    Job-Related Problems 158
    Motor-Vehicle Accidents 158
    Crime 159
    The Family 159
    Suicide 159
ALCOHOLISM 160
    What is Alcoholism? 160
    Causes of Alcoholism 166
    Women and Alcohol 166

Treatment and Rehabilitation Services   167
Treatment Approaches   169
THE MOVEMENT AGAINST DRUNK DRIVING   171
Mothers against Drunk Drivers   171
Students against Driving Drunk   172
RESPONSIBLE DRINKING   173
SUMMARY   173
NOTES   174

OPIATES

NONSYNTHETIC OPIATES   177
Morphine   178
Heroin   178
Codeine   182
SYNTHETIC OPIATES   183
Methadone   183
Propoxyphene Hydrochloride (Darvon)   184
DRUG ABUSE-RELATED LEGISLATION   184
National Addiction Rehabilitation Administration (NARA)   184
Further Legislation   186
DETOXIFICATION   187
General Effects   188
THERAPEUTIC APPROACHES   188
Small-Group Support   188
Therapeutic Communities   189
Personal Responsibility and Commitment   190
METHADONE MAINTENANCE   190
Introduction   190
Possible Hazards and Side Effects   191
The Process   192
Rate of Success   193
Social Implications of Methadone-Maintenance Programs   194
NARCOTIC ANTAGONISTS   195
Psychological Considerations   196
The Young User   196
DOES ANY TREATMENT WORK?   197
Maturing Out   197
SUMMARY   198
NOTES   199

10

HALLUCINOGENS

202

LSD   202
    Introduction   202
    Psychophysiological Effects   203
    Society   204
    Medical Research   206
MESCALINE (PEYOTE)   207
    Introduction   207
    Psychophysiological Effects   208
PSILOCYBIN   209
    Introduction   209
    Psychophysiological Effects   209
PCP   210
    Introduction   210
    Effects on Society   210
    Psychophysiological Effects   211
SUMMARY   212
NOTES   213

11

MARIJUANA
still a controversy

215

INTRODUCTION   215
    Marijuana Use in the World   215
    Marijuana Use in the United States   216
    Paraquat   217
PHARMACOLOGICAL CLASSIFICATION   218
PHYSIOLOGICAL EFFECTS   218
    Effects on Body Functions   219
    Pulmonary Effects   219
    Cardiovascular Complications   220
    Effects on the Immunology System   221
    Effects on Endocrine Functioning   221
    Psychomotor Impairment   222
    Genetic and Brian Damage   223
    Tolerance   224
PSYCHOLOGICAL EFFECTS   224
    Psychopathology   224
    Amotivational Syndrome   225

Individuals and Society 225
Flashbacks 226
THERAPEUTIC OR MEDICAL USES OF MARIJUANA 226
Glaucoma 226
Cancer 227
Anorexia Nervosa 227
Other Applications 227
SUMMARY 228
NOTES 228

12

OVER-THE-COUNTER DRUGS
what you can get
without a prescription
231

INTRODUCTION 231
Development of OTCs in the United States 232
Reform 233
SALICYLATES (ASPIRIN) 234
History 234
Physical Effects 235
Side Effects 235
Therapeutic Effectiveness 236
Toxicology 237
Acetaminophen 238
LAXATIVES 239
Introduction 239
Understanding Constipation 239
Types of Laxatives 240
Laxative Use 241
COUGH RELIEVERS (ANTITUSSIVES) 241
The Cough 241
Reducing the Severity 241
ANTIHISTAMINES 242
VITAMINS AND MINERALS 243
Introduction 243
Specific Use 244
Specific Vitamins 245
Misconceptions 248
Megavitamin Madness 248
DIET PILLS 249
SUMMARY 250
NOTES 250

13

PRESCRIPTION AND OTHER DRUGS OF INTEREST

253

PLACEBOS 253
   Introduction 253
   Individual Differences 254
   Social Environment and Situational Variables 254
   Administration, Frequency, and Cost 254
ANTIBIOTICS 256
   Classification 256
   History 256
   Effects 256
   Resistance to Antibiotics 257
   Misuse 257
ANTIDEPRESSANTS 258
   Introduction 258
   Classifications 259
   Psychophysiological Effects 259
NITROUS OXIDE (N$_2$O) 260
LITHIUM 260
   Classification 260
   Pharmacology 260
   Medical Use 261
LAETRILE 261
DIMETHYL SULFOXIDE (DMSO) 262
   History 262
   Physical Effects 263
ORAL CONTRACEPTIVES 264
   History 264
   Composition and Use 264
   Mechanism of Action 264
   Possible Side Effects 265
   Birth Defects and the Pill 266
   A Pill for Males 266
FERTILITY PILLS 267
   Introduction 267
   Method of Effect 267
   Possible Side Effects 268
   Multiple Births 268
FOOD ADDITIVES 269
   Introduction 269
   History 269
   Adverse Effects 275
SUMMARY 276
NOTES 277

14

THE CONSUMER
AND DRUG LEGISLATION

280

INTRODUCTION   280
THE PHYSICIAN'S ROLE   280
THE DRUG INDUSTRY   282
    Profit and Production   282
    Marketing and Advertising   282
    Research and Development   282
    The High Cost of Prescription Drugs   283
DRUG USE AND THE LAW   283
    Victimless Crimes   284
    Drug Education   285
A HISTORY OF MAJOR DRUG-RELATED LEGISLATION   285
    Regulation of Opiates: 1865-1905   285
    The Pure Food and Drug Act: 1906   286
    The Shanghai International Conference: 1909   286
    The Harrison Narcotic Act: 1914   286
    Prohibition: 1920   287
    Importation of Heroin Banned: 1924   287
    Linder v. United States: 1925   288
    Porter Narcotic Farms Bill: 1929   288
    Federal Bureau of Narcotics: 1930   288
    The Marijuana Tax Act: 1937   288
    The Food, Drug and Cosmetic Act: 1938   289
    The Boggs Amendment: 1951   289
    The Narcotic Drug Control Act: 1956   290
    Kefauver-Harris Amendments: 1962   290
    Robinson v. California: 1962   290
    The Community Mental Health Centers Act: 1963   291
    The Drug Abuse Control Amendments: 1965   291
    The Narcotic Addict Rehabilitation Act: 1966   291
    The Comprehensive Drug Abuse Prevention and Control Act
     (The Controlled Substances Act): 1970   292
    The Black Market: 1971   295
    Consumer Issues and Legislation: 1973   295
DECRIMINALIZATION   298
    Marijuana   298
    Opiates   299
SUMMARY   302
MILESTONES IN ATTEMPTED DRUG REGULATION   303
NOTES   304

15

ALTERNATIVES TO
PSYCHOACTIVE DRUG ABUSE

A NEW PHILOSOPHICAL PERSPECTIVE   306
    Drug Education in the Schools   307
    Accepting Potential Drug Benefits   307
ALTERNATIVES   308
    Exercise   309
    Wilderness Experiences   311
    Work   312
    Social-Political Activism   312
    Religion   313
    Biofeedback   314
    Meditation   315
SUMMARY   319
NOTES   319

INDEX

321

PREFACE

In this revised edition of *Drugs of Choice* we have attempted to retain the strong points of the first edition and update those areas where changes have occurred. The first four chapters offer the reader a basic foundation for discussion and understanding of drugs. Chapter 1 offers an overview of drugs, describes the "gray area" of drug use, and explains how difficult it is to generalize about drugs. Chapter 2 describes the delicate balance among the psychological, sociological, and biological reasons people use drugs. Chapter 3 deals with the ever-changing drug scene, describing how there are as many drug scenes as there are people. For convenience, however, it is divided into the youth, adult, and senior-citizen drug scenes as a way of discussing some of the more common types of drug use. It points out the increasing problems with drugs in athletics and the workplace. Chapter 4 provides an overview of pharmacy and physiology. A unique feature of this chapter is the inclusion of consumer-safety rules.

Chapter 5 focuses on "uppers," such as amphetamines, methamphetamines, cocaine, and caffeine. Particular attention is placed on the increasing recreational use of cocaine (especially in athletics and the workplace). Some of the findings from calls to the toll-free 800 COCAINE number are disturbing. Also discussed is methylphenidate (Ritalin) and the increase in look-alike drugs. Chapter 6 now includes several new reports on smoking and cardiovascular disease, cancer, and chronic obstructive lung disease. These reports further validate many of the findings of the 1979 surgeon general's report on the health consequences of smoking. The nonsmokers' movement and their goal of a smoke-free society by the year 2000 are highlighted. The chapter also includes a section on clove cigarettes.

Chapters 7–9 focus on "downers." Dramatic changes on alcohol use and alcoholism have been made. Also, the impact of alcohol legislation by Mothers Against Drunk Driving (MADD) and Students Against Driving Drunk (SADD) is discussed. The debate about prescribing heroin for patients with intractable pain is also included.

Chapter 10 presents LSD, mescaline, psilocybin, and phencyclidine (PCP). Special attention is given to sporadic increases of a milder LDS and the epidemic of PCP use. Chapter 11 offers a comprehensive discussion of both the research findings and the current status of the increasing popular drug Marijuana. The crop-production and distribution growth in the United States and the increased potency of the drug are newer dimensions that are addressed.

Chapter 12, on over-the-counter drugs, reveals that sizable numbers of our population self-medicate or find relief with an assortment of over 300,000 nonprescription drugs. The safety and effectiveness of these drugs and their potential problems are ongoing issues. Chapter 13, on prescription and other drugs, discusses a number of drugs (antibiotics, antihistamines, and oral contraceptives) that have been used for some time. Also, an update is given on laetrile, DMSO, and food additives (for example, NutraSweet).

The final two chapters deal with how society and individuals have attempted to control drug abuse. Chapter 14 discusses the importance of being alert and responsible drug consumers, as well as the numerous attempts to legislate drug behavior. Chapter 15 attempts to show some alternatives to drug use. Such alternatives may prove to be the most successful approach to the problem of drug abuse.

The authors would like to acknowledge the Drug Information Center (DIC) at the University of Oregon for its support during this revision.

RICHARD G. SCHLAADT
PETER T. SHANNON

DRUGS
OF CHOICE

current perspectives on drug use

1

INTRODUCTION

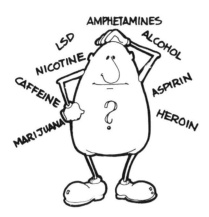

THE GRAY AREA

The United States is a drug-oriented nation. Media messages concerning the benefits—or dangers—of drug use continually bombard us. According to physician Andrew Weil,

> The use of drugs to alter consciousness is nothing new. It has been a feature of all human life in all places on the earth and in all ages of history. . . . the ubiquity of drug use is so striking that it must represent a basic human appetite. Yet many Americans seem to feel that the contemporary drug scene is something new, something qualitatively different from what has gone before. This attitude is peculiar because all that is really happening is a change in drug preference.[1]

Though the messages are frequent, they are often "gray"—a combination of fact and fiction that the listener must sort through. Half-truths and sensationalism

1

distort-drug related discussions and make accurate assessment of the drug scene difficult. Wide variation in drug use and its effects on the individual further obscures attempts to clarify the issues surrounding drug use. Worse, drug treatment programs have no fixed standards of success or failure, and different experts on drug abuse define the nature and extent of the problem differently.

Five aspects of the "gray area" of drug use need to be probed: (1) individual differences in reactions to drugs, (2) quality control—or lack of it, (3) effect of drug use on a drug user's expectations, (4) influence of setting, and (5) relation of a drug's legality to its effectiveness and to the treatment of those who use it.

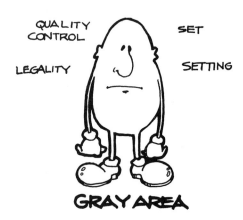

Individual Differences

Individuals are unique in their reactions to drugs. Too often we issue blanket statements about how people will react to a drug. Such generalizations must be carefully examined since most are based on "normal reaction" to a drug. Health status, size, age, sex, time of day, personal expectations, dosage, previous experience, and surroundings all influence the effect of a given drug on a given individual. For example, penicillin is valuable in combating certain diseases, but those individuals who are allergic to it experience unpleasant and adverse reactions following its use. Physicians and pharmacists anticipate that 3 to 5 percent of any given population may be allergic to a given drug. In short, not all individuals react the same way to a drug.

Quality Control

Federal Food and Drug Administration (FDA) procedures and regulations make it extremely difficult to introduce a new drug on the market.

Before a new drug can be approved, pharmaceutical companies must expend considerable time and money putting it through a series of rigorous tests to determine its safety and effectiveness. (The effects of the drug thalidomide have demonstrated the importance of such testing.) In spite of this extensive research, a few individuals will suffer complications from using the drug. For example, some women react adversely to birth control pills, experiencing nausea, blood clotting, hypertension, metabolic alterations, and associated pain. Medical drug use needs to be regulated and monitored to maximize its possible benefits.

Further down the line of quality control, the pharmacist must fill each prescription to the exact chemical amount specified. A lesser amount might be totally ineffective and a greater amount might cause adverse reactions. The final responsibility for quality control rests with the individual. Self-medication or irresponsible use of drugs is likely to result in adverse reactions. Drugs borrowed from friends may mask symptoms, confuse diagnosis, and cause the individual to defer proper medical treatment.

However, in addition to regularly prescribed and over-the-counter drugs, which have been approved for use, there are also "street drugs"—prescription drugs as well as other drugs that "street manufacturers" cut and dilute for sale. A prescription drug such as amphetamine, for example, can make its way onto the street through various illicit channels and be sold as a stimulant, perhaps cut with cocaine. Because there is no quality control on the street, one drug may be substituted for another. Caffeine-pill look-alikes can be substituted for amphetamine pills, for example, resulting in a nice profit for the "manufacturer."

Street-produced drugs are suspect for a number of reasons. First, they are often impure and adulterated. Second, some of the preferred chemical constituents may be unavailable and substitutions of less desirable components made. Third, the qualifications of the street "pharmacist" are sometimes as suspect as the equipment being used. As a result, drug potency and purity often vary from batch to batch. Finally, street manufacturers are often on the move to avoid police detection, and this leaves them little time to follow proper procedures: distillation and filtration processes that might normally occur in legal environments often do not exist on the street.

Set

Set means people's expectations of a drug and what they think it will do for them. In other words, this deals specifically with one's *internal* environment or expectations and personality characteristics. The set will not always guarantee a particular type of experience, but it can have a great effect. For example, expectations of a pleasurable experience can often bring one about, as in the case of students who thought they were taking marijuana feeling high when in actuality they had been smoking Sir Walter Raleigh tobacco.[2] At the other end of the spectrum, people feeling very depressed or frustrated prior to drug use are likely to feel more so afterward.

Setting

The setting consists of the people and the environment in which a drug is taken. Setting can greatly influence the drug's effect. It primarily involves the *external* social and physical environment. Being among friends at a festive, pleasurable New Year's Eve party may enhance the drug experience. But a tense setting, as in situations where there is anger, fighting, depression, or the fear of being arrested, can produce anxiety. Research by John Reed on controlled drinking in a simulated bar confirms this belief in the setting's influence. Reed studied three groups: group I members were given alcohol; group II members were told they were drinking alcohol but were not given any; and group III members were told they had not been given alcoholic beverages but actually had been. Group I responded in an intoxicated manner, as would be expected, but group II responded the same way, even though they had not been given alcohol. Group III exhibited traits of sobriety even though they were drinking alcoholic beverages.[3]

Legality

If a drug can be used legally, anxiety may not be associated with its use. Illegal drug use, on the other hand, can often bring with it a feeling of danger and fear. Such risk taking may enhance or decrease the effectiveness of any drug.

The heavy drug user (alcoholic, heroin dependent, etc.) is gradually being viewed as ill rather than criminal. Efforts are under way to decriminalize the use of some drugs and make sentencing for drug possession uniform. Many individuals feel that present laws actually create criminals rather than help those with problems. More emphasis is being placed on prevention and treatment, as we will see.

PERSPECTIVE ON DRUGS

In the following pages we present an overview on drugs that will set the stage for the more specific coverage in the chapters to come. This perspective portrays the total drug scene in relation to society without implying that any one drug is of greater or lesser importance to the individual. The use of drugs is not limited to any socioeconomic group. Today drugs are used in the affluent suburbs and middle class neighborhoods as well as the ghetto. The FDA distinguishes drug use, misuse, and abuse as follows. *Drug use* is the taking of a drug for its intended purpose and in an appropriate amount, frequency, strength, and manner. *Drug misuse* is the taking of a substance for a purpose, but not in the appropriate amount, frequency, strength, or manner. *Drug abuse* is the deliberate use of a substance for other than its intended purpose, in a manner that can damage health or ability to function.

The American drug-use pattern began to shift from the primary use of alcohol and tobacco toward hallucinogens, marijuana, amphetamines, and barbiturates in the early 1960s—the beginning of the period (which extended through the 1980s) commonly referred to as the Age of Anxiety. The numerous reasons for this shift are discussed throughout the book. But one general reason is the stress individuals found themselves subjected to. As mental and emotional pressures increased, millions of Americans began taking doses of stimulants, depressants, and hallucinogenic drugs regularly each day. Today, the majority of adults rarely go through a week without consuming alcohol in some form. Large numbers also regularly use sedatives to help them sleep and stimulants to keep them awake for prolonged periods.

Caffeine

Caffeine is a stimulant found in tea, coffee, cola drinks, chocolate, and aspirin. Although the use of other stimulants, such as amphetamines, is seriously discouraged, the use of beverages containing caffeine is commonly accepted. The coffee break, in fact, has become a regular part of many Americans' lives. Recently, however, greater attention has been focused on the adverse effects caffeine may have—high blood pressure, anxiety, and insomnia.

Alcohol

Alcohol still remains king of the drug scene: it is the most commonly abused drug in the United States today, often used to relieve anxiety and tension. Of the estimated 100 million people who use alcohol, approximately 10 million are classified as alcoholics.[4] Drinking problems cost society approximately $43 billion a year in lost production, medical costs, and other expenses.[5] In fact, according to some sources the economic cost of alcohol abuse and alcoholism may be as high as $120 billion annually.[6] Roughly $20 billion are spent each year on alcohol; it is a substantial element of the economy.[7]

Nicotine

"Warning: The Surgeon General Has Determined That Cigarette Smoking Is Dangerous To Your Health." This well-known warning appears on the label of every pack of cigarettes sold in the United States, yet despite it, approximately 53 million Americans smoke an estimated 590 billion cigarettes yearly.[8] The number of adults using tobacco products *has* declined in recent years, but alarming use trends continue among the young, especially teenage girls. The use of chewing tobacco has recently increased.

Tobacco is the second leading drug problem in the United States and the surgeon general has cited it as the primary cause of preventable disease. From 30 to 35 percent of the adult population smoke cigarettes, even though more than 117,000 deaths from lung cancer, 60,000 heart attacks, and numerous other respiratory ailments are attributed to tobacco smoking.[9] New strategies are currently being employed to reduce cigarette consumption: utilizing alternative ingredients, lengthening filters, and reducing tar and nicotine are meeting with limited success. Stressing alternatives to smoking and providing detoxification clinics and educational programs may prove somewhat successful as well.

Strong political debate is taking place over the rights of nonsmokers, and many states have passed laws requiring public business meetings to restrict the use of cigarettes to protect nonsmokers. The marketing and use of tobacco products is also surrounded by controversy, the tobacco industry and smokers promoting "smokers' rights" and scientists, environmental groups, health groups, and nonsmokers promoting "nonsmokers' rights." There also appears to be growing concern that society and specifically the government should *not* use tax dollars to pay medical costs incurred from smoking cigarettes. In short, people who smoke should pay their own medical bills, it is argued.

Stimulants and Sedatives

The use of stimulants and sedatives, both legal and illegal, is widespread in American society.

Stimulants   Many individuals use stimulants such as amphetamines and caffeine to remain alert, increase work capacity, alleviate fatigue, and induce a sense of euphoria. Prescription stimulants are available in a limited supply for dieting, hyperactivity, and the sleeping disorder narcolepsy. Over-the-counter stimulants containing caffeine are available from drugstores and supermarkets, and the sale of illicit stimulants to students, those working graveyard or swing shifts, and long-haul truck drivers is common. Since 1972, the federal government has attempted to restrict by law the production and dispensing of prescription stimulants by pharmaceutical houses because of the illicit routes along which the products were often diverted.

Many stimulants can be harmful. Repeated use may lead to tolerance, and increased dosages may then be required to produce the original stimulation. Intravenous use of methamphetamines, the most potent amphetamine, by "speed freaks" in San Francisco during the late 1960s often resulted in psychotic episodes brought on by the sleep deprivation experienced during the "speed run." The use of cocaine, among the most powerful of the available stimulants and in great demand as a recreational drug, may result in psychological dependence.

Sedatives   Physicians frequently prescribe sedatives to relieve a number of ills. Sedatives have sleep-inducing properties; they are also prescribed at lower dosage for daytime sedation (relaxation) and for the relief of anxiety. Valium and Librium have replaced many of the barbiturate-based sedatives. Currently, middle-aged women rely on sedatives for relief of anxiety and insomnia more than their male counterparts do. In November 1983 the Lemmon Company, the last manufacturer of methaqualone, announced that it would no longer produce the drug and would destroy its remaining stockpiles of it. The company cited as reasons the widespread illicit use of the substance and government pressures to ban its preparation.[10]

Marijuana

The use of marijuana has become commonplace in recent years because of its availability and relative inexpensiveness, and because results of medical studies indicate some of its dangers have been exaggerated. The early 1970s saw a growing movement toward the decriminalization of marijuana and possession of small amounts of marijuana was downgraded from a criminal act to a misdemeanor in several states. Since Oregon established a law in 1973 making possession of less than an ounce of marijuana a misdemeanor incurring a maximum fine of $100, eleven other states, including New York, California, Ohio, and Michigan, have passed similar legislation.[11]

Marijuana depresses the central nervous system, producing a sense of relaxation in most individuals. Although occasional disorientation and confusion may result, marijuana usually calms people and is often used recreationally as a mild sedative. Its capacity to alleviate stress and reduce tension, to produce a sense of euphoria and a feeling of lightness, to alter and intensify perceptions, and to produce minimal side effects has made it a popular drug.

Marijuana is also gaining greater medical acceptance as a potential adjunct for treatment of such ailments as glaucoma. However, its relationship to lung cancer, emphysema, and sexual fertility is still unclear.

Hallucinogens

The use of hallucinogenic, or psychedelic, drugs such as LSD was widespread in the United States among the middle-class youth in the 1960s and early 1970s. Though the use of LSD continues, its popularity seems to have declined in favor of less powerful drugs originating from organic (natural) sources (psilocybin and mescaline from mushrooms, and peyote).

Hallucinogenic drugs alter and frequently enhance the processing of sensory and emotional information in brain centers, and for this reason their use appears to coincide with a person's search for individuality and an understanding of life. Depending on the dosage, the expectations of the drug experience, and the physical and emotional settings of the individual, LSD can chemically facilitate a person's sense of well-being and greater awareness of body functions. If the dosage is too great and/or the setting is unsupportive or inappropriate, LSD may trigger distortions of the environment, causing anxiety or, in more severe forms, psychological crisis and trauma. However, evidence is still inconclusive that brain damage or major personality change results from LSD use.

Opiates

Heroin is the most widely used of the opiate drugs, but accurate figures on the extent of its use are difficult to obtain. Some studies estimate that 10 percent of heroin users are dependent on the drug and mainline (inject) it; the remaining 90 percent are weekend "chippers" who inhale or snort it as a recreational activity or inject it just underneath the skin. Heroin-dependent individuals are found in all professions, socioeconomic strata, and communities. Most are under 35.

Methadone maintenance programs have been implemented to treat opiate-dependent people. Though still controversial, methadone, a synthetic opiate that blocks the euphoria given by heroin (but that nonetheless is dependency-producing itself), coupled with a strong psychological support and counseling, can often be a viable alternative to heroin dependence. Despite the success of methadone, problems remain with illicit street diversion of the drug, inadequate funding of programs, and ethical objections to a program that substitutes one dependency for another.

Volatile Substances

The use of volatile inhalants, such as gasoline, glue, and typewriter correction fluid, is usually limited to elementary and junior high students. Regardless of the user's age, the misuse of such substances can be fatal. When death occurs, however, it is difficult to determine if it has been caused by inhalation of the fumes or suffocation from placing an inhaling aid, such as a plastic bag, over the nostrils and mouth.

DRUG TECHNOLOGY

Drug technology and the production of new drugs have grown astonishingly in recent decades. Forty years ago, physicians had at their disposal only 12 to 20 chemotherapeutic agents. Today more than 22,000 prescription "name" products are available to physicians.[12] (This figure is misleading since the same drug may be listed in the *Physician's Desk Reference* twenty or more times under different names.)

The combination of this rapid increase in prescription drugs and a growing trend among the general population to visit a physician regularly has had several notable effects. Average life expectancy has increased dramatically. New hygienic procedures, passed on from physician to patient, are reducing the incidence and severity of disease. Refinements in certain drugs have alleviated pain and suffering. Millions of people now benefit from the wise and judicious dispensation of prescription drugs by physicians.

Despite the positive changes drug use has brought about, available data suggest that adverse drug reactions afflict large portions of the population, causing hundreds of thousands of unnecessary hospitalizations and thousands of needless deaths. There are far more *iatrogenic* (medically induced) illnesses or death than is commonly realized by the general public. Evidence from the limited studies done to date indicates that between $3 and $4 billion in direct and indirect drug-induced damage is done each year. Current estimates of deaths caused by adverse drug reactions vary from 6000 per year to as many as 140,000.[13]

Some of the responsibility for these figures rests with physicians, who, "are lamentably ill-instructed in clinical pharmacology, a hardly recognized specialty for which no formal training is usually given,"[14] but who must select the correct prescription from among thousands of chemotherapeutic agents at their disposal. Furthermore, some studies have gone so far to say that "even where fully tested and established drugs are concerned, most of the adverse reactions are the direct result of the indiscriminate and overindulgent prescribing habits of physicians who often rely solely on advertisers' copy for their guidance.[15]

Current trends in prescriptive practices also invite possible adverse drug reactions or drug abuse. A substantial number of the psychoactive agents prescribed, many of them stimulants or sedatives, can be unknowingly abused. The phenomenon of *polypharmacy*—many sources supplying one person with medications that may be harmful when taken concurrently—is another cause of drug abuse.

Although doctors realize the negative effects of polypharmacy and although they are inadequately trained in giving prescriptions,

> prescribe they do, often with alacrity and apparent casualness and often without knowing that the patient may already be dosing himself with all kinds of heavily advertised medicines bought over-the-counter, which may greatly affect his reaction to the prescribed drug. . . . Certain hospital surveys have identified patients who are taking up to 30 different preparations a day. Small wonder new diseases develop, and who is to say whether the symptoms are caused by the original complaint or by the drug combination given to treat it?[16]

One study found that 40 percent of patients receive drugs prescribed by two or more physicians, and are therefore more liable to dangerous drug interactions.[17]

Patients themselves may also contribute markedly to the high rates of adverse drug reactions and drug-induced death. Noncompliance with a physician's instructions can bring about serious consequences ranging from the failure of the drug to affect the disease to intensification of the disease and even death. Studies have indicated that noncompliance in the case of prescription drugs runs as high as 85 percent, with the highest degree of noncompliance seen in nonhospitalized patients. On the other hand, many patients pressure their physician to overprescribe, particularly in the case of tranquilizers, currently one of the most frequently dispensed medication. Many drug experts, both within and outside the FDA, insist that drug abuse and adverse reactions must be combated by (1) improving physicians' training and sources of clinical drug information; (2) developing informed consent procedures that provide detailed descriptions of drug effects, proper utilization of preparations, and patient prescription monitoring; and (3) informing the public about the effects of drugs and the responsible use of any drug.

A recent trend concerning the prescription drugs could have substantial adverse effects on street drug users: drug enforcement officials are suggesting that almost half the drugs now seen on the illicit street market are diverted pharmaceutical drugs. It is estimated that approximately 13,000 physicians and pharmacists (2 percent of the registered population) are involved in this diversion.[18]

Over-the-Counter Drugs

The number of over-the-counter (OTC) drugs has also expanded dramatically. Forty years ago, only 50 to 60 products were available without prescription; currently, more than 300,000 medications are available at the local drugstore.[19] Many of these preparations are geared to minor ailments, including aspirin for headaches, laxatives for gastrointestinal upset, sleeping aids for insomnia, and antihistamines for hay fever. The public is willing to pay to obtain relief from these ailments, and consequently OTC drugs continue to be big business.

Television advertising is a key factor in OTC sales: one in every eight commercials advertises a drug.[20] But drug experts point out that advertising creates false expectations for relief by stressing drug benefits without discussing side effects or contraindications (inadvisable use of the drug). And though the public expects consistent alleviation of ailments through chemical use, physicians know all too well that a drug's benefit may be reduced by negative side effects.

OTC drugs do not possess dose strength sufficient to achieve full therapeutic potential (in which case they would be prescription medications). To obtain relief with weak OTC preparations, individuals will often consume more than the recommended dosage, thus increasing the incidence of side effects, adverse reactions, and poisoning.

Because of consumer concern about the safety and effectiveness of OTC products, the FDA engaged in an extensive review of OTC medications from 1972 to early 1984. Several FDA panels reviewed more than 700 ingredients, many of them several times because of their use in different products. The panels found that only about one-third of the ingredients are effective and safe; the rest require additional proof from manufacturers if the products containing them are to remain available for sale. This does not mean that two thirds of all OTC drug products are unsafe. Most products have safe and effective ingredients even if they contain other ingredients that are ineffective.[21]

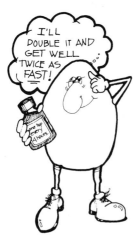

Over-the-counter drugs represent the largest drug market openly available to consumers. Yet most people who obtain OTC products rarely have the pharmacological training to ensure proper drug usage. Since noncompliance with physicians' instructions occurs frequently, one must assume it occurs with OTC product instructions at an equal or greater rate.

Commercial Drugs

Commercial drugs include food additives, industrial chemicals and inorganic wastes introduced into the atmosphere and water supply, household chemicals (cleaners, detergents, polishes, and the like), and cosmetics. Most of the commercial drugs utilized today were not available fifteen years ago.

In previous years, consumer interest focused on the danger of children being poisoned by household chemicals or factory workers being exposed to industrial chemicals. Today so many new substances have such far-reaching effects that the recognition of any risks associated with them has lagged far behind appreciation of their benefits. The general public usually becomes aware of possible dangers only when some tragic event becomes news. [22]

Exposure to chemicals in the environment has been increasingly recognized as a major cause of cancer in humans. The National Cancer Institute has reported that more than 80 percent of the cancer in humans can be prevented by the reduction of exposure to certain natural or synthetic chemicals in foods, household products, and industrial by-products found in the air and water. [23] In passing the Delaney Amendment in 1958, Congress sought to prohibit the use of substances capable of producing cancer in humans. Consumers must be warned in supermarkets and workers at work sites by special notices of hazardous and carcinogenic materials. The Environmental Protection Agency also oversees efforts under the Toxic Substances Act to ensure that exposure to carcinogens is reduced. However, scientists still warn that Americans may have to make major changes in diet (high fat) and use of tobacco products, and that rigid standards of air and water quality must be maintained to ensure reduced cancer rates.

Recreational Drugs

Recreational drugs are chemical agents that adults may legally consume, including alcohol (in beer, wine, distillates), nicotine (in cigarettes, snuff, cigars, pipe tobacco), and caffeine (in coffee, tea, soft drinks, chocolate). Large segments of the population take such substances for relaxation, stimulation, and, in some cases, social acceptance.

Advertising in the print and electronic media promotes extensive use and availability of recreational drugs. Yet despite this exposure, little effort is made to ensure that individuals are taught judicious and responsible use. Irresponsible drug consumption can result in psychological and physiological dependence, medical complications, traffic accidents, violent crimes, high treatment costs, imprisonment, court costs, loss of work productivity, broken homes, scarred interpersonal relationships, and death.

To help people make better-informed and more realistic decisions about their drug-consuming behaviors, and to help them learn what drugs can provide in terms of self-growth and recreational activity, significant educational efforts must be made, starting at the elementary school level. Adults, too, must be educated to understand appropriate alcohol levels for driving, potential drug/alcohol interactions, appropriate consumption of caffeine, and methods of reducing nicotine use.

Herbal Preparations

Herbal chemicals, those occurring naturally in plants, have been used since earliest times. Today, more than half of all available prescription and OTC products are derived from plant chemicals.[24]

When an individual obtains a preparation from a plant, he or she is obtaining all the chemicals the plant uses for its metabolism. In a pharamaceutical (synthetic) preparation, the single desired chemical has been isolated from the others and provided in the correct dosage, which is somewhat difficult to estimate when using bulk quantities of a plant. Whether a drug is organic or synthetic, it will be metabolized in the body by the same processes. Renewed public interest in herbal preparations, however, fosters from the public belief that organic drugs are inherently better than synthetic chemicals.

Among the most popular of the psychoactive substances are the peyote cactus button (mescaline), various mushroom species containing psilocybin and psilocin, and the coca plant leaf, from which cocaine is derived. Interest in these substances has caused some concern since many individuals exploring forests, pasture lands, and deserts for the plants are not able to properly identify them. Gauging appropriate dose levels and coping with side effects may also be difficult. The need for public education in responsible herbal-preparation use may grow as new drugs are derived from plants.

Illegal Drugs

Illegal drugs are those chemicals that government authorities have determined to be subject to abuse or that are capable of causing severe harm. Among them are marijuana, amphetamines, cocaine, opiates, sedatives, and tranquilizers. Laws have been passed to prevent the public from obtaining or distributing these drugs, and to deter and punish people who attempt to use them without a physician's prescription.

Despite repeated warnings from drug "experts," use of illegal drugs has continued to grow. Educational efforts aimed at exposing dangerous side effects or stressing alternatives to drugs are beginning to have a positive effect. To change this pattern, effective drug education incorporating the teaching of personal decision-making skills and alternatives to drugs needs to begin in the early grade levels and continue through elementary, middle, and high school.

SUMMARY

To gain a solid understanding of drugs and their use, one must consider several factors. The topic is highly emotionally charged; it is heavily laden with individual values and biases; it is inundated with myths and inaccurate information; it is subject to rapid change in valid data. Often these factors conflict with each other, and as a result the drug scene is a "gray area" of unanswered questions and vague issues. Individual differences, quality control, set, setting, and legal implications must all be considered. And it must be understood that it is often difficult to put drugs in a realistic and rational perspective. For example, alcohol and tobacco, both legal drugs for those of age, probably lead to more health and economic problems than do illicit drugs. A full range of drug education is therefore necessary.

Because of the increasing number of drugs available for prescription, OTC, and recreational use, an awareness of drug technology is highly important. With physicians unable to remain informed on all the drugs currently available for treatment, with billions of dollars paid each year for licit and illicit drugs, with over-the-counter drugs filling drugstores and supermarkets, and with drug advertising and promotion the big business it is, today's consumer must be informed and responsible if he or she is to use drugs rationally.

NOTES

[1]From *The Natural Mind,* by Andrew Weil. Copyright © 1972 by Andrew Weil. Reprinted by permission of the publisher, Houghton Mifflin Company.

[2]A graduate student report presented to an HEP4536 Drugs in Society class at the University of Oregon, March, 1985, Eugene, Oregon.

[3]Lecture by Peter Shannon to a Drugs in Society class at the University of Oregon, January 1978.

[4]"The Sobering Cost of Alcoholism," *Science News* 114, no. 18 (October 28, 1978):293.

[5]Ibid.

[6]Office of Technological Assessment. *The Effectiveness and Costs of Alcoholism Treatment.* Washington, D.C.: U.S. Government Printing Office, March 1983, p. 3.

[7]Bryan R. Luce, "Smoking and Alcohol Abuse: A Comparison of Their Economic Consequences," *New England Journal of Medicine* 298, no. 10 (March 9, 1978):569.

[8]National Interagency Council on Smoking and Health, "Dramatic Drop in Number of Smokers and Cigarette Production Sends Shock Waves through Tobacco Industry," *Smoking and Health Reporter* 1, no. 3 (April 1984):1. Copyright © 1984 National Interagency Council on Smoking and Health. Used with permission.

[9]Department of Health, Education, and Welfare, "Teen-age Smoking Survey," *National Institute on Education,* April 26, 1978.

[10]"Quaaludes 'Dead', Agents Claim," *Eugene Register Guard* 19 August 1984, p. 17D.

[11]*Focus on Alcohol and Drug Issues* 3m, no. 1 (January–February 1980): p.2.

[12]Lecture by Mark Miller to a Drugs in Society class at the University of Oregon, April 1980.

[13]N. S. Irey, "Deaths Due to Adverse Drug Reactions," *Journal of the American Medical Association* 231, no. 1 (January 6, 1975):22–23; J. Kock-Weser, "Fatal Reactions to Adverse Drug Reactions," *New England Journal of Medicine* 291, no. 6 (August 8, 1974):302–3.

[14]Special Commission on Internal Pollution, "Toward Assessing the Chemical Age," *Journal of the American Medical Association* 234, no. 5 (November 3, 1975):509.

[15]Ibid.

[16]Ibid.

[17]George J. Caranasos, Ronald B. Stewart, and Leighton E. Cluff, "Drug Induced Illness Leading to Hospitalization," *Journal of the American Medical Association* 228, no. 6 (May 6, 1974):716–17.

[18]*Pharmaceutical Manufacturers Association Newsletter* 25, no. 24 (July 4, 1983):2.

[19]Lecture by Mark Miller.

[20]"Television Advertising and Drug Use: Health Care Sociology," *Drug Intelligence and Clinical Pharmacy* 11, no. 8 (August 1977).

[21]"Panels' Review Completed" *FDA Consumer* (February 1984):32–33.

[22]Special Commission on Internal Pollution, "Toward Assessing the Chemical Age."

[23]American Cancer Society, *1981 Cancer Facts and Figures.*

[24]Lecture by Mark Miller.

WHY PEOPLE USE DRUGS

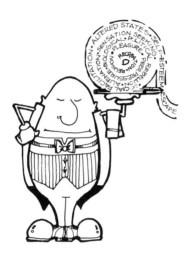

INTRODUCTION

Different individuals use different drugs for different reasons. Whereas one will use alcohol to facilitate interaction at a cocktail party, another may smoke marijuana as a political statement. The reasons individuals use psychoactive substances vary as much as the individuals themselves: to enhance sexual fulfillment, to seek spiritual enlightenment, to have fun, to produce mood fluctuations, to enhance athletic performance, to supplement behavior in bar settings, to fight boredom, to satisfy curiosity, to be "in" as opposed to "left out."

The many reasons for psychoactive substance use are similar to those causing drug dependence, but they can be broken down into two major groups: psychological (interpersonal) and sociological (environmental). The two are not mutually exclusive, since personal and societal factors work in consort to determine behavior. Theories on the nature of dependency states fall into three camps—psychological, sociological, and biological—which again are not mutually exclusive. A composite of the three areas offers an explanation of drug dependency.

PSYCHOLOGICAL FACTORS

Recreation/Social Facilitation

The American cocktail party is a setting in which drug use and the reasons for use are plentiful. Alcohol is in demand at such occasions because it facilitates interpersonal and group dynamics through its capacity to depress the central nervous system. Alcohol and other recreational drugs may foster a sense of camaraderie and co-adventure, and may fulfill the need or desire to feel good. Therefore, individuals who feel poorly and want to feel better may use these drugs; so may individuals who already feel fine.

Social Facilitation

People use drugs recreationally simply to enhance social facilitation and to feel good—at cocktail parties, at football games, on Friday at the local watering hole, in restaurants, on picnics, and during lazy afternoons. Social drug use brings people together. It helps to create an atmosphere in which openness becomes appropriate and people share more of themselves than they normally would. The character armoring, as Reich would say, may become less rigid.

Alexander Shilgin, responsible for synthesis of the hallucinogen STP, comments,

> In drinking, there is this marvelous level, somewhere during the second martini; you can't say what's happening, but suddenly everything is a little bit brighter, conversation a little bit more relaxed, the music is suddenly proper, you are fitting into the environment. That's the goal of alcohol drinking. I find it a fabulous moment.[1]

Finding that level is a goal and motive that is shared by a significant segment of the drinking population. Again, as an amplification of the cocktail party, social drug use promotes communication by allowing the possibility of sharing a common feeling or experience. In short, people use drugs to communicate and because it is ritualistic fun.

Sensation Seeking

The present emphasis on sports, the preponderance of sex and violence in films and television, video games and computers, and the level of drug dependency already displayed by millions of people give credence to the current need for stimulating experiences—the pursuit of sensation. But heightened and exciting experiences become increasingly difficult to achieve as people build up tolerance to sensation and need new regions to explore and experience. It may be that,

> football and hockey spectacles are a pallid substitute for the corny productions of the Roman Coliseum. In past centuries, war, conquest, and exploration, along with saturnalias, tournaments, public executions, and orgiastic feasts, fed the hunger for unusual and arousing experience. . . . In 19th century America, the more adventurous struck out for the frontier when life on the eastern seaboard became tame and predictable. Ever since our ancestors settled in permanent locations, boredom has been a problem that varies with the need for survival.[2]

Sensory bombardment through high technology has led to sensory numbing.

Individuals vary in their susceptibility and reaction to boredom. Security in a well-defined and repetitious lifestyle is not a goal, but a plague. Psychologist Marvin Zuckerman explains: " 'Boredom' is the term we use to describe the negative feeling produced by lack of change in the environment. . . . Boredom drives us to seek relief in the form of risky adventures, artistic creation, sex, alcohol, drugs, and even aggression. It is a demand for stimulation and varied experience."[3]

Sensory-deprivation research pioneered by John Lilly proved that in an environment where stimuli are constant, uniform, and never changing, the "bored" mind will initiate auditory and visual hallucinations to keep cognitively awake and stimulated. Describing his work with the National Institute of Mental Health in Bethesda, Maryland, Lilly wrote,

> In the absence of all stimulation it was found that one quickly makes up for this by an extremely heightened awareness and increasing sensory experience in the absence of known means of external stimulation. . . . I went through dreamlike states, trancelike states, mystical states. In all of these states, I was totally intact, centered, and there. . . . I went through experiences in which other people apparently joined me in this dark silent environment. I could actually see them, feel them and hear them. At other times I apparently tuned in on networks of communication that are normally below our levels of awareness, networks of civilizations way beyond ours. I did hours of work on my own hinderances to understanding myself, or my life situation.[4]

The need for periodic variation in sensory stimuli may be a biological function, according to Zuckerman. The basic survival needs for food, drink, and warmth must be satisfied, but following such satisfaction we do not usually sit and hibernate, waiting for the next upswing in the internal-need cycle. Human beings, like other mammals, have the urge to explore their environment. We spend a great deal of our time playing in our physical and social surroundings.

Sensation-seeking behavior may be a general trait—not restricted to any one sensory modality—experienced by all human beings to some degree. Its particular expression may depend on the range of environmental options available, and psychoactive drug expression may be one of those options.[5]

Many drug users take recreational drugs to experience heightened sensuality. Cocaine provides such intensified physiological sensations. Sigmund Freud, a famous user of cocaine, wrote to his fiancé in the mid 1800s:

> Woe to you my princess when I come. I will kiss you quite red and feed you till you are plump. And if you are forward you shall see who is the stronger, a gentle little girl who doesn't eat enough or a big wild man who has cocaine in his body. In my last severe depression I took coca again and a small dose lifted me to the heights in a wonderful fashion. I am just now busy collecting the literature for a song of praise to this magical substance.[6]

Alexander Dumas extolled the beauty of erotic sensation in his classic, *The Count of Monte Cristo:*

> . . . and then followed a dream of passion like that promised by the prophet to the elect. Lips of ice become like heated lava, so that to Franz, yielding for the first time to the sway of the drug, love was as a sorrow and voluptuousness as a torture, as burning mouths were pressing to his thirsty lips, and he was held in cool serpent-like embraces.[7]

Religious/Spiritual Factors

Some people use drugs to gain spiritual enlightenment and to enhance religious ceremonies. Medical studies have determined that psychoactive substances can produce profound perception changes that can enhance and/or facilitate spiritual experiences. The Native American church of the American Southwest and the Tarahumara and Huichol Indians of Mexico utilize the peyote cactus, whose plant buttons contain mescaline.[8] Hindu religious rites call for the use of ganja (bhang), a rich, potent tea made from cannabis.

> To the Hindu, the hemp plant is holy. A guardian lives in 'bhang' . . . bhang is the joy giver, the sky flier, the heavenly guide, the poor man's heaven, the soother of grief . . . no god of man is as good as the religious drinking of bhang. The students of the scriptures of Benares are given bhang before they sit to study. At Benares, Vjjain and other holy places, yogis take deep draughts of bhang, that they may center their thoughts on the eternal.[9]

When used in a religious setting—be it a temple or the desert—alcohol, cannabis, and psychedelic drugs can elevate the emotional intensity of a person's perceptions.

Altered States

From a strictly pharmacological standpoint, psychoactive substances increase the intensity of mood. By causing changes in the neurotransmitter levels of serotonin, dopamine, and norepinephrine, the reticular activating system (the human sensory-screening mechanism) becomes less able to selectively filter out indigenous environmental stimuli. Individuals use drugs in this way to alter thinking patterns and to experience and enhance different sensations.

From a metaphysical viewpoint, drugs are often used to enhance reflection and to find new ways of looking at oneself and the world. Ken Kesey, author of *One Flew Over the Cuckoo's Nest* and *Sometimes a Great Notion,* calls this "looking at the books." In Buddhism, everything one does is recorded in time and stored up as karma (the impact a person has during his or her existence). The books are the track record of one's life. More than a few have taken psychoactive substances to look at the books. Though some have unlocked important clues to their inner selves, others have been shattered by the experience.

Rebellion and Alienation

On college campuses in the early 1960s, students were told to "turn on, tune in, and drop out." Then Harvard professor Timothy Leary, along with fellow academician Richard Alpert (later to become Ram Dass) extolled the virtues of thinking along alternative pathways: war was wrong; conspicuous material consumption was an illusion; people should strive for harmony with nature. Young people were asked to seek new perspectives, to redefine priorities, and they were told that hallucinogens could facilitate this process. Such motives for drug use became tantamount to a cultural revolution.

Many students followed Leary's belief. They began to see and find fault with many of the standards and values of the time. To express their rejection of these middle-class values, they grew their hair long, dressed in nontraditional clothes, listened to antiestablishment music. They expressed their discontent conspicuously, and drug use was a part of that expression.

Drug use became a way people could reveal something of themselves. It also became a political act, as it was used to make social statements. In the late 1960s, marijuana was smoked openly as a counterculture flag-flying gesture; it was flaunted in the face of those who deemed it illegal. The dissident users were telling mainstream America that they were not accepting traditional American values, that a change in attitudes and laws was needed. Some changes were eventually undertaken, but many people ended up behind bars for their antiestablishment acts.

Some individuals also use drugs to cope with alienation (Who am I? Where am I going?); others use drugs to combat depression and dysphoria (feeling unwell, impatient, restless) to experience euphoria, and to remove themselves from the boredom of their existence. They may be living at a rat-race pace, competing to the point of emotional if not physical death, unable to make any sense of or to accept their existence. Therefore, they bring in the "fog"—the chemical haze that envelops their consciousness and muffles their perceptions. The fog can be delivered by alcohol, marijuana, Valium, Seconal, methaqualone, the phenothiazines, Prolixin, Dalmane, Sinequan, glue, PCP, or any number of other substances. The fog may not last long initially, but with repeated doses it will stay as long as one desires.

SOCIOLOGICAL FACTORS:
PEER PRESSURE AND GROUP ENTRY _____

Peer-group pressure influences our activity phenomenally. We copy the activities and behavior of our peers as a way of learning social behavior and as a way to gain acceptance. Behavior acquired through environmental influence is visible in the young of many species as they learn survival techniques. In humans, drug consumption is often a group-entrance requirement.

In gaining entrance to a group, we prove ourselves to the group and to ourselves. When drugs are involved, there is a challenge of strength, if not survival.

> It is not unlike the game of "chicken," but instead of testing oneself against the fear of a high speed head-on collision with another automobile, the "contest" is an internal one which tests one's ability to come as close as possible to a psychotic "crash" or even go over the line and then return unscathed.[10]

So-called primitive societies still have initiation rites. Young men go out into the woods to spend a specified amount of time on their own. If they survive to return to the group, they have passed the test of "manhood." This trial becomes more difficult if a particular task is required, such as slaying an animal or returning with an object that required hazardous efforts to obtain.

Modern society does not often provide this overt testing for group entrance. Ritualized ceremonies, where they are still practiced, now serve this purpose. Jewish bar mitzvahs, fraternity and sorority initiations, licensing tests for the professions, fraternal-club initiations, and chugging contests provide avenues for testing.

Once individuals have been accepted into the group, socialization continues. It determines their behavior, dress, skill acquisition, interests, speech, and so on. In short, the group can help establish and maintain an individual's self-concept and orientation and how he or she views and reacts to the world.[11] Such direction can include use of psychoactive substances.

The family also affects attitudes toward drug use, although its effect, more pronounced in a child's earlier years, diminishes as peer influence increases. Parent figures are powerful models, and young children model their behavior in much the same fashion individuals seeking group entrance do. For example, children born into alcoholic families are more likely to become alcohol-abusive or -dependent than those growing up in families in which alcohol use is nonexistent to moderate.

DEPENDENCY STATES:
PSYCHOLOGICAL PERSPECTIVES _____

Existential/Psychoanalytic View

There are many ways of looking at drug dependency. Some suggest that certain individuals have an "addictive personality," a constitution dis-

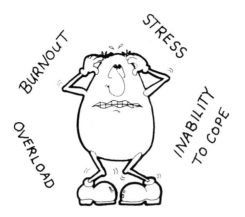

posed to the use of narcotics (or other drugs). These people argue that to end drug dependency a restructuring of the user's personality is needed. Freudians, on the other hand, argue that drug use is a case of unresolved childhood conflicts—that narcotics use is an immature response of acting out, rather than dealing with, these conflicts. Existentialists argue that life's unresolved conflicts constantly bombard people with insurmountable pressures, but offer no viable means of relief. Thus, for some, drug use may be viewed as self-treatment for internal distress.[12] Manuel M. Pearson and Ralph B. Little describe the course of addiction:

> The addict, however, has a special psychological relationship with his addicting drug—a pathological dependency upon the agent which he needs and without which he cannot deal with the stressful factors in his life situation.
>
> Later on, such a dependency produces the pathological craving, a central feature of all addiction that is reflected in the subsequent reorientation of his existence. Obtaining and taking this drug becomes his way of life.[13]

The necessary state for addiction is *preaddiction* or a *predilection* for addiction. Before using a drug, people experience certain feelings or drives that prepare them for becoming drug-dependent. The potential user may be unaware of his or her vulnerability to dependency.

People inclined toward drug use usually suffer from psychological tensions that, left unabated, become painful and may produce a state of helplessness. Such a state may bring on self-deprecation and depression, exacerbating the problem and contributing to further tension and loss of self-esteem. This cycle of negativism may continue, resulting in the use of psychoactive substances and, depending on the intensity of the predependent state, some degree of drug dependence.[14] The gratifying use of narcotics relieves the tension and may be tantamount to a return to the womb, where frustrations are nonexistent and the painful realities of existence have little impact.

Generally speaking, the personality traits of a drug abuser may include (1) difficulty handling frustration, anxiety, and depression; (2) an urge for immediate gratification of desires; (3) difficulty relating with others; (4) low self-esteem; (5) impulsiveness, risk taking, little regard for health; and (6) resistance to authority.

The Adlerian Theory of Ego Compensation

The Adlerian interpretation of drug dependency focuses on the individual's inferiority complex. The theory states that neurotic symptoms develop to safeguard an individual's self-esteem. The "perceived inferiority causes withdrawal from social participation and leads to compensatory maneuvers. Drug abuse would be such a maneuver."[15]

The person who is drug-dependent would like to succeed, but all too often can't. Drug taking becomes an act on which the blame for failure can be placed and is the excuse to relinquish responsibility for failure. It takes on the role of scapegoat, as in, "If I only didn't have this drinking problem, I could succeed."[16] Drug dependency becomes a self-fulfilling prophecy, absolving the individual from all responsibility.

Basic to the Adlerian psychiatric view of addiction is the theme of weak-ego compensation by a source other than the individual. The drug is supposedly taken to strengthen the normal defense mechanisms that have failed the user in coping with stress: the user actually believes that the drug will facilitate his or her ability to overcome the obstacles that are interfering with gratification and unlock or unleash restricted potentials and powers.[17]

DEPENDENCY STATES: SOCIOLOGICAL PERSPECTIVES

Sociological perspectives hold that humanity is responsible for drug dependency.

> The sense of hopelessness and defeat among dwellers in our city slums, the sense, among young people today, to belong to a group and their consequent drift into groups of heroin users . . . an addict relapses, according to some sociological theories, because he returns to the same neighborhood where he became addicted and associates with addicts once more.[18]

The origin of this theory can be found in the urban ghetto, where men and women have to "fight like hell" in order to stay alive, let alone enjoy themselves. The physical conditions offer visual proof and a constant reminder that the occupants are living in the dirtiest, most run-down part of the city—and not by choice, but by necessity. What's happening in the classrooms is often not what's happening in the real world. Consequently, even if there were job possibilities and access to employment related to their education, they could not avail themselves of those possibilities because by then they've quit school. The area is impoverished, legitimate employment is simply not a reality, and learning takes place in the streets. The ghetto can be a living nightmare.

Can it be any wonder, then, that people in these environments are continuously on edge, angry, depressed, and frustrated? That interpersonal relationships are at best taut and frayed, and at worst brutally violent? The familiar names include Detroit, Harlem, and, the most infamous, Watts. No money, no jobs, rats, deteriorating buildings, tremendous noise and overcrowding, garbage, and littered streets—the chain of frustration can easily lead ghetto dwellers to seek escape—in drug use. The "no hope but dope" scenario is finally enacted. But we also have the other extreme: individuals who have too much become bored and unhappy.

DEPENDENCY STATES: BIOLOGICAL MECHANISMS

Philosophical Concerns

In comparison with psychosociological theories, biological explanations of dependency states are relatively new. Such explanations emphasize that psychological and sociological causes of drug dependency are only part of the picture, and that biochemistry is also a factor, involving cellular dependency on the molecules of certain chemicals. This viewpoint is somewhat *a priori* in that it states what may occur to the chemistry of the body with repeated exposure to psychoactive substances. It also tells us that an individual may remain, or become, drug-dependent in spite of, a harmonious mental state and environment.

Explaining human behavior, maladaptive or otherwise, in terms of biological abnormalities is enticing. It has already been seen to be easier to define and correct mental disorders by biological means than by psychological and sociological ones, and test-tube solutions may be easier to secure, and less costly, than sweeping social and interpersonal change. Of course, biochemical theories gloss over and deny the idea that the world is incorrect, preferring to say that the individual is simply "out of synch," thus eliminating the need to confront and change the social order.

There is some validity to the biological argument. Even so, far too often treatment of people with problems consists of making them fit into society, rather than acknowledging that their problems stem from living in an often crazy world. Helping individuals adapt to the existing social order with pills, potions, and surgery can be a quick and inexpensive "cure." But any objective thinker must see that the biochemical perspective must address the important psychological and sociological aspects of dependency as well as its physiological aspects. The combination of the three will give a complete explanation of dependency states.

Biochemical Theory

Current trends in research may someday explain dependency conditions for all psychoactive substances in biochemical terms. Opiate dependency is presently explained in this manner as a response to repeated administrations of the opiate molecule in its natural or synthesized form (opium, morphine, heroin, demerol, dilaudid, percodan). The time required for an individual to become drug-dependent may vary from several months to a number of years, depending on the frequency of drug use and the dosage.

Simply stated, the body gradually adapts to the presence of the opiate molecule with repeated exposure to it. At some point the body becomes so adapted that the molecule becomes a necessity for proper physiological functioning. Further research may produce opiate biochemical concepts that are applicable to other psychoactive substances as well.

The foundation for a biochemical theory of opiate dependency was being set by the mid 1970s.[19] For some time it was suggested that certain areas of the brain, and the central nervous system in general, were particularly sensitive to opiates, that certain receptor mechanisms or binding sites specifically received opiate molecules administered into the body. Recent research indicates that opiate-receptor mechanisms were actually binding sites for an internally produced chemical. What, then, becomes of the body's own chemical in the presence of the opiate molecule? What is its own function? Furthermore, will it bind with the opiate-receptor mechanisms following discontinuation of opiate use? Researchers are still investigating these questions.

Enkephalins and Endorphins

The existence of the opiate-receptor mechanism was first established in an article in *Neurosciences Research Program Bulletin*. The stumbling block in identifying the receptor mechanism was that opiates, like most other compounds, bind to virtually any biological or nonbiological membrane. Research studies by Avram Goldstein at the Stanford University School of Medicine and Solomon H. Snyder and Candice B. Pert at the Johns Hopkins School of Medicine eventually broke the ice. Using membrane fragments from homogenized brain cells and radioactively labeled Naloxone (an opiate antagonist), they conducted tests that established the phenomenon of specific binding to receptor mechanisms.[20]

After the receptor mechanisms had been identified, research could be directed to how they function. Many neurotransmitter systems (systems in which chemicals released by nerve endings modulate the firing of other nerve cells, thereby transmitting messages) and brain functions were known to be distributed throughout the brain. If opiate-receptor distribution were to mirror some specific brain property, then opiate action might be implicated as a necessary component of the property. Because opiates are pain killers, the brain structures involved in pain were natural suspects. Of the two known pathways implicated in the perception of pain, the pathway for duller, more chronic, and less localized pain is relieved quite effectively by opiates. The other pathway, which transmits sharp, localized pain, is poorly relieved by opiates.[21] The paleospinothalmic (opiate-affected) pain pathway consists of many interconnected nerve cells, most of which lack a fatty myelin insulation and therefore conduct impulses rather slowly.

Distribution measurements indicated striking parallels between the opiate-affected pain pathways and opiate-receptor mechanisms. Opiate-receptor binding occurs at high density in the limbic system, which mediates emotion in humans.[22] Furthermore, this binding appears to affect memory and spatial orientation (the awareness of where one is in relation to the environment). Says Snyder:

> Clearly man was not made with morphine inside him. The existence in all vertebrates of specific opiate receptor sites strongly indicated the presence of a natural morphine like substance in the brain, possibly a neurotransmitter, that acts at these sites.
>
> Opiates, like most other drugs that affect the mind, are thought to act primarily at synapses in the brain, the specialized regions where the terminal of a nerve fiber makes a junction with the outer membrane of another nerve cell and chemically modulates its activity . . . it appears that the opiate receptor is associated with synaptic regions of the brain.
>
> Since neurotransmitters act as synapses, the opiate receptor appeared to function very much like a receptor site for a natural neurotransmitter substance in the brain.[23]

This reasoning eventually led to the discovery of the endogenous (internally produced) neurotransmitter.[24] Experiments conducted by researchers John Hughes and Hans W. Kasterlitz of the University of Aberdeen provided the evidence of a morphinelike neurotransmitter. Subsequent studies by Lars Terenius of the University of Uppsala and Pasternak and Snyder independently identified the same substance. Hughes and Kasterlitz isolated the factor from the brain of pigs and named it *enkephalin,* from the Greek word meaning "in the head." A similar peptide, beta endorphine, is also found in the pituitary gland. "Enkephalins are neurotransmitters of specific neuronal systems in the brain that mediate the integration of sensory information having to do with pain and emotional behavior, and that subserve unidentified functions as well."[25] With the discovery of enkephalin came a new theory of opiate dependence.

Years of research have thus provided a fairly clear model of the biochemistry of opiate dependence. Opiate receptor mechanisms in the body facilitate the amelioration of certain types of pain throughout the central nervous system and the gastrointestinal tract and bind with the body's own morphinelike substances,

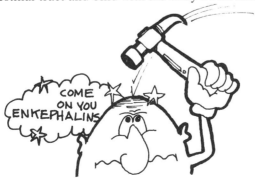

enkephalin and beta endorphine, found in the pituitary gland. Enkephalin release, in the presence of administered opiates, is reduced, though its production remains constant. But continuous opiate administration results in a complete stoppage of enkephalin release. If opiate use is discontinued, the receptor mechanisms are left without any chemical counterpart, and a series of intracellular events occur that lead to withdrawal symptoms. Eventually, enkephalin, in the absence of opiates, is gradually reintroduced into the system and begins to neutralize the elevated nucleotide levels. This return to normal chemical levels signifies the termination of the withdrawal symptoms.[26]

Sometimes, however, the desire to use opiates returns after total withdrawal. The cause for this is unclear, though it may be that enkephalin levels or the level of their release never quite returns to the predependent level. As a result the feeling remains that there should always be just a little more, and therefore the need for just a little more.

What application this model of opiate dependency has to other dependency-producing psychoactive substances is not clear at this time, but it is possible that similar situations result from the use of other mild-altering drugs. As Snyder states:

> in a formal sense the processes of tolerance and physical dependence are the same for most classes of drugs. Hence, if one could understand the biochemical mechanisms involved for one class, such as the opiates, one would know something about what was happening with drugs in other classes.[27]

SUMMARY

The reasons for the use of psychoactive drugs are as varied as the individuals who use them, but most can be categorized as either psychological (interpersonal) or sociological (environmental). These factors, which work in consort to affect human behavior, include the need for mood alterations, interpersonal and social communication, recreation, stress reduction and relaxation, religious and spiritual enlightenment, sexual enhancement, personal awareness, sensation seeking, political expression, coping with alienation, peer pressure, and parental behavior modeling. Biochemistry also enters into drug-dependency study.

NOTES

[1]Quoted in David Rorvik, "Mood Drugs," *Penthouse* 10, no. 4 (December 1978).

[2]Marvin Zuckerman, "The Search for High Sensation," *Psychology Today* 11, no. 9 (February 1978):38. Reprinted with permission from *Psychology Today Magazine*. Copyright © 1978 American Psychological Association (APA).

[3]Ibid.

[4]Reprinted from *The Center of the Cyclone* by John C. Lilly. Copyright © 1972 by John C.

Lilly. Reprinted with permission of The Julian Press, Inc. The quotation appears on pages 42–43. Crown Publishers, Inc.

[5]Zuckerman, "The Search for High Sensation," p. 40.

[6]Quoted in Edward M. Brecher et al., *Licit and Illicit Drugs* (Boston: Little, Brown, 1972), p. 273.

[7]Quoted in Solomon H. Snyder, "What We Have Forgotten about Pot: A Pharmacologist's History," *New York Times Magazine,* December 13, 1970, p. 125.

[8]Louise A. Richards, "Role of Society," in *Drug Abuse: Clinical and Basic Aspects,* ed. Sachindra N. Pradham and Samarendra N. Dutta (St. Louis: C. V. Mosby, 1977), p. 511.

[9]Snyder, "What We Have Forgotten about Pot."

[10]Lester Grinspoon, *Marijuana Reconsidered* (New York: Bantam Books, 1971), p. 202.

[11]Richards, "Role of Society," p. 506.

[12]Jerome Jaffe, "Drug Addiction and Drug Abuse," in *The Pharmacological Basis of Therapeutics,* 6th ed., ed. Alfred Goodman Gilman, Louis S. Goodman, and Alfred Gilman (New York: Macmillan, 1980), p. 543.

[13]Manuel M. Pearson and Ralph B. Little, "The Addictive Process in Unusual Addictions: A Further Elaboration of Etiology," *The American Journal of Psychiatry* vol. 125:9, pp. 1166–1171, March 1969. Copyright © 1969, The American Psychiatric Association. The quotation appears on page 1166. Used with permission.

[14]Ibid.

[15]Ronald A. Steffenhagen, "Drug Abuse and Related Phenomena: An Adlerian Approach," *Journal of Individual Psychology* 30, no. 2 (November 1974):240–41.

[16]Ibid.

[17]Pearson, "The Addictive Process," p. 1669.

[18]Jaffe, "Drug Addictions and Drug Abuse," p. 543.

[19]See, for example, Solomon Snyder and Steven Matthysse, eds., "Opiate Receptor Mechanisms," *Neurosciences Research Program Bulletin* 13, no. 1 pp. 48–53.

[20]Solomon H. Snyder, "Opiate Receptors and Internal Opiates," *Scientific American* 236, no. 3 (March 1977):53.

[21]Ibid., p. 48.

[22]Ibid.

[23]Ibid., p. 49.

[24]Snyder and Mattysse, ed., "Opiate Receptor Mechanisms," *Neurosciences Research Program Bulletin.*

[25]Snyder, "Opiate Receptors and Internal Opiates."

[26]Ibid.

[27]Ibid.

3

THE DRUG SCENE

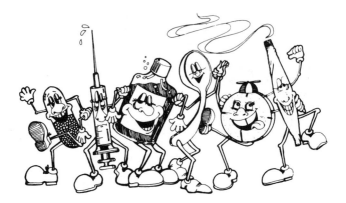

INTRODUCTION

This chapter focuses on several major groups involved in the drug scene—youths, adults, and senior citizens. We realize that there are many subgroups as well. However, these three major headings will clarify some of the general differences among youths, adults, and senior citizens. This chapter offers an overview of the drug scene; greater detail will be provided in later chapters.

Our culture frequently accepts one type of drug consumption while rejecting and often penalizing those using other types of drugs. For example, alcohol, caffeine, and nicotine are legal and often thought of as innocuous drugs, but marijuana and cocaine are classified as illegal and dangerous substances. Whatever the drug, the problem of misuse has grown to astounding proportions. Patterns of intense drug-taking have reached virtually all classes of society. The consumer can pick from many thousands of drugs now available. Furthermore, each generation seems to vary in its motivation for drug use. Youths, possessing the exuberance of young life and feeling pressures to succeed, often use drugs to satisfy the need for sensation or confidence. Adults, burdened with the pressures of family, advancing age, and the world of work, may use drugs to rest and relax. Senior citizens are motivated toward drug use to ease physical pain as well as the pain of lost family and friends, fixed incomes, and sleepless nights. Drug use is a part of most people's lives.

THE YOUTH DRUG SCENE

Background

The contemporary youth drug scene encompasses a vast number of people, from all socioeconomic classes, in their teens and early twenties. These people are confronted with rapid change, too many choices, and computerized technology that often leads to depersonalization. They face difficult and confusing decisions about education, religion, work, and the directions they will choose for their lives. Because of the tensions such decisions and situations can bring, many youths look to drugs to temporarily escape or look inward for solutions.

Conflicting reports about the physiological effects of drugs often confuse youths. A classic example of this confusion appeared in a 1969 Supreme Court decision:

> To be a confirmed drug addict is to be one of the walking dead. . . . The teeth have rotted out, the appetite is lost, and the stomach and intestines don't function properly. The gall bladder becomes inflamed; eyes and skin turn bilious yellow; in some cases membranes of the nose turn a flaming red; the partition separating the nostrils is eaten away and breathing is difficult. . . . Such is the torment of being a drug addict, such is the plague of being one of the walking dead.[1]

A recent study has found that drug users are increasingly younger, that use begins as early as elementary school. It has also been found that there is a growing propensity toward polydrug use (the use of several drugs), with younger students imitating the drug-taking behavior of classmates and friends.[2] Group acceptance plays a key role in this increasing drug-taking behavior. Many youths do not have the strength or the desire to resist peer pressure, and often find themselves involved in drug-related problems. Consistent with these facts are the yearly increases in the number of liquor- and marijuana-related arrests of those under eighteen.

Our society is based on drugs. Nearly everyone relies upon them to cure aches and pains as well as for recreational purposes. Drug use begins very early. Chemical substances are given to infants and toddlers. Children are frequently treated with prescription drugs, over-the-counter remedies, or home remedies. In addition, youngsters are often given chemicals such as vitamins. As kids enter school they continue to use prescription and over-the-counter drugs. However, there is usually a dramatic increase in the use of caffeine in the form of chocolate, cocoa, or cola drinks.

During grades 4, 5, and 6 recreational illicit drug use and abuse begin to appear. At this age level the types of drugs used to "get high" are often aerosols and inhalants. This is because these substances give a quick high and are everyday items—for example, glue—that are easily obtained. As children continue to use these subtances, they often begin to experience irritation. However, they are not willing to give up the high, so they turn to other drugs. Grade schoolers may begin using tobacco, marijuana, alcohol, or amphetamines. It is alarmingly easy for children as young as eleven or twelve to obtain drugs.[3]

Children often report their first experience with alcohol in grades 5 and 6. Many of these children have older siblings who are drinkers, or alcoholic parents. At the junior high, alcohol and marijuana use increases; it is often associated with school dances or other evening functions. The ease of buying drugs such as marijuana and speed contributes to their increased use at the junior high level. At the high school there is much greater use of a wider variety of drugs. Serious problems such as dependency and drug-related accidents and fatalities happen more frequently.

Alcohol and tobacco cigarettes continue to be widely used by high school–age and younger students, but the use of the latter appears to be leveling off or declining. Tobacco cigarettes are frequently used in emulation of adults or as a status symbol. Girls from twelve to eighteen seem to be the fastest growing group of tobacco smokers, but this increase has leveled off recently to the point that about the same percentage of boys and girls smoke.

Abuse of alcoholic beverages by youth is tolerated by some parents because they fear their child's use of other drugs and believe alcohol is not as habit-forming or dangerous. In addition, the use of alcohol does not carry a social stigma for them, and the legal consequences for its use are not as severe as those for other drugs. In effect, most parents are more familiar with alcohol than with other drugs and can identify with its effects. Alcohol is still generally thought to be the drug used in the greatest *quantity* by youth.

However, marijuana has recently been cited as the drug most *frequently* used. According to a report published by the National Institute on Drug Abuse, more than one in ten high school seniors uses marijuana daily or almost daily. Daily use of marijuana is slightly more common than daily use of alcohol among this group.[4] Getting stoned is something to talk about and becomes a ritual for some youth. Among other drugs, young people frequently consume caffeine in cola drinks, coffee, chocolate bars, and cocoa. Cocaine is increasing in popularity. Though very expensive (it is second only to heroin in this respect) it offers an exhilarating high. It is frequently found among television and movie stars, athletes, and those with high incomes who frequent resort areas. Cocaine has worked its way through various socioeconomic levels and into the youth drug scene. Heroin use can also be found among young people. However, it is still confined mostly to big-city youth, many of whom are filled with despair for the future.

TABLE 3-1   National Youth and Polydrug Study

Substance Category	Ever Used, Lifetime	Weekly Use, Lifetime[a]	Current Use[b]	Current Weekly Use[c]
Marijuana	90.4	85.9	81.8	72.4
Alcohol	89.1	79.8	80.1	58.5
Amphetamines	45	32.3	28.5	14.2
Hashish	42.4	27.4	28.2	10.9
Barbiturates	39.9	29.4	26.2	13.6
Hallucinogens	40	23.8	21.5	6.3
Phencyclidine	31.8	22.2	20.7	10.2
Nonbarbiturate sedatives	29	21.1	18.9	10.4
Inhalants	28.8	19.9	13.1	6.9
Cocaine	25.8	9.5	12.9	4.5
Other opiates	24.7	14.4	12.2	5.6
Heroin	12.5	7.8	6.7	4.3
Over-the-counter drugs	8.4	4.9	3.3	1
Methadone	3.9	1.7	1.6	0.8

[a]Weekly or more frequent use for at least four consecutive weeks.
[b]Use within the three months before admission to treatment.
[c]Current weekly use is defined as regular use.

Source: Yoav Santo and Alfred S. Friedman, "Overviews and Selected Findings from the National Youth and Polydrug Study," *Contemporary Drug Problems* 9, no. 2 (Fall 1980):285. Copyright © 1980 Federal Legal Publications, Inc., 157 Chambers Street, New York, New York, 10007.

Youth also seem to be susceptible to fad drugs such as methamphetamine (speed), methaqualone (ludes), and phencyclidine (PCP). Risk taking is very common during this period of life, and many accidental deaths, suicides, and homicides are associated with drug abuse. One of the most striking findings from the National Youth and Polydrug Study (NYPS) is the large number of *different* substances used by youth. Possibly the most important feature of these data is that the majority of young drug users report little difficulty in obtaining a variety of illicit substances such as nonbarbiturate sedatives, barbiturates, and amphetamines. The study also found that marijuana is being used at an earlier age. Finally, nearly all adolescents who seek drug treatment are involved in multiple substance abuse: on the average, it was reported, they had used more than five different substances in their lifetime and four drugs on a regular basis (at least weekly for one month or more).[5]

Table 3-1 illustrates the prevalence of drug use by those in the NYPS sample. (Tobacco use was not covered in this study.) Perhaps the most obvious finding in the data was that practically all clients had at some time in their lives used marijuana and alcohol. Next came amphetamines: almost half of the sample reported having used it some time during their lives. Another interesting finding was that almost one third of the clients reported having used PCP. PCP use was more common than the use of tranquilizers, inhalants, cocaine, and opiates.

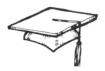

Drugs on Campus

The social values that swept the nation's campuses in the 1960s are now shared by many students and deeply influence the whole of society. According to Daniel Yankelovich, "these new values are not simply a matter of adopting a freer, more casual life style. They symbolize a profound value transformation affecting every phase of life."[6]

These values can be divided into three domains: (1) moral norms, consisting of more liberal sexual attitudes, changes in one's relation to authority institutions, different attitudes toward churches and organized religion as a behavior guide, and a change in traditional concepts of patriotism and national allegiance; (2) new values pertaining to the traditional Protestant work ethic, marriage, family, and success defined in terms of money; and (3) a vague but intense concern with self-fulfillment, which is an individual's statement that there must be more to life than just working to make ends meet.[7] Drug use is associated with each of the three areas: it is often considered an expression of political consciousness; it may cause a person to relinquish obligations to friends and country; and it may initiate dissatisfaction with work and work-related problems.

In college marijuana, alcohol, cocaine, and amphetamines are the drugs of choice. The results of a random sample of college students found that alcohol was used by 70 percent of drug users, marijuana by 60 percent, and cocaine by 28 percent.[8] Amphetamine use remains steady, but barbiturate and hallucinogen use appears to be on the decline. Drug taking has reached a higher level of sophistication now that greater knowledge has been accumulated about various drugs and their effects.

Pollster Yankelovich believes that there is a clear psychological line separating college drug users from abusers. He states that "abusers are people who go through severe bouts of depression, anxiety, and frustration far more often than either users or nonusers"[9] (see Table 3–2). In short, characteristic symptoms of college drug abusers are preoccupation with drugs, association with other drug abusers, disturbances in mood, a negative self-image, and an inability to carry on everyday life.

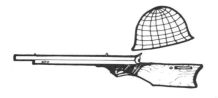

TABLE 3-2   DIFFERENCES AMONG DRUG ABUSERS, USERS, AND NONUSERS

Abusers (%)		Users (%)	Nonusers (%)
47	are unable to finish projects	26	26
48	see things as hopeless	17	19
47	feel something or someone stops any progressive move forward	21	18
42	feel angry or frustrated most of the time	24	20
36	often find it difficult to get through the day	19	18
34	have never found a group they felt they belonged to	8	8
66	have run away from home	37	—
36	reported failing classes	16	16
70	have been expelled from school	41	—
62	have purposely damaged property	43	—
89	keep drugs on hand	41	—
51	sell drugs for profit	14	—

Source: Daniel Yankelovich, "Drug Users vs. Drug Abusers: How Students Control Their Drug Crisis," *Psychology Today* 9, no. 5 (October 1975):41. Reprinted with permission from *Psychology Today Magazine.* Copyright © 1975 American Psychological Association (APA).

Drugs in the Military

In 1978, both licit and illicit drug use was shown to be higher among men in the military services than among civilians of the same age. In the early 1970s, however, drug use in the military was more than simply high—it reached epidemic proportions in Vietnam.

Drug Use in Vietnam   The unusual setting and circumstances of the Vietnam War provide a unique perspective on the drug scene. In Southeast Asia, all varieties of drugs except hallucinogens were plentiful, inexpensive, and easy to obtain.[10] Initially, marijuana was the most popular drug among American servicemen there, so much so that the rate of use grew to alarming proportions, even in the field of combat. Eventually, this extensive use became of great concern to the military and to a number of stateside politicians, resulting in rigid controls and sanctions regarding marijuana use. At that point servicemen were forced to seek drug alternatives, and they turned to opiates, which were also readily available and inexpensive. In time purified heroin became the most commonly used opiate by American GIs. Injection, the stateside method of heroin administration, was rare. Vietnam heroin, because of its high purity, was usually smoked or inhaled. Thus the geographical setting, in which heroin was easily accessible, played an important role in the Vietnam drug scene.

The Vietnam drug epidemic began in the early 1970s. An estimate supported by chemical tests as well as various military surveys showed that by 1972 approximately 7 percent of Army enlisted men were using heroin. In 1974, counselors in the Army drug program estimated that well over half of the lower-ranking enlisted men were using hashish or marijuana.[11]

Reasons for Use in Vietnam   One of the most common motivating factors for drug use in Vietnam was a desire to escape from mental and physical pain and fear. The social setting was also a factor, since military morale was generally very low, few regarded their duty as functional and useful, and off-duty time was often boring and frustrating. Since many soldiers felt that Vietnam was not part of the "real world," behavior was permitted there that would not normally have been condoned stateside.[12] There was also the cultural shock associated with combat in a foreign country. Finally, peer pressure played a significant role in a soldier's drug involvement.

Rehabilitation and Treatment for Returning Vietnam Veterans   In December 1970, the United States Army took responsibility for treatment and prevention of drug abuse. The program the Army developed consisted of diagnosis, drug-education classes, rehabilitation through group therapy and medication, cooperation with civilian authorities in reducing drug traffic, and amnesty for those who voluntarily sought treatment. The Free Radical Assay Technique (FRAT) was used to detect heroin in the urine; other tests measured barbiturate, amphetamine, opiate, and methadone involvement. Treatment centers were set up in barracks, hospitals, and prisonlike settings. Diagnosis was made by a physician, and treatment ranged from four days to two weeks.

Many soldiers, however, lacked trust in the military justice system. Consequently, they often considered amnesty a hoax and felt they would be harassed if they joined the program.[13] Servicemen participated in the program primarily out of fear of not returning home on time, or fear of punishment or prosecution. The Army's goal of total elimination of the drug problem may have been unrealistic.

Conclusion   What lessons may be learned from the Vietnam experience? First, as shown by the Army's attempt to stop marijuana use, high-pressure drug control is usually ineffective and may instead promote a switch to other drugs. Second, the belief that a drug problem can be eliminated by cutting off the drug's availability is incorrect. Third, people usually seek periodic escape as a way of coping with stressful situations; one of the means of escape can be drug use or abuse. Fourth, a high rate of drug use may be a situational response to a specific setting, as demonstrated by returning servicemen who reverted to preservice patterns of drug use, which included high marijuana use and amphetamine, barbiturate, and narcotics use, in descending order of frequency.

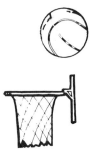

Drugs and Athletics

Introduction   Drug use has been reported throughout the sports world, from amateur athletics to professional sports. Most of the drugs used come under two headings: restorative and ergogenic (additive). Restorative drugs are used with the intent of returning the athlete to a previous level of proficiency following illness, injury, or performance anxiety. These drugs may include antiinflammatory agents, pain-killers, and tranquilizers used as muscle relaxants. Ergogenic drugs are used with the intent of enhancing an athlete's normal ability. These drugs may include anabolic steroids and amphetamines.

The use of ergogenic aids is a growing problem in today's athletic community and has led to rigid drug testing for control. An ergogenic aid is defined as any substance that will improve not only athletic performance but work level as well. Therefore, it may be inferred that industrial workers share the same interest in ergogenic aids that discus throwers might have. Athletes have used a variety of supposedly ergogenic substances in an effort to improve performance. Alcohol, amphetamines, anabolic steroids, caffeine, hormones, and protein supplements are examples.

Drug Use in College and Amateur Athletics   The reports on college athletic drug use are somewhat ambiguous. Numerous claims have been made about the pregame use of novocaine and other analgesics, amphetamines, and tranquilizers for muscle relaxation, but it is difficult to estimate the amount of drugs being used. College coach Tom Ecker, however, says, "It's a great rarity today for someone to achieve athletic success who doesn't take drugs."[14]

Distance runners sometimes used caffeine to help improve their performance. Two hundred milligrams of caffeine (there are 100 to 150 milligrams per cup of coffee) taken one hour before a race raise a runner's fat utilization from 22 percent to about 40 percent, thus allowing the runner to travel further and faster before having to utilize his or her glycogen reserve.[15] Various marathoners recommend the use of aspirin to provide relief from inflammation. Others report that aspirin prevents cartilage deterioration by inhibiting the enzymes responsible for the breakdown.[16] Don Kardong, one of America's premier marathoners, believes that aspirin helps race performance by thinning the blood (thus improving circulation) and increasing the body's ability to expel excess heat during prolonged racing.[17]

Drug Use in Olympic and Other International Competition
Amphetamines and anabolic steroids are probably the most prevalent drugs used today by athletes in international competition. "Introduced in the late 1950's, anabolic steroids are synthetic derivatives of the male hormone testosterone. They stimulate a building up, or anabolic, process in the body through synthesis of protein for muscle growth and tissue repair."[18] Athletes use steroids for a variety of reasons. "First of all, competitors have discovered that anabolic steroids allow them to recover more quickly from workout sessions, which in turn makes more intense training possible."[19] They also use them to increase

aggressiveness and build strength. Overall, athletes use steroids to gain a competitive edge.

The benefits of anabolic steroids in athletic performance may not be conclusive, but the adverse effects are certainly gaining support both theoretically and scientifically. The massive doses taken by athletes have been found to cause hair loss, heady agressiveness, and shrunken testicles in males and deepening of the voice, growth of facial hair, breast shrinkage, and clitoris enlargement in females.[20] Anabolic steroid use may also lead to a decrease in sperm production in men as well as liver damage and clogged arteries in both sexes.[21] Clogged arteries can be linked to the effect that these synthetic hormones have on transporter molecules in the blood called high-density lipoproteins (HDLs). HDLs are thought to transport cholesterol out of the blood vessels.[22] It has been found that after athletes take high-dosage steroids for four weeks, their normal HDL levels drop by about 60 percent. Therefore, less cholesterol is leaving the blood stream and remaining to clog blood vessels.[23]

Not all research concerning steroids is negative. Steroids still fulfill their original purpose of increasing the intake of protein to build muscles in patients suffering from chronic diseases and to protect blood cells from destruction by radiation and chemotherapy.[24] In addition, steroids are used in the treatment of burns, hormonal imbalances, certain bone diseases, such as osteoporosis, and some cases of effeminacy. Last, they can help control muscle-wasting diseases and certain kinds of anemia and speed healing after surgery or long illness.

How can these drugs be so useful in medicine and so dangerous in sports? The main reason is dosage. Doctors usually prescribe 5 to 15 milligrams per day of a certain steroid whereas atheletes who are self-prescribing may take from 50 to 500 milligrams per day. This increase of 10 to 100 times the prescribed dosage is where adverse side effects from steroids can be found.

At the 1984 Summer Olympics held in Los Angeles, officials went all out to make sure the competition would be the fairest in history. One of the top priorities was to crack down on drug use. Officials set up a $2 million state-of-the-art drug-testing laboratory—the only one of its kind in the United States. Located on the campus of the University of California at Los Angeles, it combines the well-established analytic technique of gas chromatography and mass spectrometry. The $30,000 gas chromatograph screens a small portion of the urine sample that an athlete provides. As a stream of helium gas sweeps the urine through a long tube, a detector registers a peak on a graph whenever it spots molecules that contain nitrogen or phosphorous—components of almost every banned drug. The time that the peak takes to appear reflects the time that the substance needs to pass through the tube, which in turn gives a strong hint as to the nature of the substance that produced the peak. When technicians see a peak that seems to correspond to an illegal drug, they run another portion of the urine sample through a mass spectrometer, a $200,000 instrument that fragments molecules into easily recognized pieces. The instrument acts like an unerring fingerprint expert: if the urine sample fits the pattern of a banned drug, which is programmed into the machine, the test is positive.[25]

In addition to the Olympic drug-testing program, colleges and universities and professional sports have stepped up the crackdown on drug use in sports. In any event, it appears that emphasis should be shifted from drugs to nutrition, training techniques, and biomechanics as means of improving athletic performance.

Professional Sports   Some professional athletes take amphetamines to "get up" and barbiturates or depressants to "come down." In general, professional football players appear to use amphetamines in three ways.[26] The first is ingestion of high doses (30 to 150 milligrams or more) only on game days for pain relief and the induction of rage. (A professional linebacker recalled a football game in which he took a little extra amphetamine: "I was bouncing all over the field. . . . I was running and jumping along the sidelines hollering, I'm a superplayer, they can't block me. No one can block me, it was really funny, I knew what I was saying but I just didn't care."[27]) The second involves taking lower doses (5 to 30 milligrams) on game days to increase speed and combat pain. The third, also used for weight control by other professional athletes, such as jockeys, boxers, and wrestlers (approximately fifteen milligrams per day), is usually confined to the first several weeks of summer camp and the preseason, when overweight players must lose weight quickly.

The results of abuse of these drugs are often dramatic and affect not only athletes on the playing field but the players' family life as well.[28] Pathological jealousy, wife abuse, drinking binges, fighting, and various physiologic ailments can be caused by such abuse, and other drugs, such as sleeping pills, may be needed to bring players down. Bob Lundy, Miami Dolphin trainer, comments, "I've seen players in a daze as late as Tuesday after Sunday's game. . . . Some need a week to come down after a game. It's a continuous cycle; pepped up, drunk (or tranquilized), hung over, and pepped up.[29]

The impact of cocaine on the professional sports arena has been incredible. A number of lives and teams have been devastated by this white powder. Interestingly, it appears that the acknowledgment of cocaine in the sporting world has been fairly recent. But the presence of this very powerful psychoactive substance has been increasingly documented since the mid 1970s. The notoriety of cocaine use in professional sports became increasingly apparent in the latter part of that decade. More and more professional athletes were linked to the use of cocaine. Indeed, the list reads like a who's who in a variety of sports, with the three major professional sports of football, basketball, and baseball grabbing the lion's share of the limelight. In the late 1970s Thomas "Hollywood" Henderson and Mercury Morris became two of the first name athletes to gain this ill-advised notoriety. At the time, Henderson was a starting linebacker for the Dallas Cowboys. Shortly thereafter he experienced several cocaine-related arrests. Perhaps no other initial drug-related incident gained more exposure than that of Mercury

Morris. Morris was one of the gifted members of the famed Miami Dolphins teams of the early 1970s. Morris was sentenced to twenty years in prison for possession of a controlled substance—cocaine.

A more recent arrest for possession of cocaine was that of E. J. Junior, linebacker for the St. Louis Cardinals. Among the creative stipulations mandated for his probation was working in a care unit for adolescent drug abusers. A number of Cincinnati Bengals players were apprehended for cocaine use. Defensive tackle Ross Browner and mammoth fullback Pete Johnson were suspended in response. Eventually, Johnson was traded to San Diego and then Miami, where he was the only running back to pass the urinalysis drug check. Teammates Chuck Muncie and Ricky Young failed the test and were released from the team. Muncie had previously had several episodes of cocaine use, detection, and treatment.

In 1985 the National Basketball Association enacted the toughest drug regulations in professional sports history. Detection of cocaine use could result in a lifetime ban from the sport. These measures were drafted in response to drug-related incidents involving a number of name players, including David Thompson of Denver, John Drew of Atlanta, Michael Ray Richardson of the New York Knicks, and John Lucas of Houston.

One of the more carefully watched cases involved Steve Howe, the gifted Los Angeles Dodger pitcher. In 1984 Howe, a cocaine user, experienced a series of treatments and relapses. He was suspended from the team and forced to sacrifice his $900,000-a-year salary. Lonnie Smith and David Green of the St. Louis Cardinals were also scrutinized by the press for their cocaine use. From 1983 to 1985 the list seemed to grow to endless proportions. Claudell Washington of the Atlanta Braves was detected. The Kansas City Royals were decimated by the loss of Willie Wilson, Willie Mays Aikens, Vida Blue, and Jerry Martin, all detected and referred to treatment.

What this points out is that over the years, professional athletes have been scrutinized by drug traffickers. This is nothing new, really. The main difference is the drugs being trafficked. Professional athletes cannot escape drug traffickers, who hang out at every arena, restaurant, and hotel making themselves available for purchases. The public is led to believe by the media that the life of professional sports is exciting, glamorous, and full of "the jazz." In reality, quite often, nothing could be further from the truth. Athletes are human and fall to the same temptations as others in our society. The endless repetition of one-night stands, hotel rooms, and restaurant food makes the travel life of the professional athlete tiring, and worse yet, boring. Cocaine use is in many instances tantamount to an antiboredom remedy.

The mandate is clear. The home offices within each professional league must continue to establish and enforce strict measures concerning drug use and abuse. There is a chance to reverse the drug-related media notoriety showered on athletes over the last decade. It is obvious that without this external motivation the status of professional athlete will continue to decline and further lessen the attractiveness of professional sports in general.

THE ADULT DRUG SCENE

Four major drug groups are used by adults: (1) alcohol, (2) barbiturates, tranquilizers, and sedatives, (3) nicotine, and (4) caffeine. Other drugs used with less frequency include aspirin, amphetamines, marijuana, and opiates. Since these drugs are associated most closely with the adult drug scene, they will be emphasized in this section.

Alcohol

Alcohol use is widespread among adults: approximately 70 to 75 percent use it. Though most adults are moderate drinkers, some become alcohol-dependent. The majority of these are males, though more and more women are now drinking.

The problem drinker and the alcoholic encounter many problems. They may expect a ten- to twelve-year decrease in life expectancy. They may experience personal problems including love-relationship difficulties. A tremendous economic loss may result from their drinking, affecting them and their families as well as the nation. In addition, approximately half of all fatal motor-vehicle accidents and one third of all suicides are alcohol-related.[30]

Alcohol is also responsible for half of adult deaths by fire and plays a significant role in drowning. The economic costs of alcoholism are difficult to estimate. In terms of lost production, health expenses, violent crimes, and traffic accidents, alcoholism and alcohol misuse have been estimated to cost from $43 billion a year to $120 billion a year.[31]

Tranquilizers and Sedative-Hypnotics

According to the National Clearinghouse for Drug Abuse Information, studies of the late 1960s and early 1970s showed widespread adult use of both tranquilizers and sedative-hypnotics (barbiturates and nonbarbiturates), with the former more popular.[32] Seventy percent of all adults in a 1974 California study frequently used sedative-hypnotics and 10 percent used minor tranquilizers. Almost twice as many women as men are frequent tranquilizer users, and Caucasians, people from middle socioeconomic classes and between 30 and 60, and people with higher education levels are most likely to be regular users.[33]

What complications arise from heavy depressant use? The short-term psychological and behavioral effects of barbiturates are similar to those of alcohol.[34] Depending on conditions, a low dose can either relax or excite a person. Heavy use, however, may cause apathy, reduced drive, and reduced ambition. It may also cause death (often in combination with alcohol), from accidental overdose or suicide.[35] Such abuse occurs more frequently among women (80 percent) than among men (20 percent). If barbiturates are used in high enough doses to cause tolerance and dependence, withdrawal may lead to convulsions severe enough to be life-threatening.

Nicotine

Generally speaking, cigarette smoking is more common among males than females, in cities than in small towns, among people from twenty to forty-four, and among alcoholics than nonalcoholics. It is least common among people sixty-five and older. As the hazards of smoking have become better known, more and more people have succeeded in quitting the habit. Doctors have been leaders—less than 21 percent now smoke. Still, many Americans die each year of cigarette-induced heart attacks, lung cancer, chronic bronchitis, and emphysema.[36] The amount of cigarette-induced illness and loss of work, money, and enjoyment of life is proportionately heavy.

Caffeine

Although caffeine is found in chocolate and cola drinks, most adults in the United States ingest it through coffee. The National Center for Health Statistics reports that adult Americans currently average about three cups of coffee per day, or about twelve pounds per year.[37]

Alfred Gilman and Louis Goodman report that:

> over indulgence in xanthine* beverages may lead to a condition that might be considered one of chronic poisoning. Central nervous stimulation results in restlessness and disturbed sleep; myocardial stimulation is reflected in cardio-irregularities; essential oils of coffee may cause some gastro intestinal irritation; and diarrhea is a common symptom.[38]

Quite frequently a dependent caffeine user experiences prolonged headaches during periods of abstinence from caffeine, only to find relief several minutes after drinking one cup of coffee.

The morning cup of coffee and coffee breaks are definitely part of the American lifestyle. And because so many people drink coffee, it has somehow become legitimate to consume the stimulant it contains. With its relatively low cost and easy availability, coffee consumption has become an accepted ritual of socialization.

Aspirin

According to Oakley Ray, "there are over 300 aspirin-containing products on the American market. Each day Americans gobble down about 44 million aspirin tablets. Twenty-one tons of aspirin (acetylsalicylic acid) a day."[39] If we consider the tremendous availability and use of aspirin, the high incidence of toxic reactions (salicylate poisoning) that may result in death (the number one cause of poisoning in children under five) and the incidence of aspirin-related gastrointestinal disorders should come as no surprise. The toxicity of the salicylates

*Xanthines are alkaloids (chemicals capable of neutralizing acids) found in a variety of plants throughout the world. The chemical family Xanthines include caffeine, theophylline, and theobromine.

in aspirin is underestimated, and they should not be viewed as a harmless household remedy. Aspirin would have great difficulty being approved by the FDA as an over-the-counter drug on the basis of today's knowledge and standards.

Amphetamines

At one time, overweight adults used amphetamines to control their appetite and decrease hunger. Others used them to overcome fatigue and to keep alert while driving. However, amphetamine use is not nearly as widespread among American adults as it was several years ago. Production and prescription rates dropped dramatically in the mid-1970s. Still, adults with long working hours or taxing schedules may find the temporary relief offered by amphetamines extremely desirable. In 1972 federal regulatory agencies began to act to reduce production of amphetamines by pharmaceutical companies. In 1978 the FDA removed amphetamines as a medication for obesity, and the legitimate medical use of amphetamines (for such conditions as narcolepsy) is much lower today.[40]

Marijuana

The use of marijuana as a psychoactive substance has become more and more popular with adults. Many of those who began as youthful marijuana users have continued their use into their adult years. Lessening fear of physical harm caused by marijuana and the lessening legal penalties for possession of it have made the drug more acceptable.

Opiates

For most adults, narcotic abuse begins in response to pain. Adults also take opiates to relieve anxiety and to enjoy the strong euphoric effect the drugs offer. Once tolerance develops, though, it becomes necessary to increase the amount taken to achieve the desired effect: continued use and increased amounts may lead to dependence. According to the National Clearinghouse for Drug Information,

figures show that more than half [of narcotic dependents] are under 30 years of age. . . . All narcotic addiction in the United States is not limited to heroin users. Some middle-aged and older people who take narcotic drugs regularly to relieve pain can also become addicted. So do some people who can obtain opiates easily, such as doctors and nurses. They take injections to keep going under pressure and eventually find themselves locked into narcotic addiction.[41]

The Workplace

Drug use has become very widespread in business and industry. The problem has drawn increased awareness and growing concern among business leaders and the public in general. American industry doubled its referrals to federal drug programs between 1977 and 1979, and this trend continues. The number of company-sponsored employee assistance programs (EAPs) has increased dramatically in recent years to over 3000.

Business and industry are concerned not only by the increased use of drugs on the job but by the wider acceptance of drug use, the greater availability of drugs, and the increased variety of drugs taken. Alcohol is still the most abused drug on the job, followed by marijuana and cocaine. Here is one illustration of the wider acceptance of drugs in the workplace:

> "I've been on jobs where the foreman actually passes out stuff to make sure the work gets done," says John E. Neece, a building union leader in California. "Sometimes 90 percent of the crew have been doing uppers."[42]

Cocaine use is extensive, accepted, and steadily growing in financial centers from coast to coast. "One reason for the increase in use and acceptance is that the increase in use and acceptance in the generation of people who used drugs other than alcohol in the 60's and 70's are growing older and taking their drug habits to the workplace."[43]

Industry is finally realizing that it has a very real and costly problem on its hands. Though some companies choose to ignore the problem, others, with an extremely limited understanding of drugs, are nevertheless attempting to confront it. It is a difficult situation for industry, since very few companies have established drug policies and many supervisors lack training in dealing with drug users. It is also difficult for a supervisor who has a two-martini lunch to discipline an employee for smoking a joint during lunch. Even so, companies are starting to spell out drug policies stating what will happen to those caught using drugs.

Drug use on the job causes many problems. The most talked about is lost productivity. Industrial workers, stockbrokers, doctors and nurses, and electronics employees are all affected. Directly related to lower productivity and poor quality are an increase in production costs, breakage costs, health insurance, and other insurance costs. There is also the extra cost of training replacements to fill posts left vacant by drug-using personnel. The direct cost to employers in lost productivity due to drug use on the job is estimated to be at least $16.8 billion a year.[44] Some suggest that alcohol use alone costs employers that much.[45] A large number of employers are therefore attempting to rehabilitate their drug-using employees.

A Firestone Tire and Rubber Company study completed in mid 1983 found that drug users were thirty-six times as likely to be involved in a plant accident and 2.5 times more likely to require absences lasting more than a week than employees who didn't use drugs.[46] The increased concern over industrial accidents directly caused by employees using drugs has spread to the public. For example, in September 1982, in Livingston, Louisiana, a freight train derailed and two tank cars carrying chemicals exploded and burned. About 3000 people who lived within five miles of the accident site had to be evacuated for up to two weeks, and environmental damage was extensive. The National Transportation

Safety Board found that impairment of the engineer's faculties by alcohol contributed to the accident.[47]

An increasing number of companies are searching employees and company grounds for drugs. Shell Oil Company uses trained dogs to search all employees leaving and going to work on offshore oil rigs![48] An increasing number of companies are using undercover security personnel and local police to arrest employees violating laws.

As we have seen, the use of EAPs seems to be a growing trend among companies. A number of companies immediately fire anyone who fails a test of drug use. However, employees who admit to a drug problem before taking the test are granted leave to seek treatment, which is kept confidential. EAPs are being expanded to include therapy for all types of drug use. Many companies are funding EAPs to save money in the long run and they find that these employees so served are extremely productive. "When you're able to help an employee save his life," says Frank Price, head of Owens-Illinois EAP, Program in Atlanta, "there's dedication that dollars and cents can't buy."[49] Business and industry are starting to deal with their growing drug problem through a variety of approaches. With more experience, it is hoped, they will be able to improve these approaches.

THE SENIOR CITIZEN DRUG SCENE

Though limited attention is given to drug use by people fifty-five and older, it is known that the elderly make up 11.5 percent of the population (as of 1982) and use about 25 to 30 percent of all medications.[50] The average healthy senior citizen takes at least eleven different prescription medicines in a year. The cost of drug-induced hospital visits for people of all ages is $21 billion, and a person over sixty is two to seven times as likely as a younger person to suffer adverse side effects.[51] Seniors also spend three times more money, proportionately, than the rest of the population.

As recently as the turn of the century, the average life span in the United States was approximately forty-nine years; by 1980 it had risen to seventy-three years. Furthermore, it is estimated that by the year 2000 there will be 31 million Americans over sixty-five, representing almost 13 percent of the population. Drug technology has contributed to this increase in longevity by eliminating and/or helping control many infectious and chronic diseases.[52]

In the past, elderly drug dependents were not considered drug abusers by professionals because long-term drug dependents generally die before age sixty and those who survive have given up drugs.[53] But senior citizens show a dramatic lack of drug knowledge, considering it of little benefit to them, and this often causes drug abuse. In a recent study of the level of drug knowledge and misconceptions among senior citizens, half of the subjects thought there were risks involved in taking prescribed medicine; 60 percent believed some medications should not be mixed with certain foods; and the majority believed that drugs could be habit-forming. In addition, over 70 percent were unaware of the side effects of aspirin and 60 percent used laxatives to stimulate a bowel movement.[54]

Where age makes a difference in how well a drug does its job is in drug distribution—the process by which a drug is delivered to various sites in the body.[55] Drug distribution in the elderly is partly altered because of changes in their body's composition. Body water and lean body mass (muscle and bone) decrease and fat increases, even though there is no increase in weight. This means that some of the drug normally distributed in lean body tissue will end up in the blood stream. On the other hand, some drugs, such as barbiturates and diazepam (Valium), are stored in fatty tissues. The increased fat in the elderly can serve as reservoirs for these drugs and prolong their working time.

Types of Drug Use

To better understand the senior citizen drug scene, we will consider four ways in which seniors use drugs: (1) proper use of drugs, (2) misuse of drugs, (3) accidental abuse of drugs, and (4) purposeful use of dependency-causing drugs. As for every other age group, there are many problems that involve older citizens in drug use. But for some seniors, several of the problems become pronounced. Many older people are socially isolated and their main source of communication and enjoyment may be the mass media, where they are constantly bombarded with drug advertising. Furthermore, according to Ruth Weg, "eighty-six percent of the aged have one or more chronic conditions," many of which require medical drug treatment.[56]

Proper Use   Proper drug use involves taking prescription and over-the-counter drugs according to the directions given. The physician plays a key role in the drug use of the elderly. He or she should be the primary source of clear, understandable instructions. A 1982 survey by the Food and Drug Administration of persons sixty and older, however, revealed the following:

44% stated doctors did not tell them how much medication to take.
42% stated doctors did not tell them how often to use medication.
87% were not advised about refills.
72% were not given information on precautions.
73% were not told about possible side effects.[57]

Small wonder that the pharmacist is becoming the primary adviser to the elderly on both prescription and over-the-counter drugs.

Proper drug use also involves refraining from taking several drugs that may have been prescribed by different physicians for different conditions. A doctor will often write a prescription without knowing that other physicians are treating the same patient. The elderly often dwell upon the increasingly debilitated condition of their bodies, and many ingest multitudes of drugs to help themselves feel young again. Illness and the approach of death often cause extreme depression, and seniors also take drugs to alleviate this condition, as well as loss of appetite and weight, sleep disturbances, and constipation.

Misuse of Drugs   Senior patients may become drug-dependent without their physician's or their own knowledge. They may visit several physicians at a time, each for a different condition, and be prescribed a different drug by each. They may also "repeatedly self-administer drugs and . . . eventually come to feel that they cannot carry on normal everyday activities unless they take drugs."[58] As tolerance to the drugs occurs, elderly patients sometimes increase the dosage at will.

Noncompliance is another dimension of the misuse and abuse of drugs by the elderly. A recent study showed that "only 22 percent of prescriptions were being taken properly—and 31 percent were being misused in a manner which posed a serious threat to the patient's health."[59] Many of the elderly fail to understand that many medications are prescribed to prevent problems from developing and they will often stop taking them when symptoms do not appear or, if present, when they are alleviated or become less observable. "Various studies of older patients indicated that 50 to 60 percent of them make medication errors or simply don't take their medicine at all."[60]

Though some nursing-home staffs may overmedicate their patients in an attempt to keep them quiet or happy, sometimes producing undesirable mental conditions as well as adverse physical problems, there is no indication that all or even most physicians are unconcerned about their elderly patients. Most of those physicians who do incorrectly prescribe do so out of frustration and/or lack of knowledge about the aged patient and the drugs themselves. They may prescribe medications without realizing the undesirable side effects they can produce. This may lead to a vicious cycle of drug-induced diseases, including fainting spells, slurred speech, rashes, constipation, and an increased tendency to bruise easily.

Accidental Abuse of Drugs   Many cases of accidental abuse of drugs are caused by improper self-administration. The elderly person may not have enough information to take a certain drug wisely. He or she may not be able to read the label or remember to take the medication at the proper time. Or there may be so many drugs in the medicine cabinet that selecting the appropriate one is confusing and difficult.

As many as 25 percent of patients eighty or over experience adverse drug reactions, compared with 9.9 percent for younger adults.[61] Another study stated that adverse drug reaction occurred in 3 percent to 8 percent of hospitalized patients under fifty-nine. In patients over sixty, 11 percent to 21 percent exhibited drug reactions.[62]

Accidental drug abuse may also be caused by self-diagnosis and self-prescription—over-the-counter drugs, drugs used for past illnesses, or drugs obtained from a friend. In these cases, errors can be made not only in "diagnosis and prescription" but also in the use of outdated drugs and/or drugs that may interact adversely with other drugs being taken at the same time. Many people overdose themselves, thinking that if a little is good, more must be better. Other patients may take too little of a prescribed drug because they lack the funds to purchase the drug, forget to take the drug, or simply stop taking it when they feel better, instead of stopping after the recommended course of treatment.

Purposeful Use of Dependency-Causing Drugs   Until recently, it was assumed that drug dependency was almost nonexistent among the elderly. However, several reports and studies now reveal that drug dependency is not so rare in the older segment of the population. In 1970, the oldest patient in an Oregon methadone program was in his 80s and had been dependent on codeine for years. At the beginning of another methadone maintenance program, the administrators "were surprised to discover that a disproportionately large number of first applicants for help were men and women over sixty years of age. They comprised perhaps fifteen to twenty percent of all patients coming in off the streets."[63] After the program began, however, the number of older addicts attending dropped and leveled off at about $2\frac{1}{2}$ percent. It was speculated that the reason for the decline was that older dependents did not like methadone and were not committed to its use. The real number of older opiate dependents can only be guessed at.

A problem once neglected but now of concern is alcohol abuse among the elderly. As one physician observed,

> looking back on my experience with elderly patients in a variety of settings . . . I begin to see that there always were more aged alcoholics around than I recognized at the time. By conservative estimate they comprised at least ten percent of the elderly patients with whom I had some contact.[64]

As with other age groups, alcohol is a commonly used drug by the elderly too. Alcohol related problems, such as health or marital problems, affect about 10 percent of the elderly. Male Caucasians are more likely to drink, and drink heavily, than members of other racial groups. Late onset of alcoholism seems to correspond to losses of loved ones, social deprivation, and loss of status and boredom. The man who is seventy-five or older and has lost his wife seems to be the most vulnerable to alcohol dependency. Elderly alcoholics usually began drinking heavily in their forties or fifties, but receive voluntary treatment more often than younger alcoholics, and consequently respond to and complete therapy programs much more frequently. Perhaps this is because they experience more alcohol-induced health problems.

Alcoholism among the elderly may increase, inasmuch as people are living longer, there is a per-capita increase in alcohol consumption, and alcohol-treatment services for the elderly are greatly lacking. But since alcohol is often used as a mechanism for coping with a number of physical, social, and emotional problems, geriatric alcoholics

> respond readily to a therapeutic regime combining antidepressant medication with resocialization. They just stop drinking, and they do it without the assis-

tance of Alcoholics Anonymous or Antabuse [a substance used in the treatment of alcoholism].

The geriatric alcoholic's problems are clearly reactive. He responds readily when he finds a sympathetic ear for his problem, when he feels that someone is concerned about him. Once his depression lifts, he discovers that he doesn't need alcohol to adapt gracefully and effectively to the stress of aging.[65]

SUMMARY

We are a drug-oriented society, with many types of drugs and reasons for drug use. For young people, alcohol, nicotine, and marijuana are very popular. There is also continued use of various hallucinogens, volatile substances, and amphetamines. Initiation to cocaine and heroin usually begins in youth and may continue into the early adult years as well. Youths take drugs to get high or relax, and take them while going to school, during social activities, in military service, and in athletics. Drug abuse in athletics has reached such a high level that greater restrictions and punitive action is being taken to confront the problem. Some school districts are even planning drug testing of students in public schools.

Adult drug use focuses very heavily on tranquilizers, alcohol, nicotine, and caffeine. Though males still constitute most of the alcohol-dependent population, there has been a large increase in the number of female alcoholics during the past few years, and the numbers appear to be growing rapidly. Adults also smoke marijuana, a behavior they have carried over from their youth. Amphetamine use has dropped in recent years, but cocaine use has become prevalent among a growing number of adults. Heroin continues to be the most notorious illicit drug. Business and industry now find it necessary to monitor many of their employees and executives because of great financial losses associated with drug abuse on the job.

Among senior citizens, we find a disproportionate amount of prescription drugs being used. Older people also have more problems with misuse and accidental use of medicines than do the other groups. Another area of growing concern is nursing homes and convalescent centers, where drugs are frequently overprescribed to quiet patients or make them happy.

NOTES

[1]Quoted in Herman W. Land, *What You Can Do about Drugs and Your Child* (New York: Hart, 1969).

[2]Lawrence Ziomkowski, Rodney Mulder, and Donald Williams, "Drug Use between Delinquent and Non-Delinquent Youth, *Intellect* 104, no. 2367 (July–August 1975):36.

[3]See, for example, "1983 Drug Use Questionnaire," issued by Youth Help, Inc., Hoquiam, Washington.

[4]*Marijuana and Health,* Ninth Report to the U.S. Congress from the Secretary of Health and Human Services (Rockville, Md.: National Institute on Drug Abuse, 1982), pp. 1–20.

[5]Yoav Santo and Alfred S. Friedman, "Overviews and Selected Findings from the National Youth and Polydrug Study," *Contemporary Drug Problems* 9, no. 2 (Fall 1980):285.

[6]Daniel Yankelovich, "Drug Users vs. Drug Abusers: How Students Control Their Drug Crisis," *Psychology Today* 9, no. 5 (October 1975):39. Reprinted from *Psychology Today Magazine.* Copyright © 1975 Ziff-Davis Publishing Company.

[7]Ibid., p. 41.

[8]Lee H. Bower, "The Relationship between Sex, Drugs, and Sexual Behavior on a College Campus," *Drug Forum: The Journal of Human Issues* 7, no. 1 (1978–1979):69.

[9]Yankelovich, "Drug Users vs. Drug Abusers," p. 41.

[10]"Vietnam Heroin Abuse Drops, but Problem Still Severe," *Journal of the American Medical Association* 219, no. 10 (March 6, 1972):1280.

[11]Cited in Ibid.

[12]"Vietnam Heroin Abuse Drops."

[13]See John F. Greden and Donald W. Morgan, "Amnesty's Impact upon Drug Use: A Pre/Post Study," *American Journal of Psychiatry* 129, no. 4 (October 1972):123–25.

[14]Quoted in Jack Scott, "It's Not How You Play the Game but the Pill You Take," *New York Times Magazine,* October 1971, p. 12.

[15]"Coffee Makes Longer Easier," *Runner's World* 13, no. 7 (July 1978):52.

[16]See Elbert Glover, "Aspirin: Is It the Next Wonder Drug for Everyone," *Runner's World* 15, no. 4 (April 1979):67–70.

[17]Cited in Ibid. p. 67.

[18]Jack C. Horn, "A Dangerous Edge," *Psychology Today* 17 (November 1983):68.

[19]"The Doping of Amateur Sports," *Macleans,* 95:41 June 21, 1982.

[20]"Athletes and Steroids," *Macleans,* November 14, 1983, p. 60.

[21]Hal Quinn, "The Science of Winning," *Macleans,* January 12, 1981, p. 38.

[22]Ian Anderson, "Drugs and the Olympics," *World Press Review,* March 1984, p. 61.

[23]D. Franklin, "Steroids Heft Heart Risks in Iron Pumpers," *Science News* 126, no. 6 (July 21, 1984):38. Reprinted with permission from *Science News,* the weekly newsmagazine of science, copyright © 1984 by Science-Service, Inc.

[24]"The Doping of Amateur Sports," p. 41.

[25]Robert O. Voy, "The Science of Fair Play," *Technological Review* 87, no. 6 (August/September 1984):34. Reprinted with permission.

[26]Arnold J. Mandell, "The Sunday Syndrome," *Journal of Psychedelic Drugs* 10, no. 4 (October/December 1978):379–84.

[27]Quoted in Bil Gilbert, "Drugs in Sports," *Sports Illustrated* 30, no. 25 (June 23, 1969):27.

[28]Mandell, "The Sunday Syndrome."

[29]Quoted in Bil Gilbert, "Problems in a Turned on World," *Sports Illustrated* 30, no. 26 (June 30, 1969):30.

[30]Secretary of Health, Education and Welfare, *Alcohol and Health Report* (New York: Scribner's, 1970), pp. 417–19.

[31]Office of Technological Assessment: *The Effectiveness and Costs of Alcoholism Treatment* (Washington, D.C.: U.S. Government Printing Office, March 1983), p. 3.

[32]Department of Health, Education and Welfare, *CNS Depressants* (Washington D.C. National Clearinghouse for Drug Abuse Information, 1974), pp. 7–8.

[33]Cited in ibid.

[34]*Commission of Inquiry into the Non-Medical Use of Drugs: Final Report* (Ottawa: Crown, 1973), pp. 417–19.

[35]American Cancer Society, *1980 Facts and Figures* (New York, 1980), p. 144.

[36]American Cancer Society, *Dangers of Smoking: Benefits of Quitting and Relative Risks of Reduced Exposure* (New York, 1980).

[37]Jill Andresky, "The Caffeine Controversy," *Consumer Digest* 20, no. 6 (1981):31–34.

[38]Alfred Gilman and Louis S. Goodman, eds., *The Pharmacological Basis of Therapeutics,* 4th ed. (London and Toronto: Macmillan, 1971), pp. 367–68.

[39]Oakley S. Ray, *Drugs, Society and Human Behavior* (St. Louis: C. V. Mosby, 1978), p. 208.

[40]Michael Dolan, "Clamping Down on 'Uppers'," *American Pharmacy* 18 (new series), no. 4 (April 1978):18.

[41]Department of Health, Education and Welfare, *Fact Sheet 6,* no. 1 (Washington, D.C.: National Clearinghouse for Drug Abuse Information, 1974), p. 2.

[42]Quoted in Jo Brecher et al., "Taking Drugs on the Job," *Newsweek,* August 22, 1983, p. 52.

[43]Quoted in Stephen J. Sanswee, Thomas Petzinger, Jr., and Gary Putka "High Fliers: Use of Cocaine Grows Among Top Trades in Financial Centers," *Wall Street Journal,* Sept. 12, 1983. Reprinted by permission of *Wall Street Journal,* © Dow Jones & Company, Inc. 1983. All Rights Reserved.

[44]Bensinger, "Drugs in the Workplace."

[45]Tobin Quereau and Les Virgil, "Whose Business Is It? Chemical Dependency in the Work Place," *Focus* 6, no. 4 (July/August 1983).

[46]Sidney Cohen, *Drug Abuse and Alcoholism Newsletter* 12, no. 6 (1983):1.

[47]Bill Paul, "Danger Signal: Alcohol and Drug Use by Railroad Crewman Poses Threat to Safety," *Wall Street Journal,* August 16, 1983, p. 1.

[48]Bensinger, "Drugs in the Workplace."

[49]Brecher et. al., "Taking Drugs on the Job,".

[50]William Sampson, *Medications and the Elderly* (Rockville, Aspen, 1984), p. 150.

[51]A. D. Gilman, "Grandma Junkies," *Health* 16 (January 1984):150.

[52]"Drugs and the Elderly," *OPEN: Oregon Prevention and Education Newsletter* 2, no. 1 (January–February 1980).

[53]Emil Pascarelli, "Old Drug Addicts Do Not Die, nor Do They Just Fade Away," *Geriatric Focus* 11, no. 5 (1972):1.

[54]Emil Pascarelli et al., "Drug-Related Behavior, Knowledge and Misconceptions among a Selected Group of Senior Citizens," *Journal of Drug Education* 8, no. 2 (1978):85–92.

[55]A. Hecht, "Medicine and the Elderly," *FDA Consumer* 17 (S' 1983):20–27.

[56]Ruth Weg, "Drug Interaction with the Changing Physiology of the Aged: Practice and Potential," in *Drugs and the Elderly,* ed. R. H. Davis and W. K. Smith, (Los Angeles: University of Southern California Press, 1973), p. 73.

[57]Cited in Chris W. Ledos, "Diet and the Elderly," *FDA Consumer* 19 (December 1984–January 1985):7–9.

[58]Walter L. Way, *The Drug Scene: Help or Hang Up?* (Englewood Cliffs, N.J.: Prentice-Hall, 1970), p. 17.

[59]William Nolen, "Doctor's Orders: Why Patients Should Never Ignore Them," *Fifty Plus,* April 1984, p. 52.

[60]Hecht, "Medicine and the Elderly," p. 2.

[61]Beverly G. Clark and Robert E. Vestal, "Adverse Drug Reactions in the Elderly: Case Studies," *Geriatrics* 39, no. 12 (December 1984):53.

[62]William G. Berlinger and Ronald Spector, "Adverse Drug Reactions in the Elderly," *Geriatrics* 39, no. 5 (May 1984):40

[63]George M. Anderson, "Alcoholism and the Aging," *American* 143 (September 1980):139.

[64]Pascarelli, "Old Drug Addicts Do Not Die," p. 1.

[65]Sheldon Zimberg, "The Geriatric Alcoholic on a Psychiatric Couch," *Geriatric Focus* 2, no. 5 (1972):1.

PHARMACOLOGY
basic concepts of drug activity

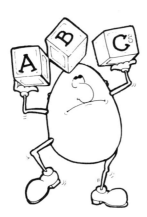

SPECIFIC PHARMACOLOGY _____

Without knowledge of the pharmacological properties of drugs, it is hard for people who have taken drugs to understand why the mind and body change during the drug experience. Scientists are constantly presenting new discoveries to the public. For example, in 1975 neuroscientists discovered enkephalin and endorphin.[1] These hormones are thought to be the body's own source of relief from pain and disabling emotions, binding with receptors in the brain and inhibiting pain signals there.[2] They may also improve memory. Furthermore, they may offer an explanation for acupuncture analgesia.[3] In addition to reducing pain, enkephalin and endorphin may effectively treat depression and schizophrenia.[4]

CONSUMER SAFETY

Responsible consumer safety requires one to consider seven basic points in deciding whether or not to take a drug:

1. the chemical being considered
2. the receptor mechanisms affected
3. the dosage and the method of administration
4. the kinds of drug interactions that will likely take place
5. the potential for allergic reactions
6. the potential for tolerance
7. the potential for physical dependence[5]

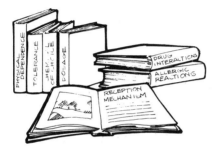

The Chemical (Drug) Being Considered

A drug is a compound that, when taken into the body, affects the chemical functioning of the organism. It may cause changes in bodily processes or behaviors. The water we drink, the air we breathe, and the food we eat are all chemicals producing various effects in our bodies.

To maintain life, an organism must produce, or otherwise obtain, various chemicals. When a chemical must be obtained from substances taken into the body, it must be determined how the chemical will affect the system.

The Receptor Mechanisms Affected

The chief determinant of the effects of a drug is its site of action within the body. Current theories on drug action suggest that chemical receptors within the body provide chemical sites coded to receive specific chemical substances. When a drug finds it chemical receptor mechanism (binding site), which is part of a large chemometabolic pathway, the interaction of the drug with that chemical-receptor mechanism will alter the eventual function of the pathway. Chemicals that bind to one or more of these binding sites will either fulfill normal biochemical functions or alter them and thus our bodily activities as well.

As a drug is distributed throughout the system, it acts only at those sites where complementary chemical-receptor mechanisms are available. Any given chemical receptor may be found throughout the body and may be involved in many systems or functions. Similar drugs may end up at a variety of binding sites. Thus, a drug, binding at these scattered receptors, can have a wide variety of actions and effects. When these are beneficial, they define a drug's therapeutic or medical use. An *adverse reaction* occurs when a drug produces unexpected or undesirable effects. The desired effect is usually considered the main effect; the unwanted responses are labeled the *side effects*. Apart from side effects, drugs can occasionally induce more serious adverse reactions, such as toxic manifestations and elevated or lowered blood pressure.[6]

The Dosage and Method of Administration

The amount of a drug present at a binding site determines the intensity or depth of response to the drug's characteristic actions. Therapeutic effects are obtained only when specific concentrations of the drug are present at the appropriate receptors. Incorrect concentrations can result in a lack of action, toxic reactions, or other alterations in the expected effects.

How much of a chemical must be taken for it to be effective? Surprisingly, the best effects of many drugs are achieved at low dosages, but each drug has its own optimum dose that will act to achieve maximum benefits with minimal side effects. In order to determine how effective a drug will be, a person should know how the action of a drug is affected by body mass (weight). (Convert pounds to kilograms [2.2 pounds equals 1 kilogram] and multiply by the amount of the drug that has been determined through research to produce the maximum beneficial effects and minimum side effects. Then compare the resulting figure with the specified dosage.)

The way a drug is administered affects the onset of the drug's effects, the duration of its action, and its potency. In general, substances injected into the bloodstream go into effect quickly, last a short time, and produce a great effect. Inhalation, ingestion, or inunction (rubbing into the skin to achieve a systemic effect) are means of administration that may be used when an immediate high dosage is not required.

Like the method of administration, absorption is an important pharmacological factor in drug activity. Drugs must be lipid-soluble (soluble in fat but insoluble in water) in order to cross cell membranes, which contain substantial amounts of lipid fats. Nonlipid-soluble chemicals may not penetrate cell membranes in sufficient quantities to affect the cells. As a drug enters the system it will usually move from a region of higher concentration of molecular volume per specific surface area to a region of lower concentration; when it is unable to do this, special transport mechanisms (such as the binding of a drug to a protein molecule, which can enter a cell) go into effect. The body continually releases energy-stored nutrients and uses them to maintain balance or equilibrium. Depending on the drug and the transport mechanism it is using, more or less energy will be required to absorb the drug before sufficient concentrations have been reached to produce the desired effect.

Distribution of a drug is dependent on absorption. The blood vessels of the brain, however, are surrounded by a fatty sheath that limits the entry of many drugs into the brain. This decreased permeability of the capillaries of the brain to certain substances is frequently called the *blood-brain barrier.* This term is widely used for distinguishing drugs that can penetrate the brain from those that cannot.[7]

Many areas of the body store drugs rather than distributing them. Some of these storage depots are fat reservoirs (for drugs with high lipid solubility), bones (for heavy metals and tetracyclines), and plasma proteins (for drugs with an affinity for albumin).

Some drugs become active only after the liver transforms them biologically; others are initially active and become inactive after biotransformation. Still others may be active at one site in the body, go through biotransformation to become inactive at that site, then transfer to another site where they become active again. These transformation factors add to some of the unpredictable effects a drug can have, but after transformation the metabolites (a substance produced by metabolism) of the drug are usually filtered out and excreted by the liver and kidney.

The dose–response curve, a fundamental concept in pharmacology, illustrates how different levels of a drug in the body can produce different behavioral effects.[8] This S-shaped curve (see Figure 4–1) shows that up to a certain level (the bottom of the curve), the concentration of a drug does not produce suitable effects to warrant continued administration at that level. The dose–time curve (Figure 4–2), which is usually bell-shaped, shows that increasing the dose beyond a certain level may prolong the effects, but the effects themselves will not increase. What may increase are the side effects.

Body weight and sex are also important factors in drug activity. A specific dosage, given both to a large person and to a small person, will affect the smaller person more strongly (other factors being equal) since he or she has less tissue and blood to absorb it. Also, a woman will respond differently to a drug than will a man of the same size because her body contains a higher ratio of fat. Drugs that have an affinity for stored fat may thus have prolonged effects in women.

The route of administration, body weight, and individual metabolism affect the concentration of a drug at its receptor and the rate at which that concentration is reached. Thus, these factors also help determine a drug's effects. The possible routes of administration are ingestion, inhalation, injection, and inunction.

FIGURE 4–1   Dose–Response Curve

FIGURE 4–2   Dose–Time Curve

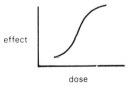

effect

dose

Dose-Response or S-Curve

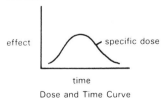

effect

specific dose

time

Dose and Time Curve

Ingestion   Drugs that are ingested are normally taken in pill or liquid form. Once swallowed, the drug goes mainly to the stomach, where some of the chemical will be broken down, then to the small intestine, bloodstream, liver, and so on. It can take twenty to forty minutes for a drug to enter the bloodstream and finally reach the receptor site, and the original dosage may be diluted and changed somewhat by the time it finally arrives. Certain drugs may not have the proper chemical charge and shape to enter the bloodstream when ingested and will be eliminated as waste. Those drugs must therefore be taken through oral inhalation or intravenously.

Inhalation   Inhalation is a drawing in through the nasal passage, oral inhalation a drawing in through the mouth. Though almost any nonliquid form of a chemical can be inhaled, only a few psychoactive substances are generally taken in this fashion. The most common of these are cocaine and, to a lesser extent, amphetamines, heroin, and volatile substances such as glue; marijuana and cigarettes, and, again, some volatile substances are orally inhaled. Drugs that are inhaled are fat-soluble (lipid) and can pass quickly into the bloodstream. However, since there is only a small amount of blood in the lungs, drugs need to be inhaled often to obtain the desired effects.

Injection

INTRAVENOUS (IV).   Drugs administered intravenously are placed directly into the bloodstream. Because of the immediate absorption and rapid distribution throughout the circulatory system this process provides, the full potency of the drug is felt very quickly. It is sometimes difficult to treat a person who has intravenously injected a lethal dose of a drug such as heroin, since the person receives full dosage in a very short time.

INTRAMUSCULAR (IM).   Here the drug is injected directly into the muscle tissue and then gradually filters out into the bloodstream. This form of injection usually takes more time than an intravenous injection to reach the binding sites, since absorption is slower. This prevents an inundation of the drug at the receptors.

SUBCUTANEOUS.   Subcutaneous injections are injections into the dermal layers of the skin. Since such shots have a slower absorption rate than intramuscular injections, they can slow the onset of effects, depending on the solubility of the drug.

Inunction   A drug administered by inunction is rubbed into the skin, and from there it works its way into the bloodstream.

The Kinds of Drug Interactions That Will Likely Take Place

A drug interaction occurs when two or more drugs are administered concomitantly; the responses are unexpected, unusual, or amplified. Such responses are the results of one drug altering the actions of another. One chemical may, for instance, affect another's absorption into the bloodstream, its distribution to receptor sites, or its rate of elimination from the body. The actions of any administered drug, as well as normal bodily processes, may be changed in these ways. Any chemical taken into the body, moreover, may compete with those already present in the body.

There are many drug interactions that can occur. Table 4–1 details the most common of these.

The Potential for Allergic Reactions

Because every person has a unique biochemical makeup, each administration of a drug is much like an experiment. Occasionally, drugs interact with bodily chemicals to produce allergic reactions. These *hypersensitivity* reactions may not present themselves initially, or even every time the drug is used.

Hypersensitivity is difficult to predict. By taking a lower dose of a drug upon first use, a person has a greater chance of avoiding a possible allergic reaction. The initial sign of hypersensitivity may be a skin rash or development of an asthmatic condition. A severe reaction may result in anaphalactic shock, respiratory depression, convulsions, or death.

Though some 3 to 5 percent of our population are hypersensitive, reacting very quickly to very small amounts of a drug, some individuals are *hyposensitive:* they require extra amounts of a drug to gain the desired effects. Other people may experience a *synergistic* response. In this case a combination of two drugs, such as alcohol and barbiturates, may have geometric rather than arithmetic effects.

The Potential for Tolerance and the Potential for Physical Dependence

The continued presence of a drug can cause its receptor site to lose sensitivity. In addition, when drugs are put into the body, the liver responds with enzymes to break them down. Increasing amounts are then required to exceed the liver's efficiency and produce the desired effects. *Tolerance* is the body's ability to adapt to existing drug dosage, thereby reducing or eliminating the desired effects; dose increases are then needed to produce these effects. Physical dependence occurs when certain drugs, in higher concentrations made necessary by tolerance, cause various biochemical transformations that in turn cause the system to become dependent on their presence. Under these circumstances, if the drug is not taken or does not reach its receptor site in sufficient concentration, a syndrome of physical responses (withdrawal) will occur.

TABLE 4–1   A Guide to Common Drug Interactions
This is only a sample of some of the most common drug interactions.
Take no action without checking with your own doctor.

Tranquilizers	Combined With	Interaction
Diazepam derivatives (Librium, Valium, Serax, etc.) and meprobamate (Miltown)	alcohol	increases effects of both
	barbiturate	increases effects of both
	MAO-inhibiting antidepressants (Nardil, Parnate, Marplan, Eutonyl)	oversedation
	phenothiazine tranquilizers (Thorazine, Compazine, etc.)	increases effects of both
	tricyclic antidepressants (Elavil, Aventyl, Tofranil, Pertofrane)	increases effects of both
Phenothiazines (Thorazine, Mellaril, Compazine, etc.)	alcohol	oversedation
	antihistamine	increases effects of both
	antihypertensive drugs	increases blood-pressure-lowering action
	barbiturate	increases sedation
	MAO-inhibiting antidepressants (Nardil, Parnate, Marplan, Eutonyl)	makes antidepressant less effective
	Demerol	increases sedation
	diazepam derivatives (Librium, Valium, etc.)	increases action of both
	thiazide diuretics (Diuril, Hydrodiuril)	causes shock
	tricyclic antidepressants (Elavil, Aventyl, Tofranil, Pertofrane)	increases action of both

Analgesics	Combined With	Interaction
Aspirin	anticoagulant	increases the blood-thinning effect and could cause bleeding
	para amonosalicylic acid (PAS)	makes PAS toxic
Meperidine (Demerol)	MAO-inhibiting antidepressants (Nardil, Parnate,	increases action of Demerol

Analgesics	Combined With	Interaction
	Marplan, Eutonyl) phenothiazine tranquilizers (Thorazine, Compazine, etc.)	increases sedation
Phenylbutazone	anticoagulant	increases the blood-thinning effect and could cause bleeding
	oral antidiabetic drugs (Orinase, Diabenese)	may make the blood sugar too low

Antihistamines	Combined With	Interaction
Diphenhydramine (Benadryl), chlorphenira- mine (Chlor-Trimeton) dimenhydrinate (Dramamine), promethazine (Phenergan), and others	alcohol	increases sedation
	barbiturate	nullifies both
	hydrocortisone	lessens effect of hydrocortisone
	phenothiazine tranquilizers (Thorazine, Compazine, etc.)	increases effects of both
	reserpine	depresses central nervous system
	anticholinergics (slows intestinal movement	makes the anticholinergic more potent

Antidepressants	Combined With	Interaction
MAO-inhibitors (Marplan, Nardil, Parnate, Eutonyl)	alcohol	increases depression of central nervous system
	amphetamine	increases effect of amphet- amine
	barbiturate	makes barbiturate more potent
	Demerol	makes Demerol more potent
	diazepam tranquilizers (Librium, Valium, etc.)	increases effect of tranquil- izer markedly
	thiazide diuretics (Diuril, Hydrodiuril)	lowers blood pressure and increases action of MAO- inhibitor
	tricyclic antidepressants (Elavil, Aventyl, Tofranil, Pertofrane)	increases effects of both
Tricyclic antidepressants (Elavil, Tofranil, Aventyl, Pertofrane, etc.)	diazepam derivatives (Librium, Valium, etc.)	increases effects of both
	phenothiazine tranquilizers (Thorazine, Compazine, etc.)	increases effects of both
	reserpine	lessens effect of reserpine

Antibiotics	Combined With	Interaction
Tetracycline	penicillin, antacid, or milk	makes tetracycline less effective
Penicillin G	chloramphenicol (Chloromycetin), antacid, or tetracycline	makes penicillin less effective
Griseofulvin (Fulvicin, Grisactin, Grifulvin)	anticoagulant	may make the anticoagulant less effective
	phenobarbital	makes griseofulvin less effective
Sulfonamide	antacid	makes sulfa less effective
	anticoagulant	makes the anticoagulant more potent
	antidiabetics (Dymelor, Orinase, Diabenese)	makes antidiabetics too powerful
Furazolidone (Furoxone)	alcohol	lessens bacterial action of drug and could skyrocket blood pressure
	amphetamine	increases effect of amphetamine
	barbiturate	increases action of the barbiturate
	MAO-inhibitor antidepressants (Nardil, Parnate, Marplan, Eutonyl)	increases effects of both
	phenothiazine tranquilizers (Thorazine, Compazine etc.)	increases effects of tranquilizers
	tricyclic antidepressants (Elavil, Aventyl, Tofranil, Pertofrane)	increases effects of antidepressant

DRUGS THAT MAY INTERACT WITH ALCOHOL

Antibacterials: inhibits germ-killing action of antibacterials.
Antidiabetic agents (including insulin): may lower blood sugar to dangerous levels. Insulin also increases the effects of alcohol.
Antihistamines: depresses central nervous system.
Antihypertensives: increases the blood-pressure-lowering effect of drugs.
Antidepressants: increases the effect of alcohol and depresses the central nervous system.
Tranquilizers: affects coordination and depresses the central nervous system.
Sedatives and hypnotics: causes oversedation and depression of the central nervous system.

FOOD INTERACTIONS

Milk and *other dairy products* combined with antibacterials (such as tetracycline) make the antibacterial less effective.
Aged cheese, broad beans, chocolate, bananas, passion fruit, pineapples, tomatoes, and *lemon* combined with MAO-inhibiting antidepressants cause blood pressure to increase to dangerous levels.

Soybean preparations, Brussels sprouts, cabbage, cauliflower, kale, turnips, peaches, carrots and *pears* may enlarge thyroid glands in susceptible people and make thyroid tests inaccurate.

DRUGS THAT MAY CAUSE SKIN ERUPTIONS WHEN PATIENT IS EXPOSED TO THE SUN

Antibacterial sulfas.
Antidiabetic drugs such as Orinase and Diabenese.
Thiazide diuretics such as Diuril and Hydrodiuril.
Tranquilizers, including Librium and Compazine.
Antihistamines, particularly Benadryl.
Antiitching preparations.
Antibiotics, including Aureomycin and Terramycin.
Antifungal agents.
Birth-control pills.

Source: FDA Consumer, Government Printing Office, 581.

THE NERVOUS SYSTEM
AS AN ELECTRICAL SYSTEM

To better understand how drugs can affect the body, we need to first understand how the nervous system works (see Figure 4–3). The nervous system consists of billions of *neurons* (nerve cells). A neuron usually consists of dendrites, a cell body (soma), and an axon with its terminals. The dendrites receive signals from other neurons, summarize the information, and transfer it to the soma for production of a nerve impulse. After the impulse is generated, it travels down the axon to the terminals, which contact the dendrites of other neurons or other terminals. The gap between a terminal and another neuron is called a synapse, and when a signal has jumped this gap it migrates to a receptor site. A neuron will not fire, however, unless sufficient excitatory receptor sites in the dendrites bring the cell to an electrochemical threshold, where it will start an impulse of its own.

In an unstimulated state, a nerve's membrane (the layer surrounding the neuron) normally has many more potassium ions inside it than outside, and many more sodium and chloride ions outside than inside. Ions are atoms with a positive or negative charge, and when they move, they form a current, which is simply a flow of charges.[9] When allowed to move freely, the ions travel from a region where they are of higher concentration to a region where they are less concentrated; if the difference in concentration between the two areas is large, more ions flow (producing a greater electrical current) than if the difference is small. As ions travel along a neuron, the membrane becomes selectively permeable, opening certain "channels" or "gates" to allow some of the ions to pass through; it is this flow of ions that constitutes the electrical signal we call an impulse, or *action potential.* Drugs that affect the sodium and potassium levels in and around a neuron might alter the quality of the impulse by making the cell capable of firing faster or slower. Coding of information in the nervous system usually rests on the frequency of firing rather than on the amplitude of the impulse.

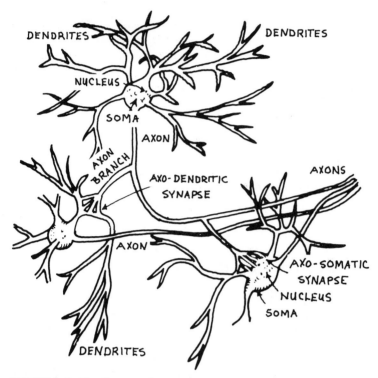

FIGURE 4–3   The Nervous System

Consequently, each receptor site (which is either excitatory, bringing the cell closer to threshold, or inhibitory, sending it farther away) will have only a partial influence on the readiness of the neuron to fire. In this sense, the excitatory and inhibitory signals from other cells are summarized, and this information is transformed into the all-or-nothing impulse.

The neuron membrane is semipermeable, allowing only certain molecules and atoms to move through it (notably, potassium, sodium, and chloride ions). Physicians closely monitor a patient's sodium and potassium levels in surgery to prevent shock. As an impulse travels along, the membrane changes its permeability so as to allow sodium ions and then potassium ions, each flowing in a different direction, and these local ion flows, or currents, actually constitute the impulse. The way a drug alters the body's pH level (its acid–alkaline balance) is very important. Drugs can thus affect currents by changing the sodium or potassium levels, and hence the degree to which they pass through neuron membranes, or by altering the permeability of the membrane itself.

Most drugs, however, do not affect nerve currents through the membrane. The great majority of psychoactive drugs alter the signal at the synapse. When an impulse comes along, vesicles in the terminal release neurotransmitters into the gap, which migrate to receptor sites in a few thousandths of a second. The transmitters activate the receptor, which then releases the transmitters back into the gap, where they are either taken into the terminal again for reuse or deactivated by a special chemical (monoamine oxidase) residing in the synapse.

When a drug is taken, it can change an impulse by altering the release, activation, re-uptake, or deactivation of transmitters. Since a drug can affect impulses throughout the nervous system, which includes the brain and the spinal cord, it can affect all life functions, memory, and personality.

There may be as many as thirty different types of neurotransmitters; we will deal only with the most prevalent. *Acetylcholine* (ACH) is an excitatory transmitter in skeletal muscles and an inhibitory one in heart muscle. Appropriately, neurons that use ACH are called *cholinergic*. *Serotonin* acts as a transmitter in many parts of the central nervous system; neurons using it are termed *serotonergic*. *Adrenergic* neurons use *dopamine* or *norepinephrine* (NE) as transmitters.

ANATOMY AND PHYSIOLOGY

There are two major divisions of the nervous system: the central nervous system and the peripheral nervous system.

Central Nervous System

The central nervous system (Figure 4–4) includes the brain and the spinal cord. There are several substructures in the brain that are significant in the actions of certain drugs.

The Hypothalamus and the Pituitary Gland The hypothalamus is like the central processing unit of a computer. It is the foundation of the mammalian brain, originating some 30,000 years ago. Also known as the *prehistoric brain,* the hypothalamus is the seat of many major life-support functions. In a sense, because of its neurological design, we can also think of it as a switchboard. Communication between the brain and the pituitary gland, which secretes hormones, occurs through the hypothalamus. Because of this, what affects the brain can affect the pituitary.

The hypothalamus regulates many of the functions of *homeostasis*—the body's need to keep its biological systems in balance. The sleep–waking cycle is housed here, as are hunger, thirst, sexual behavior, blood pressure, and body temperature. This tiny cerebral component also coordinates and selects which major pathways will be affected by analgesics, and appears to be a factor in many behavioral and chemical dependencies, such as alcoholism and other drug abuse, compulsive gambling, sexual offenses, and obesity. Many of these dependencies are influenced by the relationship between the hypothalamus and the rest of the limbic/endocrinal system (the system that regulates hormone levels, which in turn affect emotions). The general adaptation syndrome or stress response is likewise housed by the hypothalamus.

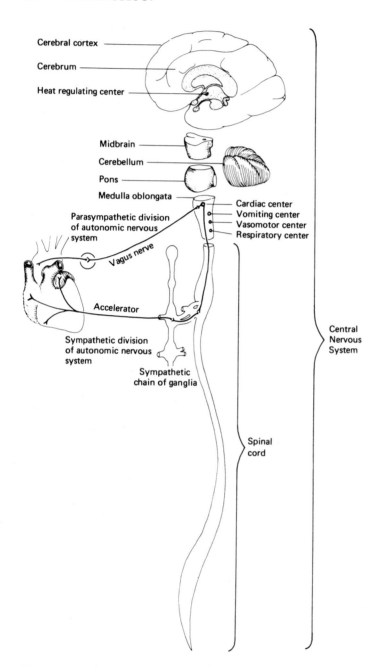

FIGURE 4–4 The Central Nervous System

Figure (p. 15) from DRUGS AND ALCOHOL by Kenneth L. Jones, Louis W. Schainberg, and Curtis O. Byer. Copyright © 1969 by Kenneth L. Jones, Louis W. Schainberg, and Curtis O. Byer. Reprinted by permission of Harper & Row, Publishers, Inc.

Medial Forebrain Bundle   A tract of nerve fibers runs through both sides of the hypothalamus. When electrodes implanted in this area are stimulated, humans report pleasurable sensations and will do work, such as pressing a lever, to receive them. This area of the brain is sometimes referred to as the pleasure center.

Periventricular System   The major part of the periventricular system consists of the periventricular nuclei, located above and to either side of the hypothalamus. The system is mainly cholingeric—that is, it transmits acetylcholine. Electrical stimulation of the area produces sensations of displeasure in humans, leading to the view that the system is a punishment center.

Reticular Formation (Ascending Reticular Activating System) This structure is located in the brain stem (see Figure 4–5), just behind the hypothalamus. It receives all types of internal and external stimuli and in turn projects messages to many parts of the cerebral cortex. The reticular formation acts as a switchboard, helping to sort impulses and direct them to the appropriate area of the brain. Many of the neurons in the reticular formation have collaterals (branches) from their axons. Each neuron can then send its signals to more than one area of the brain. One primary function of the formation is to regulate the *arousal level* of the cortex, which varies from alertness to sleep, by performing what might be called an evaluation of incoming stimuli. That is, it prepares the appropriate areas of the brain to receive the stimuli that it has already received. The reticular formation is primarily adrenergic (utilizing norepinephrine).

Medulla   The medulla oblongata is located in the lower part of the brain stem (which comprises all parts of the brain except the cerebellum and the cerebral hemispheres). The medulla has intimate connections with the reticular formation and is hence involved to some extent with the regulation of arousal. The medulla also receives inputs from the vestibular apparatus for balance and initiates reflex responses of the head position. When an individual hears a noise, the information is sent simultaneously to both the reticular formation and the medulla. The reticular formation might arouse the cortex to pay attention to that sound and to prepare for more information; the medulla would initiate a reflex response of turning the head toward the sound.

The medulla works with the hypothalamus to regulate many autonomic (automatic) functions of the body—breathing, heart rate, blood pressure, and pupil dilation. When an individual dies from an overdose of a depressant drug, the cause is usually depression of the medulla. The speed at which food moves through the digestive system and the vomiting reflex are also mediated by the medulla. The medulla is influenced by both the cortex and the internal status of the body. In short, it is involved in motor responses and homeostasis.

Raphae Nuclei   The raphae nuclei are clusters of cell bodies lying above the medulla and just behind the hypothalamus. Like the cells in the reticular formation, these cells act on the ability of the cortex to receive sensory input, but they use serotonin as a transmitter substance instead of norepine-

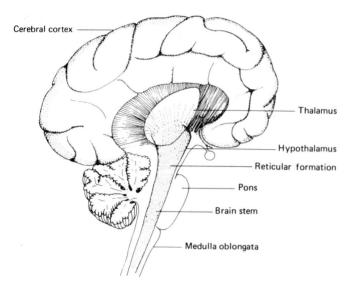

Cerebral cortex

Thalamus

Hypothalamus

Reticular formation

Pons

Brain stem

Medulla oblongata

FIGURE 4–5   The Brain

Figure (p. 16) from DRUGS AND ALCOHOL by Kenneth L. Jones, Louis W. Schainberg, and Curtis O. Byer. Copyright © 1969 by Kenneth L. Jones, Louis W. Schainberg, and Curtis O. Byer. Reprinted by permission of Harper & Row, Publishers, Inc.

phrine. According to one theory, the raphae nuclei inhibit the arousal of the reticular formation and the cortex, producing a state of light sleep.[10] Since most serotonergic neurons in the CNS are located in the raphae, drugs that affect serotonin levels (LSD, for example) will alter the functioning of these nuclei and perhaps cause new behaviors.

Cerebral Cortex   The cerebral cortex is one of the newest structures in the original mammalian brain, and its existence distinguishes mammals from other vertebrates. However, no enormous differences separate humans from other mammals. Man may have more *nuclei* (nerve cell centers) than the rat, but both brains are organized similarly. The cerebral cortex covers all other structures in a series of convolutions, or folds, to conserve space. Fully half the cells of the nervous system reside in the cortex.[11]

Language, abstract thought, personality, and the more subtle influences on how we interpret emotion seem to reside in the cerebral cortex. Learning and memory, on the other hand, are situated throughout the brain.

Several bands of accumulated nerve tracts, the corpus collosum, lie along the midline of the brain. The cerebral hemispheres communicate with each other by sending impulses along the fibers running through the corpus collosum. When these bands are cut, the individual suddenly has two completely separate brains, each capable of independent thought and independent response. Testing of epileptic patients who have had this operation reveals a functional diversity. In most people, the left hemisphere is found to be very good at language and linear

TABLE 4–2   Effects of the Sympathetic and Parasympathetic Nervous Systems on Selected Body Structures

Structure	Sympathetic Effect	Parasympathetic Effect
Heart rate	increase	decrease
Blood pressure	increase	decrease
Respiration	increase	decrease
Digestive system	inhibition	activation
Pupils	dilation	constriction
Salivary glands	decrease in secretion	secretion
Skin blood vessels	constriction	dilation
Sweat glands	secretion (ACH)	(no effect)

Source: Oakley S. Ray, *Drugs, Society, and Human Behavior,* 3rd ed. (St. Louis: The C. V. Mosby, 1983).

thought but very bad at interpreting spatial images. Just the opposite occurs in the right hemisphere. These findings have led to the speculation that one side of the brain functions linearly while the other is adept at perceiving things in their entirety.[12]

Specific cerebral functions are indigenous to specific cerebral components. On the other hand, there are systemwide memory and personality influences, which are not restricted to the left or the right hemisphere. Thus, we can view a single thought as involving billions of neurons firing in immensely complicated circuits, or we can view a thought as the firing of a single cell. Research on the vision of monkeys brought on the discovery that some neurons fire only when they "see" a line in their visual field. Other neurons are most excited when a series of lines appears in a certain pattern. A cell was found to fire most frequently when the stimulus was a monkey paw (a human hand gave a lower response).[13]

Peripheral Nervous System

Many of the nerves in the peripheral nervous system constitute the autonomic nervous system, which mediates the automatic functions of the body, such as heart rate and digestion. Two further divisions of the autonomic nervous system are the *sympathetic* and the *parasympathetic* systems.

Most body organs have nerves structured for innervation (arousal) according to Walter Cannon's "fight or flight" hypothesis. When the sympathetic division dominates, heart rate, blood pressure, respiration, and perspiration increase; pupils dilate to allow wider peripheral vision; blood is diverted from the digestive system to the skeletal muscles; and adrenaline is released. In peripheral-skeletal-muscle blood vessels and in sweat glands, the sympathetic transmitter is ACH. All other nerve innervation utilizes norepinephrine.

The parasympathetic system is very specific in its innervation: it seems to work toward maintenance and repair of the body. When the parasympathetic supersedes the sympathetic, heart rate, blood pressure, and respiration become

TABLE 4–3 Summary of Drug Information

	Effects	Side Effects	Adverse Effects	Potential for Addiction	Withdrawal Symptoms
STIMULANTS Benzedrine, Dexedrine, methamphetamines, methadrine, Ritalin, etc.)	increased wakefulness, reversal of fatigue, depressed appetite, reduction of narcolepsy	dryness of the mouth, increased perspiration, enlarged pupils, talkativeness, nervousness, involuntary trembling, restlessness, excitability, tension, anxiety, nausea, hot flashes, and bruxism; cramps, increased heart rate, and stimulation of force of heart contractions and breathing	headaches, palpitations, delirium, circulatory collapse, vomiting, malnutrition, and paranoia; depletion of the body's energy stores, GI disorders, liver and stomach disorders, and nerve damage	slowly increasing tolerance, high potential for psychological addiction, possible mild physical dependence	renewed desire to take more of the drug; overwhelming fatigue; severe depression; occasional suicidal tendencies
COCAINE	numbness—used as a local anesthetic in surgery; dilated pupils; strong stimulation of the CNS; increased motor activity	increased heart rate and blood pressure; increased respiration rate and depth of respiration *From free basing:* chest pain, sore throat, hoarse voice, shortness of breath	*Large dosage:* tremors, convulsive movements, respiratory and cardiac failure *Excessive dosage:* hallucinations, paranoid delusions, cocaine "bugs," insomnia, weight loss, financial extinction, and accidental OD	very rapidly increasing tolerance, very high potential for psychological addiction	irritability, discomfort, strong desire to repeat use; physical exhaustion, severe depression possibly leading to suicide

	Effects	Side Effects	Adverse Effects	Potential for Addiction	Withdrawal Symptoms
SEDATIVE-HYPNOTICS (Barbiturates: Seconal, Tuinal, Nembutal, etc.)	relaxation and sleep	range from subtle changes in mood and sedation to sleep and coma; typical effects are a reduction in attention span, less awareness of external stimuli, and a decrease in the ability to perform intellectual tasks	nausea, dizziness, confusion, an impaired mental state, and allergic reactions such as swelling of the face, dermatitis, skin lesions, fever, delirium, convulsions, and degenerative changes in liver	rapidly increasing tolerance, high physical and psychological potential for addiction	sweating, insomnia, vomiting, tremors, paranoia, and a short temper; excessive dreaming, nightmares, and in extreme cases hallucinations and seizures
QUAALUDE	relief of nervous tension, promotion of sleep	dreamy moods, lowered inhibitions	headache, hangover, menstrual disturbance, tongue changes, dry mouth, rashing at the angles of the mouth, nosebleeds, depersonalization, dizziness, skin eruption, pain in the extremities, diarrhea, anorexia, anxiety, nausea, and restlessness	increasing tolerance, high physical and psychological potential for addiction, plus high potential for accidental OD	irritability, vomiting, headaches, seizures, cramps, tremors, sleeplessness, mania, convulsions, and death

	Effects	Side Effects	Adverse Effects	Potential for Addiction	Withdrawal Symptoms
MINOR TRANQUILIZER (Valium, Librium, Miltown, Serax, etc.)	reduction in neuromuscular activity and thereby a reduction in environmental awareness and easier relaxation	motor impairment, speech disturbance, shortened attention span, and reduced sex drive; reduced feelings of aggression, increased sociability, and drowsiness progressing towards sleep	apathy, illogical fears, low blood pressure, fainting, chills, rashes, upset stomach, disorientation, blurred vision; bladder, menstrual and ovulary irregularities, and sleep disturbances; if taken with alcohol, toxic or fatal reaction can occur	rapidly increasing tolerance with high potential for cross-tolerance; high physical and psychological potential for addiction	anxiety, muscle twitches, insomnia, headache, fever, nausea, vomiting, abdominal cramps, sweating, and convulsions; death is possible
ALCOHOL	relaxation, euphoria, and lessened inhibitions	slight increase in heart rate, sweating, dilation of blood vessels, moderately lower blood pressure, appetite stimulation, increased production of gastric secretion, and increased urine production; levels of fat and protein affected	inability to perform simple motor activities, blackout, facilitation of hypothermia, irritation and inflammation of the linings of oral cavity, esophagus, and stomach, violent behavior, fetal alcohol syndrome, cirrhosis of the liver, permanent kidney damage, brain damage, congestive heart failure, unconsciousness, and death	tolerance increases depending on amount consumed and period of time of consumption. Very high potential for physiological and psychological addiction	irritability, sleeplessness, tremors, sweating, hallucinations, seizures, delirium, tachycardia, and low-grade fever

	Effects	Side Effects	Adverse Effects	Potential for Addiction	Withdrawal Symptoms
OPIATES (heroin, codeine, morphine, Darvon, Dilaudid, Percodan, Talwin, methadone, Demerol)	relief of pain and promotion of sleep	constricted pupils, reduced respiration and pulse, drowsiness, loss of appetite, sweating, elevated blood-sugar level, constipation, and impotence	hepatitis, blood poisoning, inflammation of the membranes lining the heart, dizziness, headache, and possible coma or death	Extremely rapidly increasing tolerance, very high physical and psychological potential for addiction	*12–24 hours:* restlessness *24–48 hours:* dilated pupils, anorexia, gooseflesh, restlessness, irritability, and tremors *48–72 hours:* increasing irritability, insomnia, marked anorexia, violent yawning, severe sneezing, lacrimation, weakness, vomiting, intestinal spasm, and diarrhea; elevated blood pressure, marked chilliness alternated with flushing
HALLUCINOGENS (LSD, mescaline, psilocybin)	altered sensory perception, stimulation of the sympathetic nervous system leading to heightened sensitivity to stimuli; synesthesia (blending of senses)	dilated pupils, rise in body temperature and blood pressure, increased heartbeat, possible moderate rise in blood sugar, nausea, headache, loss of appetite, dizziness, and mild tremors; visual distortions, distorted depth perception	hallucinations, severe paranoia, "bad trips," accidental or deliberate death	rise in tolerance not likely unless taken on a continued basis over a long period of time—increased dosage then needed to achieve desired effects; psychological addiction very possible	

	Effects	Side Effects	Adverse Effects	Potential for Addiction	Withdrawal Symptoms
PCP	anesthesia	*Moderate dose:* numbness, blurred vision, muscular dysfunction, dizziness, profuse sweating, flushing, increased blood pressure, and rapid heartbeat; spaciness, problems with perception and coordination, bloodshot eyes, impaired speech	anxiety, depression, sporadic outbreaks of violent behavior, and accidental death	definite possibility of psychological addiction	
MARIJUANA	intoxication, euphoria, enhanced congeniality, relaxed passivity	mild dilation of the blood vessels in the extremities, slight increase in blood flow to the arms and legs, reduction of body temperature; slightly elevated blood pressure, dry mouth, appetite stimulation	Irritation of the throat and lungs; cardiovascular complications; possible damage to the immune system; alteration of endocrine function; psychomotor impairment	possible tolerance; potential for addiction depending on frequency of use and amount used	short-term anxiety, panic, impairment of short-term memory, disturbance in thought patterns, lapses in attention, depersonalization, mental confusion, flashbacks, paranoid thoughts, anxiety

Source: Martin Chess, Drug Counselor, Serenity Lane, Inc., Alcohol Treatment Center, Eugene, Oregon 97401. Reprinted with permission.

slow and regular; blood is diverted from the skeletal muscles to the digestive glands (where motility is increased); and pupils constrict. Sweat glands are not affected because they are innervated only by the sympathetic system. The neurotransmitter involved in the parasympathetic reactions is always ACH. A special condition exists in the heart: it makes rhythmic contractions without outside intervention, because of a spontaneous release of potassium. Here ACH has an inhibitory effect. (The excitatory or inhibitory effect of a transmitter depends on the nature of the receptor site.) If the majority of receptor sites are excitatory or ACH, then ACH may be described as an excitatory transmitter, but not all receptors are excited—some may be inhibited by the transmitter. Some of the effects of the sympathetic and parasympathetic nervous systems are listed in Table 4–2.

Table 4–3 describes the effects, side effects, adverse effects, potential for addiction, and withdrawal symptoms for several drugs that are commonly abused.

SUMMARY

How drugs affect the human body is a fascinating process. Neuron cells and synapses relay drug messages, but the human body is able to alter the effects of drugs on the various parts of the nervous system. It can also manufacture its own drugs, such as enkephalin and endorphin, to meet its specific needs.

We must consider several basic factors if we are to be safe consumers of drugs, whether prescription, over-the-counter, or recreational. These factors include the chemical being considered; the receptor mechanisms to be affected; the dosage; the kinds of drug interactions that will likely take place; and the potential for allergic reactions, tolerance, and physical dependence. Additional pharmacological knowledge and more understanding of the physiological effects of drugs will give us more insight into what happens when we take various drugs.

NOTES

[1]David N. Leff, "Brain Chemistry May Influence Feeling, Behavior," *Smithsonian* 9, no. 3 (June 1978):64.

[2]David N. Leff, "The Pain Killers," *Time* 112, no. 23 (December 4, 1978):96.

[3]Elizabeth Frost, "Acupuncture and Hypnosis," *New York State Journal of Medicine* 78, no. 1 (September 1978).

[4]Elizabeth Frost, "Endorphin for Emotions: A Good Beta," *Science News* 114, no. 20 (November 11, 1978):326.

[5]Elizabeth Frost, "Consumer Safety Rules," in *Drug Information Center (DIC) Handout* (Eugene: University of Oregon, 1979).

[6]Robert M. Julien, *A Primer of Drug Action,* 3rd ed. (San Francisco: W. H. Freeman & Company Publishers, 1981), 75–76.

[7]Ibid., p. 76.

[8]See A. Goth, *Medical Pharmacology* (St. Louis: C. V. Mosby, 1972), p. 8.

[9]A. Goth, *Drug Information Primer* (Eugene, Ore: Drug Information Center, 1975), p. 6.

[10]M. Jouvet, "The States of Sleep," *Scientific American* 216, no. 2 (February 1967):14.

[11]D. Kimble, *Psychology as a Biological Science* (Pacific Palisades, Calif.: Goodyear, 1973).

[12]M. Gazzaniga, "The Split Brain in Man," *Scientific American* 211, no. 2 (August 1967): 24–29.

[13]C. Gross et al., "Visual Properties of Neurons in Inferotemporal Cortex of the Macaque," *Journal of Neurophysiology* 35, no. 1 (January 1972): 96–111.

5

STIMULANTS

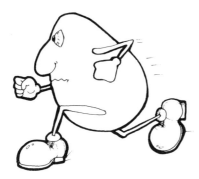

AMPHETAMINES

Introduction

The most common amphetamine derivatives currently available are amphetamine (Benzedrine), dextroamphetamine (Dexedrine), and methamphetamine (Methedrine or Desoxyn). The following information pertains to all these derivatives, unless otherwise noted.

Description and History Amphetamines are powerful CNS stimulants, particularly effective on the reticular formation and the cerebral cortex. They are synthetic drugs belonging to a class of drugs known as sympathomimetics—drugs that mimic actions of the sympathetic nervous system, or the division of the autonomic nervous system that increases the rate of body functions.

Amphetamines and all other sympathomimetics have the following actions:

1. excitatory action on smooth muscles, such as those in blood vessels supplying the skin and mucous membrane, and on secretions from the salivary glands
2. inhibitory action on other smooth muscles, such as those in the intestinal wall, the bronchial tubes, and blood vessels supplying skeletal muscles
3. excitation of heart action, resulting in increased heart rate and force of contraction
4. metabolic actions, such as an increase in the conversion of glycogen into sugar in the liver and muscles, and the liberation of free fatty acids from fatty tissues
5. excitatory action on the central nervous system resulting in respiratory stimulation, increased wakefulness, and prevention as well as reversal of fatigue
6. reduction in appetite[1]

Amphetamines may also cause dryness of the mouth, loss of appetite, increased perspiration, enlarged pupils, talkativeness, nervousness, involuntary trembling, restlessness, excitability, aggressive behavior, tension, anxiety, insomnia, nausea, hot flashes, and bruxism (grinding of the teeth).

Though amphetamines were synthesized as long ago as 1887, the first significant investigation into their pharmacology and therapeutic application was begun in 1927. Ten years later, amphetamines became available as prescription drugs. They were used to treat narcolepsy, a disease producing an uncontrollable urge to sleep, and, paradoxically, to alleviate hyperactivity in children. With continued clinical use, amphetamines were eventually found to produce other major effects including appetite suppression and stimulation.

In the early 1930s, the pharmaceutical company of Smith, Kline and French used Benzedrine in decongestant inhalers that were sold to the public.[2] The stimulating effect of the drug was first recognized when some people began chewing the wicks of the inhalers for kicks. Laws were soon passed prohibiting over-the-counter sale of Benzedrine, but in 1937 the drug was approved by the American Medical Association as a prescription medication.[3] The most popular illicit use of amphetamines is in the form of ingestion of Dexedrine tablets. Intravenous methamphetamine use, though more notorious, is much less frequent, as it spread throughout the United States in the late 1950s and 1960s. Injectable amphetamine was an alternative to opiate dependency, and unethical distribution of the drug by a few physicians made amphetamines easy to obtain.

Although closer legal controls were eventually placed on amphetamine prescriptions, a black market developed. In 1970 and 1971 amphetamines and methamphetamines were placed under strict federal controls.[4] Continued federal concern was evident in Senate hearings in 1971 and 1972, which focused on high-dose intravenous use, misuse of prescription amphetamines, and illicit diversion of legally produced amphetamines.

Physical and Psychological Effects   The stimulating effects of amphetamines occur at the brain's synaptic sites.[5] These may last from four to fourteen hours, depending on the dosage. Although rapidly assimilated into the bloodstream, large amounts of the drug may be excreted unchanged in the urine up to seventy-two hours after ingestion.

Amphetamines suppress hunger by inhibiting the appetite-control center in the hypothalamus and by depressing gastrointestinal activity.[6] Though initially helpful in weight loss, amphetamines lose effectiveness as rapid tolerance develops, and lost weight usually returns unless the dieter has increased the dose or changed daily eating and exercise habits.

Amphetamines instill alertness in the user as well as providing temporary mood elevation. However, the drug itself is not the *source* of such stimulation: as amphetamines chemically interact with the central nervous system, they release stored energy from the body's mitochondria cellular reserves. Continued use of amphetamines leads to depletion of these energy stores.

If amphetamines and other stimulants are used regularly at high dosages, tolerance will occur. Tolerance builds slowly but steadily as an adaptation at the cellular level in the CNS makes the user less sensitive to the drug's effects. Serious gastrointestinal, liver, and stomach disorders can occur since the mechanism in the liver that metabolizes amphetamines is impaired with continued use. Another mechanism of tolerance may be that high doses of amphetamines inhibit appetite markedly, causing the urine to be strongly acid. Since excretion of amphetamines is much faster when the urine is acidic, a heavy user must keep increasing his or her dose to obtain the desired effects.[7]

Prolonged use of large doses of amphetamines can lead to severe anxiety reactions, overaggressiveness, and paranoia.[8] Recent medical evidence suggests that over time they may also cause severe arterial degeneration.[9]

Abrupt cessation of high doses of amphetamines creates no classic *physiological* withdrawal syndrome. It does produce marked *psychological* changes, however, including renewed desire for the drug, overwhelming fatigue, weariness, and severe depression (occasionally provoking suicide).[10] If amphetamines have been self-prescribed to combat depression, the "crash" that follows abrupt cessation of use will generally result in an even deeper depression.

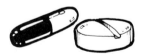

Medical Use Until recently, amphetamines were often prescribed to help overweight people reduce. However, many physicians are currently limiting such usage because of the drug's side effects. Additionally, as tolerance develops, increased dosage is necessary. Following discontinuation of amphetamines, previous eating habits often return and lost weight is gained back. Furthermore, amphetamines have little effect in suppressing the appetite of individuals whose major substance of *misuse* is food.

As we have noted, amphetamines have also been used in the treatment of narcolepsy. By increasing alertness they reduce the need to sleep that this disorder creates. On the other hand, they have been used in the treatment of certain hyperkinetic disorders in children. Hyperactivity and/or minimal brain dysfunction in children are primarily treated with amphetamine and its derivative methylphenidate (the generic name for Ritalin), but there is dispute over such use of these drugs. Though the drugs are calming in some instances, it remains unclear why amphetamines produce this effect.[11]

Amphetamines are also useful in treating brain damage or "senility" in geriatric patients. In patients with cellular damage, the drug stimulates and improves the function of the remaining cells. It also increases *epinephrine* (an adrenalin transmitter) in those whose natural level of adrenalin has diminished with age.

Misuse and Abuse   Many people are still taking amphetamines for the wrong reasons: quick pep-me-ups, extended wakefulness, weight control, and recreation.[12] The FDA is attempting to prevent such use by recommending that prescriptions of amphetamines be limited to those who have minimal brain dysfunction or narcolepsy. In general, the FDA feels that misuse of amphetamines will decrease if fewer amphetamines are produced.

Dexedrine

Dexedrine stimulates the cerebral cortex, having no action on the peripheral or autonomic nervous system, but does increase the blood pressure.[13] The drug depresses the sense of smell and the ability to taste sweet food. It suppresses appetite and can produce euphoria. Used to treat Parkinson's disease, it helps increase epinephrine availability in geriatrics, perception skill, and judgment capabilities and performance, and decreases the need for sleep. Often obtained illicitly, the pills are sometimes known as Dexies or cross-tops, because of the cross that divides each pill into four sections.

Methamphetamine

Introduction   Methamphetamine hydrochloride (Methedrine), commonly known as speed or *crank,* is usually taken orally or intravenously, occasionally in large doses. The drug depresses the appetite, is used in treating narcolepsy, relieves symptoms of Parkinson's disease, and has been used in the treatment of obesity.[14] Methamphetamine produces greater cortical stimulation than other amphetamines, has a more rapid and prolonged onset, and has less intense effects on the peripheral system and the heart. When abused, however, it can cause progressive inflammation of the medium and small arteries throughout the body, resulting in permanent damage to the kidneys, intestines, liver, and pancreas.

The Speed-Taking Ritual   Most people begin by taking amphetamine orally. Initial doses range from 10 to 20 milligrams, but a compulsive user may eventually increase to 250 to 1000 milligrams per day, since tolerance develops rapidly. Once doses get this high, intravenous injections may begin. The term *crystal* is often used in illicit preparation of speed because of the appearance of the powder. Similar to Benzedrine, methamphetamine is more

potent. The term *speed freak* refers to an individual using large doses of amphetamines for days at a time. In the early stages of intravenous use, the user
finds that three or four doses (20 to 30 milligrams each) are enough. In time, this
dose may elevate to 200 milligrams or more. (Most pills on the legal market
contain 5 to 10 milligrams of an active amphetamine.) The average patient with
amphetamine psychosis began with pills, usually Benzedrine (Bennies) or Dexedrine. As tolerance rapidly increases, the user increases the potency of the pills
and decreases intervals between pills to maintain the same level of effectiveness.
Soon the user switches from pills to injections.

Even before a user withdraws the needle, she or he feels an intense and
buzzing euphoria. Elation and hyperactivity last for several hours, and there is
no desire for food or sleep. The user will feel a sense of markedly enhanced
physical strength and increased mental capacity. She or he may "shoot up" every
three to four hours for five to six days until crashing from lack of sleep and
exhaustion. Sleep can last anywhere from twelve hours to four days, depending
on the intensity of the trip. Extreme hunger usually follows sleep. Once this
hunger is satisfied, however, a profound depression can occur.[15]

Increased doses and frequent use of methamphetamines lead to toxicity
and potential amphetamine psychosis. Various signs of these conditions are
bruxism[16] and touching and picking at the extremities, especially the face.[17] A
first sign of amphetamine psychosis is fear or suspicion: the user feels uneasy but
is not quite sure why. The fear soon becomes intense, causing paranoia and a
specific delusion. This amphetamine-induced paranoia causes a high rate of
violence among speed freaks. Users feel they are the specific target of some sort
of surveillance, that they are being watched by the police or by friends. They feel
that friends are no longer trustworthy and are "out to get them." Consequently
users often arm themselves "for their own protection" and try to assault those
who are threatening them. In this sense, the expression "speed kills" is most
appropriate.

Another unique personality trait of amphetamine users is compulsive,
repetitious behavior. Users can repeat the same action hour after hour without
fatigue or boredom. Patients who suffer from full-blown psychosis (schizophrenic mimicization) are preoccupied with taking apart complex mechanical
structures. They are usually so confused, however, that they cannot reassemble
them.[18]

A fully developed toxic syndrome is characterized by vivid visual, auditory,
and sometimes tactile hallucinations. In amphetamine psychosis, imaginary
snakes or insects crawling on or under the skin are envisioned,[19] and the sense of
reality is greatly changed. Because of such symptoms, it is extremely difficult to
distinguish amphetamine psychosis from true schizophrenia. However, rapid
recovery usually occurs with the discontinuation of amphetamine use if the toxic
and psychotic state has not lasted too long.

The relapse rate of amphetamine users after withdrawal seems to be high.
A small percentage of amphetamine users seem to be able to function socially
and professionally by restricting intake, but others show progressive impairment
punctuated by hospitalization.

Adverse Effects   A number of adverse effects can result from methamphetamine use. Needle contamination from intravenous use can lead to serious complications, including serum hepatitis, endocarditis, thrombophlebitis, and other forms of infection.[20] Users have a false sense of unlimited energy, which may result in improper self-care or create or reinforce medical and psychiatric problems.[21] There are also a number of side effects that the excessive user may experience. Among these are headaches, irritability, palpitations, delirium, circulatory collapses, nausea, vomiting, diarrhea, and abdominal cramps.[22] Nonhealing ulcers, brittle fingernails, bruxism, liver disease, and hypersensitivity have also been associated with massive doses of the drug.[23] Malnutrition and weight loss are other major concerns, since speed decreases the desire for food and increases energy output.

Treatment   Treatment for the methamphetamine user, particularly one experiencing psychosis, should include hospitalization. Psychiatric hospitalization at the point of crashing may help to avert a further cycle of amphetamine highs and withdrawal crashes. Chlorpromazine, a tranquilizer, is often used in the treatment of psychosis and may be used to block the central and peripheral effects of amphetamines.

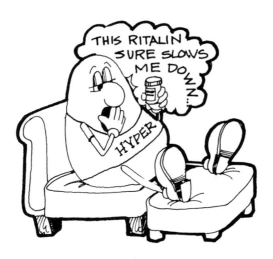

METHYLPHENIDATE (RITALIN)

Ritalin increases blood pressure, stimulates the central nervous system, and has been used in treating epileptic seizures. It has also been used for a wide variety of clinical conditions, such as obesity, depression, hypoactivity, behavioral disorders in children, and excessive sleepiness. Ritalin is less potent than amphetamines but more potent than caffeine. Its effectiveness has still not been fully evaluated and remains controversial.

Physical and Psychological Effects

Side Effects   The side effects of Ritalin are similar to, though less severe than, the adverse reactions caused by amphetamines. Side effects may consist of nausea, dry mouth, nervousness, restlessness, dizziness, headache, and palpitations. More common reactions are loss of appetite, abdominal pain, weight loss during long-term therapy, insomnia, and tachycardia (accelerated heartbeat).[24] The long-term use of Ritalin to control hyperactivity is under debate since continuous medication suppresses growth and causes weight loss.

Tolerance   Because of the length of time Ritalin stays in the body, a hyperactive child being treated with the drug must receive the dosage around noon if he or she is to sleep at night. It takes the liver approximately twenty-four hours to break down Ritalin, which is somewhat shorter than the time other drugs take to be eliminated. Thus tolerance can develop more readily with Ritalin than with other drugs.

Dependence   Most available evidence indicates that the use of Ritalin in the treatment of hyperactive children does not cause psychological dependence. Of particular concern, however, following the cessation of hyperactivity and Ritalin use, is whether the child will want to use other drugs to cope with the stresses of adolescence.[25]

Hyperkinesis

Ritalin is one of the most commonly used drugs in the treatment of hyperkinesis. This condition (hyperactivity but no academic difficulty) has been identified as one of the most common problems among school-age children in the United States. In 1975, it was estimated that 300,000 children in this country were receiving stimulant drugs for treatment of this condition. Approximately 5 percent of elementary school children have been diagnosed as hyperactive, the problem occurring more frequently in boys.[26]

Hyperactivity is the most common complaint of parents who bring their children to mental-health facilities; some say this complaint is voiced in 40 percent of all cases.[27] Robert Smith and John Netsworth believe this condition is based on some kind of inborn error of metabolism, but organic brain damage is usually not detectable.[28]

Childhood hyperactivity is characterized by a combination of behaviors: short attention span and distractability, restlessness, poor impulse control, excessive motor activity, learning difficulties, and emotional liability. The child may be easily frustrated, aggressive, destructive, and apparently antisocial. Behavioral problems may come about from poor verbal skills and problems with conception, perception, memory, attention, and impulse/motor functions (jumping, running or moving about somewhat out of control). Although the mechanism of treatment is not understood, hyperactive children do respond to stimulant medication.

There are two points to consider when treating a hyperactive child: the child is difficult to cope with and has difficulty coping.[29] One must be sure which of these problems to deal with and what approach is appropriate. Giving a child Ritalin to help him or her cope may be justifiable, but doing so to help others cope with the child is an infringement on his or her rights.

Educating the Hyperkinetic Child

Behaviors associated with hyperactivity are usually not noticed or are not much of a problem until the child begins school. In the classroom, however, such behaviors can create a classroom management problem, and learning difficulties may occur. As parent, teacher, and physician work with the hyperkinetic child they should examine their roles, since their tensions, feelings, and attitudes are altered by the behaviors they are judging.

Children who use Ritalin will frequently be identified by their teachers because of the learning deficiencies they exhibit. When instructors recognize these symptoms, they should be prepared to alter their teaching materials to meet the children's needs. Expressing negative attitudes about the children or the use of Ritalin may seriously impair the course of the medical treatment and reduce the drug's usefulness in the school environment.

Alternative Treatments for Hyperactivity There are other ways, besides using Ritalin, to treat hyperactivity: (1) behavior modification, (2) caffeine, (3) reduction of food additives, and (4) electromyographic biofeedback. Behavior modification is an attractive alternative because it is nonchemical. A study of hyperactive elementary school children was done in 1978 to find out if stimulant drugs could be withdrawn immediately, or at least reduced gradually, and be replaced with behavioral therapy; parent and teacher feedback was used in evaluating the progress of the children. The study showed that behavioral treatment improved the condition of unmedicated children by over 33 percent. Social behavior significantly improved and was related to the amount of the parents' commitment to the treatment group.[30] Another study, conducted in Atlanta and Chicago, found behavior modification of definite value in reducing symptoms of minimal brain dysfunction and hyperkinetic syndromes. This study focused on rewarding positive school performance in math and reading activities. Results indicated that schoolwork as well as behavior skills improved with behavior-modification.[31]

The second alternative to Ritalin is caffeine. "A pilot study substituting caffeine in the form of two cups of regular coffee a day suggests that caffeine may be an alternative to a Schedule II [Ritalin-based] drug."[32] (Schedule II drugs include opium, codeine, morphine, methadone, cocaine, and amphetamines.) Caffeine has a calming effect on some hyperkinetic children, and treatment with it is free. The theory behind caffeine use in hyperactivity came to light when Robert Schnacker noted an unusually high rate of coffee drinking in young hyperkinetic children. When asked why they drank so much coffee, the children replied, "It calms me down" or "I can do better in school."

Benjamin Feingold found that food additives in hyperkinetic children's diets affected their behavior. When the children ate only food containing no food additives, their hyperactivity would markedly decrease or disappear entirely. Dr. Feingold designed a diet that eliminated artificial colors and flavors and certain preservatives, including those in breakfast cereals, desserts, meats, soft drinks, flavored yogurt, colored cheeses, butter, margarine, gum, vitamins, toothpastes, cough drops, and candy.[33] Fruits such as apples, apricots, berries, cherries, currants, grapes, raisins, nectarines, oranges, and peaches, once thought to contain naturally occurring salicylates, were also banned from the diet, but recent analysis has found little or no salicylate in some of these fruits. Salicylate-containing foods are now permitted in some Feingold diets. Despite the diets' successes, however, results of several recent studies have questioned the idea that diet control is the ultimate panacea for hyperactivity.[34]

The fourth and last alternative is electromyographic biofeedback training for the reduction of muscle tension and hyperactivity. Such training

> involves the use of electronic equipment to monitor a subject's physiological processes (which are normally not attended to and not under "voluntary" control) and then making these processes known to the subject by means of some external stimulus such as a light or tone. This "externalization" of information about internal functioning ultimately allows the subject to gain voluntary control over his internal physiological systems.[35]

This alternative is relatively new, and further research is needed before it can be employed extensively in the schools.

COCAINE

Introduction

Cocaine is a potent and rapid-acting stimulant, an alkaloid derived from the leaves of the *Erythroxylon* coca plant. Coca paste is extracted from the leaves of the plant where it grows high in the Andes mountains and is then smuggled to northern Chile, Argentina, or southern Colombia, where it is processed. A typical processing compound employs 1000 people, may have as many as nineteen separate laboratories, and is capable of producing 300 tons of cocaine a year. Pure cocaine is fine, opalescent, white, fluffy, odorless, and bitter-tasting.

Cocaine has become the most popular illegal stimulant over the last decade. A recent medical-journal report estimated that over 25 million Americans had tried the drug and that another 5000 experiment with their first dose every day.[36] Until the early 1980s cocaine was used mainly by the wealthy. Now cocaine is also used by students, by heroin addicts who use it for an extra lift, and by lower-income groups.

The nationwide epidemic of cocaine addiction appears not only to have swept all socioeconomic levels but is an increasing problem for women. More women are turning up at drug-treatment centers and joining self-help groups.

According to Ronald Dougherty, director of the chemical-abuse recovery service at Benjamin Rush Hospital, a psychiatric institution in Syracuse, New York, 53 percent of women referred for treatment for cocaine abuse are younger than thirty, compared with 25 percent of the men. Women tend to use cocaine in greater quantity, between $500 and $1000 worth a week, compared with $300 for men. The price of cocaine is moving downward, depending on supply and demand, and ranges from approximately $60 to $150 per gram. "Women start earlier and are into larger amounts," said Dougherty. "With increased use, and increasing problems, women are getting into trouble with the law, with their employers and with their families."[37]

History

It is thought that a pre-Inca tribe learned to cultivate the coca plant because the wild leaves were unfit for chewing. By the end of the fourteenth century, use of the plant by the peasantry was widespread as a means of relieving hunger while increasing strength and endurance.[38] To this day, Indians living in the mountainous environment of Peru and Bolivia use cocaine to help tolerate the cold and to suppress hunger.

In 1884 young Sigmund Freud became interested in cocaine. He had read of the substance's beneficial effects and purchased a quantity of it for use in his practice with patients suffering from heart disease and nervous exhaustion. Eventually Freud was to experiment with it himself, since he suffered from depression, chronic fatigue, and various neurotic symptoms. After using the drug, he found that a mood of disfavor turned to one of cheer.

Freud continued to experiment with cocaine for three years. At that point, however, he discontinued the drug's use and no longer prescribed it for patients. During experimentations he, as well as a number of colleagues, had become concerned about prolonged and excessive uses of the drug.

The same year Freud became interested in cocaine, an ophthalmologist friend of his, Karl Koller, did intensive experimental studies on its numbing effect. The drug became popular immediately and was used in eye surgery and dentistry. William Halsted, the father of modern American surgery and one of the founders of Johns Hopkins Medical School, was the first to use cocaine extensively as a local anesthetic in surgery. The drug caught on with writers. In one of his stories Sir Arthur Conan Doyle had Sherlock Holmes injecting cocaine three times a day, and speculation has it that Robert Louis Stevenson wrote *The Strange Case of Dr. Jekyll and Mr. Hyde* with the help of the drug.[39]

In 1888 Asa G. Chandler took a momentous step in the history of popular beverages when he bought the rights to an almost completely unknown proprietary elixir called Coca-Cola. Initially very few knew that cocaine was an additive to the drink (giving a new meaning to "the pause that refreshes"), but eventually Chandler's company became worried about its corporate image when the slang term for Coca-Cola became *dope*. Passage of the Pure Food and Drug Law in 1906 forced elimination of cocaine from Coke, and in 1914 the Harrison Narcotic Act made cocaine use illegal except for limited medical purposes.

In the late 1960s illicit use of "coke" began to spread, especially among rock and movie performers. The Grateful Dead went so far as to popularize cocaine use in their song "Casey Jones." Today, it is one of the most popular drugs for those able to afford it. Heroin is the only street drug more expensive.

In recent years, efforts have been made to eradicate the excess coca fields in South America by spraying them with poisons. According to Robert DuPont, former director of the National Institute on Drug Abuse (NIDA) and a promoter of both marijuana- and cocaine-eradication operations, NIDA would eliminate all coca production in excess of that needed for local Indian consumption and legitimate exports, such as to cola companies that still use coca leaves for flavoring. DuPont claims that coca eradication would be easier and more efficient than either opium or marijuana eradication because coca is a perennial crop and requires four years of cultivation before it can be harvested. Therefore, eradication would take place only once every four years.[40]

Physiological and Pharmacological Effects

Cocaine strongly stimulates the central nervous system, and the effects may last from twenty minutes to several hours, depending on the contents and purity of the drug. Some of the first signs of this stimulation are increased motor activity, tachycardia (fast heartbeat), and high blood pressure. Since cocaine affects the medulla, increased respiration also occurs. As the dose is increased, so do the depth of respiration and the heart rate. Large doses may cause tremors and convulsive movements, medullary depression, and respiratory and cardiac failure.

Cocaine numbs the sensory- and motor-nerve endings and causes blood vessels to contract, resulting in decreased stimulation. Euphoria is felt, accompanied by an increase in mental alertness, dilated pupils, heightened muscular strength, a decrease in hunger, and an increase in talkativeness and sexual stimulation. Cocaine works on the peripheral nervous system, which releases the neurotransmitter norepinephrine. With excessive dosages, cocaine can produce hallucinations and paranoid delusions, including itching of the skin, cocaine bugs (the sensation of insects moving under or on the skin, clinically known as formication), the sensation of people brushing against the body, smelling of smoke, gasoline, feces, and other foul odors, and voices calling and whispering. Such hallucinations may be caused by seizurelike electrical discharges in the temporal lobe and increased activity coupled with selective depression of inhibitory areas of the brain.[41]

There are several ways to take cocaine. It may be swallowed, but this is not as effective as other methods because of poor absorption in the gastrointestinal tract. The most common method is to snort the drug (sniff it through the nose). The powder is first chopped fine with a razor blade and arranged into lines or columns on a piece of glass. The user may then inhale the cocaine through a rolled-up dollar bill, an empty pen cartridge, a straw, or a "coke spoon." In some cases, a tightly rolled hundred dollar bill (chic!), a diamond-studded straw, or a gold tooter become part of the ritual.

When the powder is sniffed, the blood vessels in the nose are constricted and their blood supply is reduced. Chronic rhinitis (inflammation of the sinus membrane) and, in general, greater vulnerability to upper respiratory infection are adverse effects of snorting.[42] Furthermore, less experienced and less meticulous sniffers will incur damage to the nasal pathways from their less thoroughly chopped cocaine. (Some of the materials added to cocaine, such as sugars, especially mannitol, cause clumping, and the synthetic lidocaine, with which cocaine is cut (mixed), makes the crystals harder to chop.) Recreational use of cocaine has also been linked to coronary-artery spasms and myocardial infarction.[43] In addition, cellulose granulomas have been found in the lungs of the recreational sniffer.

Finally, in 1979 two doctors (one of them the deputy chief medical examiner for Miami's Dade County) found cases in which inhalation of cocaine resulted in a symptom-free interval lasting an hour, followed suddenly by generalized seizures and death.[44] A follow-up report in 1981 showed an increase in the number of people dying after merely snorting cocaine. The key point is that the people who are dying are not snorting any more cocaine than usual. It is important to know that unexpected seizures, respiratory failure, and cardiovascular collapse one to five hours *after* cocaine sniffing can occur in recreational users. Two important findings were mentioned in the 1979 study. First, post-mortem examination showed *no* specific anatomic effects of cocaine. Second, toxicological analysis could not pinpoint adulterants in cocaine as the reason for violent reactions and death. These findings should dispel the myth that there are no dangers associated with recreational use of cocaine. Another very important consideration is that those who are at risk of heart disease or seizures or who have high blood pressure should realize the danger they place themselves in when using cocaine, even if only recreationally.

Injecting cocaine produces an intense and exhilarating rush, but one that is short-lived because of the drug's rapid metabolization by the liver. When injection is employed, there is the possibility that the active ingredients have been cut with inert ingredients. Such nondrug cuts are usually insoluble in the blood and when injected into the vein become emboli that lodge in the arterioles and capillary beds.[45] Intravenous administration provides the highest plasma concentration (gets directly into the blood stream and in a higher concentration) in the shortest period and carries the added risk of contaminated needles. Oral/muscular/etc. take longer and become diluted before entering the blood. Moreover, deaths from the acquired immune deficiency syndrome (AIDS) have been reported among intravenous cocaine shooters in the San Francisco area.[46]

Recent articles have highlighted a relatively new and more intense form of cocaine known as free-base, which is being used in affluent social circles of the United States. It is unique in its dramatic effects, cost, and possible health hazards. Free-base cocaine is popular because it produces a stronger high and because the process by which it is made eliminates some of the cutting agents. Cocaine hydrochloride (street-market cocaine) is dissolved in water and a solvent (usually petroleum ether or ammonia) is added to release the cocaine alkaloid from the salt and other adulterants. A stronger base is then added to neutralize the acid content. The solvent rises to the top where it can be filtered or drawn off. As the solvent evaporates, the cocaine salt oxidizes off, and what is left is cocaine base. The volatile nature of this process sometimes has explosive consequences.

This method gets rid of most, but not all, possible cuts in cocaine. Sugars such as mannitol and lactose are eliminated. However, other cocainelike salts remain. Since most cocaine sold on the streets is far from pure, what is left after the free-base process is often less than half the original amount.

Free-base cocaine is water-soluble, and can be smoked or injected. The high is rapid, powerful, and short-lived, much like the high from injection. Feelings of euphoria and energy last only a few minutes, but effects on the autonomic nervous system include prolonged pupil dilation, increased blood pressure, and increased heart and respiratory rates. The euphoria is quickly followed by feelings of irritability and discomfort. This extreme shift creates a strong desire to continue free basing. Some people have turned to heroin or other depressants to relieve the aftereffects. Side effects from chronic free basing include chest pains, sore throat, hoarse voice, shortness of breath, swollen mouth glands, and an aching, flulike feeling. The increased heart rate and blood pressure caused by cocaine could cause problems for people with high blood pressure. Some users have been hospitalized for ammonia poisoning when they haven't taken the time to rinse the ammonia-soaked powder in water during the final extraction stage. A few instances of bronchitis have occurred, but exactly what constant use of free-base will do to the lungs remains to be seen.

The greatest danger is the possibility of overdose, since in smoking free-base, as in injecting, a high blood level of the drug is assimilated quickly. Although individual tolerance levels vary, any more than 20 milligrams of cocaine per kilogram of body weight will severely impair the respiratory control center in the brain and the user may die of cardiorespiratory arrest.[47]

As we have noted, users often feel compelled to continue free basing in order to keep the euphoria and avoid the postuse depression, and therefore find themselves physically and financially exhausted. Heavy users experience insomnia, weight loss, and paranoia.

Although cocaine is not considered physically addictive, it induces psychological dependence and chemical tolerance. There are no major physiological withdrawal symptoms when the drug is discontinued, but severe depression may occur. As with most psychoactive substances, excessive cocaine use increases the possibility of overdose, which can result from ingesting one gram or less. However, the lethal dose fatal to 50 percent of users is said to be 500 milligrams, although deaths have been reported from lower doses.[48] In the Dade County, Florida, study previously mentioned, most cocaine deaths were found to be due to respiratory collapse immediately following intravenous injection. Ingestion or inhalation resulted in other fatalities: a symptom-free interval lasting as long as one hour would be followed by a generalized seizure and death. Seizures resembled *grand mal* epilepsy attacks, with death occurring from a few minutes to an hour after a seizure. In deaths attributed to cocaine, two or more other drugs are often detected as well, the most common of which are heroin, barbiturates, alcohol, amphetamines, and methadone.[49]

Psychological and Sociological Effects

Cocaine's popularity in years past has returned. Surveys have shown that its use is more widespread than that of heroin, and growing numbers of Americans are becoming psychologically addicted to it. The use of cocaine has permeated all classes of people. It appears to be on the increase among the young, and the drug is being used by bankers, lawyers, politicians, policemen, professional athletes, entertainers, and, in general, the workforce. Cocaine has a high potential for compulsive use because of the intense mood swings it induces. After a few lines the user feels on top of the world. But the drug runs a short course and as we have seen, leaves the user with intense cravings for more cocaine, not to mention irritability and depression. Researchers have detected minor withdrawal signs on electroencephalograms and in sleep patterns, but these "are quite undramatic when compared with the withdrawal syndromes associated with opiates, barbiturates or alcohol."[50] However, there is increasing evidence to accept a "crash" with depression and sleep as part of the cocaine withdrawal syndrome.

In the Haight-Ashbury district of San Francisco cocaine is called the "champagne of sexual drugs." It is identified as the premier enhancer of sexuality and sexual pleasure among the young and sexually sophisticated inhabitants of this area.[51]

The effect on family and friends of habitual use of a drug, particularly cocaine, which is characteristically used with other drugs (typically alcohol and heroin), can be devastating. Mark Gold, director of research at Fair Oaks Hospital in Summit, New Jersey, set up a national hotline, 1–800–CO–CAINE, in 1983. Calls range between 625 to 1200 per day. The average cocaine user is estimated to be twenty-eight to thirty years old, with fourteen years of education, an annual income of $25,000, and no previous criminal record. Among these using cocaine, 36 percent reported dealing in cocaine and 20 percent were stealing from friends, family, and employers to support their drug habit.[52]

One study reported that in many work settings the "coke break" has replaced the coffee break, although it did not list the types of employment in question.[53] Clearly, productivity is reduced by the side effects of sleeplessness, irritability, and inability to concentrate and get along with co-workers, which users have reported to 1–800–CO–CAINE. Over forty percent of the calls received are from spouses or parents concerned about the erratic and antisocial behavior that characterizes the addict. Forty percent of the callers also reported that they had lost all their money assets because of cocaine use. Cocaine is definitely taking its toll on society.

Medical Use

Cocaine has been useful as a local anesthetic since 1884, though by the 1890s the medical community had begun to feel that its use was often more harmful than therapeutic. In the early 1900s a number of cocaine derivatives were synthesized to improve the drug's medical usefulness. These cocaine synthetics (Novocaine [procaine] and Xylocaine) did not stimulate the nervous system as cocaine did and were extensively used as a topical (local) anesthetic. Despite its drawbacks, cocaine is still used in specific cases by many ophthalmologists and ear, nose, and throat specialists. It is used to dilate the pupil in certain inflammatory diseases of the eye and is sometimes used following cataract surgery to prevent perforations in the vitreous body. During a tear-duct operation, gauze is often saturated in cocaine crystals before being applied as a local anesthetic and to control bleeding.

The effects and potential use of cocaine for treatment of depressed patients were studied by Robert Post and Frederick Goodwin at the National Institute of Mental Health in Bethesda, Maryland.[54] They concluded that although cocaine was capable of eliciting positive changes, such as elation, it also elicited feelings of ambivalence and deep depression, leading them to dismiss its use as an antidepressant.

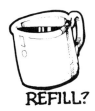

REFILL?

CAFFEINE (XANTHINES)

Introduction

If we had to identify the drug that has had the greatest impact on civilization, caffeine would be a top contender. Xanthines, the family of chemicals of which caffeine is a part, are the oldest stimulants known. Today, caffeine is perhaps the most widely used drug, constituting a regular portion of the American diet. The drug can be found in many substances, the most common of which are listed in Tables 5–1, 5–2, and 5–3.

Although down from a peak in 1945, Americans presently consume about 2.7 billion pounds of coffee per year. Americans drink three to five cups every day, for a total of 400 million cups of coffee daily. Three quarters of the caffeine in our diets is found in coffee. However, coffee is just one source of caffeine. The caffeine taken out of coffee (in the process of making decaffeinated coffee) is bought by the soft-drink industry. Soft drinks come in second, ahead of tea and chocolate, as contributors of caffeine to our diet. Cola drinks contain some caffeine naturally, but more is added during the manufacturing process. Noncola drinks may also contain large quantities of caffeine—a fact not always realized when these are given to children. Caffeine can also be found in prescription drugs (APC, Darvon, etc.) and over-the-counter drugs (Emperin, Anacin, etc.). It has been estimated that an American's daily intake of caffeine from all sources is 210 milligrams per day.

As a member of the methylate xanthines, caffeine has stimulating effects that are often pleasant:

TABLE 5–1   Caffeine Content Of Beverages And Foods

Item	Milligrams Caffeine	
	Average	Range
Coffee (5-oz. cup)		
Brewed, drip method	115	60–180
Brewed, percolator	80	40–170
Instant	65	30–120
Decaffeinated, brewed	3	2–5
Decaffeinated, instant	2	1–5
Tea (5-oz. cup)		
Brewed, major U.S. brands	40	20–90
Brewed, imported brands	60	25–110
Instant	30	25–50
Iced (12-oz. glass)	70	67–76
Cocoa beverage (5-oz. cup)	4	2–20
Chocolate milk beverage (8 oz.)	5	2–7
Milk chocolate (1 oz.)	6	1–15
Dark chocolate, semi-sweet (1 oz.)	20	5–35
Baker's chocolate (1 oz.)	26	26
Chocolate-flavored syrup (1 oz.)	4	4

Source: FDA, Food Additive Chemistry Evaluation Branch, based on evaluations of existing literature on caffeine levels, Federal Publication FDA Consumer, Spring 1983.

After taking caffeine, one is capable of greater sustained intellectual effort and a more perfect association of ideas. There is also a keener appreciation of sensory stimuli, and reaction time to them is appreciably diminished. This accounts for the hyperesthesia, sometimes unpleasant, which some people experience after drinking too much coffee. In addition, motor activity is increased; typists, for example, work faster and with fewer errors. However, recently acquired motor skill in a task involving delicate muscular coordination and accurate timing may . . . be adversely affected. These effects may be brought on by the administration of 150 to 250 milligrams of caffeine, the amount contained in one or two cups of coffee or tea.[55]

Americans may have more of a physiological and/or psychological dependence on caffeine than on all other drugs combined. Some individuals experience a jittery feeling, a slight loss of motor coordination, and insomnia after consuming it. Even small dosages increase anxiety, irritate the stomach lining, and may be undesirable for certain cardiac patients. However, the morning cup of coffee is so much a part of America that we seldom look upon its consumption as a drug habit.

As you can see in Table 5–3, caffeine is also found in many common medications. It is added to cold, headache, allergy, stay-awake, and other remedies, both prescription and nonprescription. The Food and Drug Administration's National Center for Drugs and Biologics reports that more than 1000 OTC drugs list caffeine as an ingredient.[56]

TABLE 5-2   Caffeine Content Of Soft Drinks

Brand	Milligrams Caffeine (12-oz. serving)
Sugar-Free Mr. PIBB	58.8
Mountain Dew	54.0
Mello Yello	52.8
TAB	46.8
Coca-Cola	45.6
Diet Coke	45.6
Shasta Cola	44.4
Shasta Cherry Cola	44.4
Shasta Diet Cola	44.4
Mr. PIBB	40.8
Dr. Pepper	39.6
Sugar-Free Dr. Pepper	39.6
Big Red	38.4
Sugar-Free Big Red	38.4
Pepsi-Cola	38.4
Aspen	36.0
Diet Pepsi	36.0
Pepsi Light	36.0
RC Cola	36.0
Diet Rite	36.0
Kick	31.2
Canada Dry Jamaica Cola	30.0
Canada Dry Diet Cola	1.2

Source: Institute of Food Technologists (IFT), April 1983, based on data from National Soft Drink Association, Washington, D.C. IFT also reports that there are at least 68 flavors and varieties of soft drinks produced by 12 leading bottlers that have no caffeine.

History

Caffeine has a long history, dating back thousands of years, as the world's most commonly used psychotropic drug. There are many reports of Stone Age people making beverages from caffeine-containing plants.

The history of caffeine use, like that of many other drugs, is surrounded by myth and supposition. Legend has it that coffee was discovered by a friar in an Arabian convent after he witnessed the stimulating effect the berries of a coffee plant had on goats.[57] Actually, coffee was first introduced as a medicine in England and Europe but became popular as a nonalcoholic drink. The "medicine" became so popular that about the middle of the seventeenth century coffeehouses (known as "penny universities") were established where people could listen to learned and literary figures as well as politicians for a cup of coffee bought for a penny. Despite its popularity, coffee drinking was outlawed at various times in both Arabia and England because it was considered an intoxicating beverage that often led to discussions of rebellion and slander of those in power.

**TABLE 5–3 Caffeine Content of Prescription
and Over-the-Counter Drugs**

Prescription Drugs	Milligrams Caffeine
Cafergot (for migraine headache)	100
Fiorinal (for tension headache)	40
Soma Compound (pain relief, muscle relaxant)	32
Darvon Compound (pain relief)	32.4

Nonprescription Drugs	
Weight-Control Aids	
Codexin	
Dex-A-Diet II	200
Dexatrim, Dexatrim Extra Strength	200
Dietac capsules	200
Maximum Strength Appedrine	100
Prolamine	140
Alertness Tablets	
Nodoz	100
Vivarin	200
Analgesic/Pain Relief	
Anacin, Maximum Strength Anacin	32
Excedrin	65
Midol	32.4
Vanquish	33
Diuretics	
Aqua-Ban	100
Maximum Strength Aqua-Ban Plus	200
Permathene H2 Off	200
Cold/Allergy Remedies	
Coryban-D capsules	30
Triaminicin tablets	30
Dristan Decongestant tablets and Dristan A–F Decongestant tablets	16.2
Duradyne-Forte	30

Source: FDA's National Center for Drugs and Biologics.

Tea was first known of in China, where it was used primarily as a medicine, as early as 4700 B.C. Later it was introduced as a beverage, and around 1600 it was shipped by the Dutch and British from their colonies in the East to Europe. By the 1700s, tea was being shipped to America, where it eventually became involved in the infamous battle over taxation. Participants in the Boston Tea Party deposited many cases of the herb into the waters of Boston Harbor in a statement that eventually resulted in war.

Coca, obtained from the seeds of the theobroma tree, also contains caffeine. Coca drinking spread during the sixteenth century in Spain and Mexico, and today the major coca supplier is Africa. Chocolate, first manufactured by the Dutch in the early 1800s, also contains caffeine, although the active ingredient is theobromine, a methylated xanthine.

Physical Effects

When a person drinks two cups of coffee (150–300 milligrams of caffeine), the effects begin in 15 to 30 minutes. Metabolism, body temperature, and blood pressure increase. Other effects include increased urine production, higher blood-sugar levels, hand tremors, a loss of coordination, decreased appetite, and delayed sleep. Extremely high doses may cause nausea, diarrhea, sleeplessness, trembling, headache, and nervousness. Poisonous doses of caffeine occur occasionally and may result in convulsions, breathing failure, and death.[58]

Caffeine may also present a risk for growing children. The Federation of American Societies for Experimental Biology released a report expressing concern about the levels of caffeine being consumed by children and its possible ill effects.[59] Small children are at extra risk because of their small size.

Central Nervous System

ALERTNESS AND WAKEFULNESS. The general conclusions from research on alertness indicate that caffeine users (not abstainers) require caffeine in the morning to achieve a sufficient state of alertness and readiness to face the day's tasks. Also, in the absence of caffeine, users may experience symptoms of mild withdrawal, which are relieved dramatically by caffeine intake.[60] Symptoms may appear approximately twelve to sixteen hours after the last dose of caffeine.

The results of a study of the wakefulness effects of caffeine on 230 medical students contained the following information: (1) caffeine prolonged the time required to fall asleep and disturbed the soundness of sleep when administered in a dose of 150 to 200 milligrams of caffeinated coffee before bedtime; (2) caffeine caused distinctly less wakefulness in subjects who habitually drank a great deal of coffee; and (3) some subjects, among those who drank the most coffee, experienced morning headache after about eighteen hours without caffeine—if a single dose of 150 milligrams was given the previous evening, the headache was prevented.[61] In a study of 1500 undergraduate college students, it was found that the group consuming the most caffeine had a higher frequency of psychophysiological disorders and lower academic performance.[62]

Caffeinism

Caffeine may not fit technical definitions of addiction, but "withdrawal headache" from a decrease in caffeine consumption is well documented.[63] There is also a measurable, temporary depression that occurs with caffeine abstinence. Although the literature is divided on the potential of caffeine to produce tolerance and dependence, it is evident that the substance has a hold over a large number of people. A high dose of caffeine (over 600 milligrams, less for some), perhaps in the form of five cups of coffee or more, can cause anxiety, nervousness and, insomnia and these have been recognized as symptoms of caffeinism.[64] Some feel tolerance may develop with use of over 500 or 600 milligrams of caffeine per day. A regular user of caffeine develops a tolerance and may crave the drug in order to "get going." A person going through withdrawal may be accident-prone and irritable.

OTHER CNS EFFECTS.   A large dose of caffeine stimulates the central nervous system at all levels. The drug's effect on the cortex allows the user a clearer, more productive, and more rapid flow of thought, increased cerebral efficiency, and no drowsiness or fatigue. As a result of cortical stimulation, the individual is more alert, faster, has a better memory, forms judgments more quickly, learns faster (temporarily), and has a decreased reaction time. The sense of touch may be more discriminating and the sense of pain more keen.[65] However, insomnia, restlessness, and excitement may occur, sometimes progressing to sensory disturbances such as ringing in the ears and flashing lights. Tachycardia and respiratory quickening can also occur,[66] although death is quite unlikely since the toxic dose in humans is over ten grams, or 70 to 100 cups of coffee.

Heart and Circulatory System   Xanthines directly stimulate the myocardium of the heart, causing an increase in the force of contraction, heartbeat, and cardiac output. Caffeine also acts on the blood vessels in a similar way, dilating the coronary, pulmonary, and general systemic blood vessels that act directly on the vascular musculature. However, caffeine also constricts the blood vessels by its stimulation of the medullary vasomotor center. With excessive doses, the vasodilator action predominates. Cerebral blood flow is reduced, as well as oxygen availability.

HEART DISEASE.   A study conducted in collaboration with the Boston Drug Surveillance Program was carried out in twenty-four Boston-area hospitals on the incidence of myocardial infarction and coffee consumption. In the study,

> a positive association between coffee consumption and acute myocardial infarction was confirmed by analysis of data from a multipurpose survey of 12,759 hospitalized patients, including 440 with a diagnosis of acute myocardial infarction. As compared with those who drink no coffee, the risk of infarction among those drinking one to five or six or more cups of coffee per day are estimated to be increased by 60 to 120 percent, respectively. This association could not be attributed to compounding by age, sex, past coronary heart disease, hypertension, congestive heart failure, obesity, diabetes, smoking or occupation, nor could it be explained by the use of sugar with coffee.[67]

Constant stimulation of the nervous and cardiac systems by caffeine may be a factor in cardiac problems. Caffeine ingestion also causes a significant rise in serum-free fatty acids (or triglyceride level) in the blood, causing further heart problems.

Liver and Pancreas The body normally releases glucose reserves in the liver as energy for physiological functioning. This release of glucose leads to increased availability of insulin from the pancreas, which reduces elevated blood-sugar levels.[68] When blood sugar is lowered, fatigue often results. Thus the desire for the time-honored coffee break. Several cups of coffee and a donut will raise the glucose level again. Then insulin will be released to bring the blood-sugar level back down. This process is continuous in the body's attempt to establish a balance among its chemical constituents. But with excessive fluctuations in daily functions, the liver's reserve, the pancreas, the nervous system, and the cardiac system will be subject to strain.

Caffeine also markedly affects the body's sugar metabolism: excesses of the drug have been linked to hypoglycemia (deficient glucose levels). This low sugar level can result in weakness, marked perspiration, fatigue, and fainting.

The metabolic half-life of caffeine averages from several hours to several days, depending upon age, sex, hormonal status, medications being taken, and smoking habits. Infants and children do not metabolize and eliminate caffeine as rapidly as adults, so the effects of the substance last longer in them—as much as three to four days in newborns.[69]

Diuretic Actions and Gastric Upset Caffeine is a diuretic: it causes an increased production of urine. Persons with a predisposition toward ulcers may exhibit an abnormal response to caffeine ingestion and suffer some gastric upset.

Use with Children Twelve ounces of a cola drink can produce significant reactions in children. Walter Silver, of the Maimonides Medical Center in New York, found tachycardia and insomnia in otherwise healthy preadolescent cola drinkers. Both of these complaints disappeared when the beverage was withdrawn. Silver claims that "children are more susceptible than adults to excitation by xanthines, [and that] we should . . . withdraw these beverages from our children's diet."[70]

Skeletal Muscles The xanthines, particularly caffeine, make skeletal muscles less susceptible to fatigue by increasing their capacity for muscular activity.

Birth defects A recent study indicated that 23.2 percent of mothers who gave birth to abnormal babies drank eight or more cups of coffee a day, compared with only 12.9 percent of mothers of normal babies.[71] The FDA has yet to recommend that pregnant women stop using caffeine, but the March of Dimes has recommended that pregnant women drink only moderate amounts of coffee or other caffeine-containing substances.

Fibrocystic Breast Disease   Fibrocystic breast disease is a common and worrisome complaint of many women. The characteristic lumps, nodules, and thickenings in the breast tissue are benign yet hard to distinguish from cancerous tissue, and may impede the diagnosis of cancer. Furthermore, women with fibrocystic breast disease have an increased risk of developing breast cancer.

Caffeine and related substances are suspected of increasing the supply of *Camp,* a growth-promoting compound in breast tissue. Levels of Camp are 50 percent higher in the breast tissue of women with fibrocystic disease, although it is not clear whether the elevated enzyme levels are a cause or a result of breast disease.

John Minton and his colleagues at the Ohio State University's College of Medicine advised forty-seven women with fibrocystic breast disease to eliminate coffee, tea, cola, and chocolate from their diet. Of the twenty women who complied with his advice, thirteen (65 percent) "experienced complete disappearance of all palpable breast nodules and other symptoms within 1–6 months."[72]

Decaffeinated Coffee

Since recent research has suggested that caffeine may cause birth defects, many women have switched to decaffeinated coffee. But is decaffeinated coffee safe? Decaffeination is a process using water, heat, and solvent. A hot-water solution removes the caffeine from the beans and an organic solvent removes the caffeine from the water, which is then reused. From the standpoint of taste, the process has advantages. From the standpoint of safety, however, the use of a solvent is questionable.

Trichloroethylene was used as the solvent until the National Cancer Institute announced that that substance was possibly carcinogenic (cancer-producing). A switch was then made to methylene chloride, a widely used industrial chemical best known to the public as the active ingredient in paint remover. This additive has not been tested thoroughly as an ingested chemical additive, though a recent study suggests that it too is carcinogenic.[73] The FDA is permitting no more than ten parts per million. For the time being, it may be safe to say that the risk of caffeinated coffee probably far exceeds the risk of decaffeinated coffee for pregnant women.[74] However, additional information is needed to make accurate conclusions.

MDA (METHYLENEDIOXYAMPHETAMINE) _____

Experienced LSD users have confirmed clinical evidence that MDA (euphemistically known as Mellow Drug of America) produces LSD-like effects without the accompanying hallucinations.[75] The drug produces a sensation of joy, feelings of peace, tranquility, and gentleness, but no despair or remorse. Also absent are visual distortions or misperceptions. Reactions such as anger, aggression, confusion, disorientation, paranoia, loneliness, and isolation occur infrequently. MDA gained popularity in the mid to late 1960s and early 1970s as a number of people, particularly at rock concerts, used it as a pseudoaphrodisiac.

Though there are pleasant effects, there are also negative physiological effects from the drug's use. These include increased pulse rate, fluctuating blood pressure, dilation of pupils, overstimulation, loss of appetite, and insomnia. The average street dose (100 to 150 milligrams) takes effect within an hour, with peak effects occurring within the first two hours. Depending on the dosage and the user's state of mind, MDA's effects can last up to twelve hours.

MDA is called a psychomimetic amphetamine because it produces both stimulation and various forms and degrees of hallucinations. Look-alikes have stimulatory side effects and can harm individuals vulnerable to high blood pressure.

LOOK-ALIKE DRUGS

After restrictions were placed on production and distribution of amphetamines in the early 1970s there was an initial disruption of the flow of these drugs to the illicit street market. In the late 1970s, however, new, nontraditional companies started manufacturing and distributing what have since been called look-alike stimulants. These companies usually use three over-the-counter cold preparations: caffeine, ephedrine, and phenylpropanolamine. When these three ingredients are combined into a single preparation they produce stimulatory side effects that are somewhat similar to the arousal and alertness caused by amphetamines. The drugs obtained the title of *look-alikes* because their manufacturers packaged them in a variety of pills and capsules whose letters and markings gave them the appearance of prescription medications.

Large numbers of these preparations are now consumed each year in the United States, and they are frequently advertised in drug-oriented magazines and other publications. Side effects can include high blood pressure, which could make sensitive individuals more prone to strokes. More routine side effects consist of a mild to severe headache and possibly mild to moderate stomach irritation. With continued frequent use over time, tolerance can develop such that large amounts taken over time are required to obtain the original effects of the drug.[76]

SUMMARY

A number of stimulants are currently used in the United States. Amphetamines, for example, may be used to help people overcome fatigue, improve performance, prevent narcolepsy, or lose weight. For some, methamphetamine is used to experience intense exhilaration. However, intravenous injection of these drugs can lead to serious health hazards as well as deleterious social consequences.

Methylphenidate (Ritalin) is sometimes used to calm hyperactive children or people with minimal brain damage. This particular use has led to considerable controversy, some claiming that behavioral modification, use of caffeine, reduction of food additives, or electromyographic biofeedback could accomplish the same goal without the possibility of the child becoming dependent on drugs as a coping mechanism.

Cocaine has seen limited medical application as an aesthetic for various surgical operations. Because of its euphoria-producing properties, however, it has gained great street popularity. However recent research has indicated that cocaine may not be a safe drug because of the increasing number of heart attacks it causes in healthy users.

Another drug that millions of Americans use on a regular basis is caffeine, found in beverages such as coffee, tea, and cocoa. Caffeine can also be found in prescription and over-the-counter analgesics (headache and pain relievers).

NOTES

[1]Stanley Einstein, *Beyond Drugs* (New York: Pergamon Press, 1975), p. 52.

[2]"*Amphetamine: Alcohol and Drug Fact Sheet*," in *Drug Information Center* (*DIC*) (Eugene Ore.: University of Oregon, 1979). p. 1.

[3]Ibid.

[4]Ibid.

[5]Ibid.

[6]Ibid.

[7]Peter Ognibere, "Amphetamines and Barbiturates," *New Republic* 168, no. 5 (February 3, 1973):130.

[8]Department of Health, Education and Welfare, *Amphetamine*, Report Series 28, no. 1 (Washington, D.C., National Clearinghouse for Drug Abuse Information, 1974). p.3.

[9]*Amphetamine: Alcohol and Drug Fact Sheet*, p. 1.

[10]Thomas Weisman, *Drug Abuse and Drug Counseling* (Cleveland: Press of Case Western Reserve University, 1972), p. 90.

[11]"Clinical Aspects of Amphetamine Abuse," *Journal of the American Medical Association* 240, no. 21 (November 17, 1978):2317–19.

[12]Michael Dolan, "Clamping Down on Uppers," *American Pharmacy* 18, no. 4 (April 1978): 18–23.

[13]"*Amphetamine: Alcohol and Drug Fact Sheet*," p. 1.

[14]Ibid.

[15]Louis S. Goodman and Alfred Gilman, eds., *The Pharmacological Basis of Therapeutics*, 4th ed. (New York: Macmillan, 1970), p. 294.

[16]*Dorland's Illustrated Medical Dictionary*, 24th ed. (Philadelphia: Saunders, 1965), p. 245.

[17]Goodman and Gilman, *The Pharmacological Basis of Therapeutics*, p. 294.

[18]Ibid., p. 295.

[19]Edward Brecher et al., *Licit and Illicit Drugs* (Boston: Little, Brown, 1972), p. 285.

[20]"*Amphetamine: Alcohol and Drug Fact Sheet*," p. 1.

[21]Einstein, *Beyond Drugs*, p. 54.

[22]Ibid.

[23]*The Nonmedical Use of Drugs: An Interim Report of the Canadian Government Commission on Inquiry* (Ottawa: Penguin, 1970), p. 85.

[24]"*Amphetamine: Alcohol and Drug Fact Sheet,*" p. 1.

[25]A. F. Charles, "Case of Ritalin: Drugs for Hyperactive Children," *New Republic* 165, no. 17 (October 23, 1971):17–19.

[26]Alexander Lucas and Morris Weiss, "Methylphenidate Hallucinesis," *Journal of the American Medical Association* 217, no. 8 (August 23, 1971):377.

[27]Robert L. Sprague, Kenneth R. Barnes, and John Werry, "Methylphenidate and Thorazine: Learning, Reaction Time, Activity and Classroom Behavior in Disturbed Children," *American Journal of Orthopsychiatry* 40, no. 4 (July 1970).

[28]Robert M. Smith and John Netsworth, *The Exceptional Child: A Functional Approach* (New York: McGraw-Hill, 1975).

[29]C. J. Weithorn and R. Ross, "Stimulant Drugs for Hyperactivity: Some Disturbing Questions," *American Journal of Orthopsychiatry* 46, no. 1 (January 1976):171.

[30]Susan G. O'Leary and William E. Pelham, "Behavior Therapy and Withdrawal of Stimulant Medication in Hyperactive Children," *Pediatrics* 61, no. 2 (February 1978):211–17.

[31]Garnun Gray, "Order in the Classroom: Drugging for Deportment," *Nation* 221, no. 14 (November 1, 1975):424.

[32]Robert C. Schnacker, "Caffeine as a Substitute for Schedule II Stimulants in Hyperkinetic Children," *American Journal of Psychiatry* 130, no. 7 (July 1973): pp 297–316.

[33]"The Feingold Diet for Hyperactive Children," *Medical Letter* 20, no. 12 (June 16, 1978):56.

[34]J. Preston Harley and Charles G. Mathews, "The Hyperactive Child and the Feingold Controversy," *American Pharmacy* 18, no. 6 (June 1978):44–46; C. K. Connors and C. H. Goyette, "The Effects of Certified Food Dyes on Behavior: A Challenge Test," *Clinical Drug Evaluation Unit Program* 7 (1977):18–19; Jeffrey Mattes and Rachel Gittleman-Klein, "A Cross-Over Study of Artificial Food Colorings in a Hyperkinetic Child," *American Journal of Psychiatry* 135, no. 8 (August 1978):987–88.

[35]Reprinted from *Journal of Learning Disabilities,* "Use of Electromyographic Biofeedback in Control of Hyperactivity," by Lendell Brand and Lupin, Volume 8, Number 7, September, 1975. The Professional Press, Inc. 101 E. Ontario Street, Chicago, IL 60611.

[36]A. Washton, and N. Stone, "The Human Cost of Cocaine Use," *Medical Aspects of Human Sexuality* 18, no. 11 (November 1984): 122–30.

[37]Cited in "Cocaine Addiction: A Growing Problem for Women," *Register Guard* (Eugene, Oregon), February 18, 1985, p. 5b.

[38]"Cocaine: Alcohol and Drug Fact Sheet," in *Drug Information Center (DIC)* (Eugene: University of Oregon, 1979). p. 298.

[39]"Dr. Jekyll and Mr. Cocaine," *Science News* 99, no. 16 (April 17, 1971):264.

[40]Cited in Fred Gardner, "Beyond Paraquat: Cocaine Eradication," *New Times* 10, no. 11 (May 29, 1978):17–19.

[41]Ronald K. Siegel, "Cocaine Hallucinations," *American Journal of Psychiatry* 1 (March 1978):309–14.

[42]G. Gay, "You've Come a Long Way, Baby! Coke Time for the New American Lady of the Eighties," *Journal of Psychoactive Drugs* 13, no. 4 (October–December 1981): 297–316.

[43]J. Schachne et al., "Coronary-Artery Spasm and Myocardial Infarction Associated with Cocaine Use," *New England Journal of Medicine* 13, no. 4 (June 1983): 297–316.

[44]Charles V. Wetli and Ronald K. Wright, "Death Caused by Recreational Use of Cocaine," *Journal of the American Medical Association* 241, no. 23 (June 8, 1979):2519–22. Copyright © 1979, American Medical Association.

[45]*The Gourmet Cokebook* (White Mountain Press, 1972), p. 78.

[46]*Pharmaceutical Chemical Newsletter* 12, no. 5 (September–October 1983):p. 1.

[47]"Cocaine," p. 78.

[48]Welti and Wright, "Death Caused by Recreational Use of Cocaine," 2520.

[49]Ibid.

[50]Craig Van Dyke and Robert Byck, "Cocaine," *Scientific American* 226, no. 3 (March 1982):132.

[51]G. R. Gay et al., "The Sensuous Hippie: Drug/Sex Practice in the Haight-Ashbury," *Drug Forum* 6, no. (1) (1977–78):27–47.

[52]Editorial, *U.S. Journal* 7, no. 9 (September 1983).

[53]Washton and Stone, "The Human Cost of Cocaine Use," p. 125

[54]Robert M. Post, Joel Kotin, and Frederick K. Goodman, "The Effects of Cocaine on Depressed Patients," *American Journal of Psychiatry* 1 (March 1978):411.

[55]Louis Goodman and Alfred Gilman, "Xanthines," in *The Pharmacological Basis of Therapeutics*, 4th ed., ed. Goodman and Gilman, (New York: Macmillan, 1970),pp. 358–370.

[56]Chris Lecos, "The Latest Caffeine Scorecard," *FDA Consumer*, OHHS Publication No. (FDA) 84-2184 (Washington, D.C.: Department of Health and Human Services, 1984).

[57]Goodman and Gilman, "Xanthines," p. 199.

[58]National Institute on Drug Abuse. *Stimulants and Cocaine*, DHHS Publication No. (ADM) 83-1304 (Washington, D.C. U.S. Government Printing Office 1983).

[59]G. N. Fuller, P. Divakaran, and R. C. Wiggins, "The Effect of Postnatal Caffeine Administration on Brain Myelination," *Brain Research* 249 (October 1982):189–91.

[60]Brecher, *Licit and Illicit Drugs*, p. 202.

[61]A. Goldstein, "Wakefulness Caused by Caffeine," *Naunyn-Schmiedebergs Arch in Pathopharmacology* 248 (1964):269–78.

[62]Gilliland and D. Andress, "Ad Lib Caffeine Consumption, Symptoms of Caffeinism, and Academic Performance," *American Journal of Psychiatry* 138, no. 4 (April 1981):512–14.

[63]D. Sawyer, H. Julia, and A. Turin, "Caffeine and Human Behavior: Arousal, Anxiety, and Performance Effects," *Journal of Behavioral Medicine* 5, no. 4 (1982):415–39.

[64]F. W. Furlong, "Possible Psychiatric Significance of Excessive Coffee Consumption," *Canadian Psychiatric Association Journal* 20 (1975).

[65]Betty Bergerson and Elsie E. Krug, *Pharmacology in Nursing*, 14th ed. (St. Louis: C. V. Mosby, 1979), p. 360.

[66]Ibid.

[67]Hershel Jick et al., "Coffee and Myocardial Infarction," *New England Journal of Medicine* 289, no. 2 (July 12, 1973):63–67.

[68]J. Lin Boniface and Reginald E. Haist, "Effects of Some Modifiers of Insulin on Insulin Biosynthesis," *Endocrinology* 92, no. 3 (March 1973):735–42.

[69]"Caffeine," *Contemporary Nutrition Newsletter* 9, no. 5 (May 1984).

[70]Walter Silver, "Insomnia, Tachycardia, and Cola Drinkers," *Pediatrics* 47, no. 3 (March 1971):35.

[71]Michael Jacobson, "Caffeine's Role in Birth Defects," *Nutrition Action*, October 1978, p. 8.

[72]John P. Minton, "Response of Fibrocystic Disease to Caffeine Withdrawal and Correlation of Cyclic Nucleotides with Breast Disease," *American Journal of Obstetrics and Gynecology* 135, no. 1 (September 1979):157–58.

[73]Grant Bunin, "More Doubts Brewing in the Coffee Pot," *Nutrition Action*, January 1979, p. 10.

[74]Ibid.

[75]See "MDA: Alcohol and Drug Fact Sheet," in *Drug Information Center (DIC)* (Eugene: University of Oregon, 1980).

[76]See "Look-Alike Drugs: Information Fact Sheet," in *Drug Information Center (DIC)* (Eugene: University of Oregon, 1981).

TOBACCO
america's number one
preventable hazard

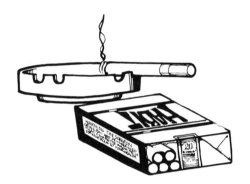

HISTORY

In the almost 500 years since European explorers first saw American Indians smoking tobacco, a great segment of the world population has become dependent on the extremely harmful products made from this plant. Ironically, tobacco first became popular in Europe for its supposed curative powers and was looked upon by some as a panacea for health problems. The smoking of tobacco spread rapidly across Europe and eventually the entire world.

Early on, tobacco was smoked through a pipe. But in the mid nineteenth century, this form of tobacco use decreased in Europe and the United States and was replaced by chewing tobacco. Spittoons became an accepted part of the era, and by the end of the nineteenth century half of all the tobacco consumed in the United States was chewed. Later, cigars and cigarettes were introduced. Their consumption increased steadily, and in 1885 over one billion cigarettes per year were sold.

According to the Maxwell Report, the production of cigarettes has dramatically decreased since 1983. Moreover, production had already dropped from 624 billion in 1982 to about 590 billion in 1983 (slightly under 3000 per person). Since the 1964 Surgeon General's Report, over 35 million Americans have voluntarily quit smoking.[1]

CHEMISTRY

Cigarette smoke from burning tobacco consists of a mixture of approximately 3000 chemical substances that are dangerous to living tissue.[2] These substances include (1) droplets of tars and other compounds, which form 40 percent of the smoke; (2) nicotine, a drug that is poisonous in higher concentrations; and (3) a dozen gases, including carbon monoxide, hydrogen cyanide, and nitrous oxides. The toxicity of these gases and compounds, coupled with nicotine, is responsible for many of the cigarette-related premature deaths that occur each year in the United States.

Tar and nicotine in cigarettes are usually present in the ratio of ten to one.[3] Research has shown tobacco tars to be carcinogenic (cancer-producing) when applied to the skin or bronchial tubes of mice and other laboratory animals. Other chemicals in tobacco tar are co-carcinogens (substances that do not themselves cause cancer, but stimulate the growth of certain cancers when combined with other chemicals). For example, the phenols present in tar are not inherently carcinogenic but may combine with benzopyrene, another substance in the tar, to produce cancer.

A combination of hydrogen cyanide, tars, and the drying effect of cigarette smoke paralyzes or destroys the action of the cilia, the mucous-covered hairlike structures that keep the lungs free from mucous, germs, and dirt. Eventually, the bronchial tubes become saturated with a brown, sticky coating of hydrogen cyanide, tars, etc., and, in attempting to dislodge this matter many smokers develop a "smoker's cough" or "hack."[4]

Pharmacologically, nicotine, which is liberated from tobacco by the heat produced by combustion, is classified as a stimulant. Cigarettes contain significantly large amounts of nicotine alkaloid, and clinical findings indicate that the major nicotine effects on the body are respiratory stimulation and gastrointestinal hyperactivity, since nicotine is readily absorbed from oral and gastrointestinal mucosa, the respiratory tract, and the skin.[5] Because deeper inhaling takes place in cigarette smoking, more tars, nicotine, and carbon monoxide are inhaled by smoking cigarettes than by smoking cigars or pipes. Nicotine in snuff and chewing tobacco is absorbed through buccal (cheek and mouth) membranes, rather than from inhalation.

Cigarettes contain from 0.7 to 3.0 percent nicotine, or 0.5 to 2.0 milligrams per cigarette,[6] depending on the type of tobacco used. The amount absorbed varies with the moisture content of the tobacco, the amount of filter added, the length of the cigarette, heat, rapidity of smoking, and depth of inhalation, but conservative estimates indicate that approximately 90 percent (0.45 to 1.8 milligrams) will actually be inhaled and absorbed into the bloodstream. Though 60 milligrams is considered a lethal dose, 4 milligrams may occasionally produce alarming symptoms in novice or infrequent users. These symptoms may include giddiness, nausea, vomiting, abdominal cramping, a cold sweat, and vasomotor collapse.[7]

Smoke is readily absorbed by the body, andd some of its nicotine goes directly to the brain. Eighty to ninety percent of the nicotine absorbed is metabolized by the liver before it is excreted by the kidneys.[8] The amount excreted depends on the pH of the urine; four times as much is excreted when the urine is acid. Absorbed nicotine can be transferred to infants during breast feeding by lactating mothers who smoke.

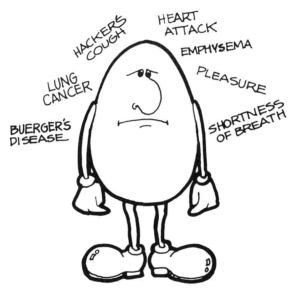

THE 1979 SURGEON GENERAL'S REPORT _____

In 1979, the surgeon general reported "overwhelming" evidence that smoking contributes directly to disease and death.[9] Surgeon General Julius Richmond noted that this conclusion was based on a 1200-page report of a "review and reappraisal" of research accumulated over the previous fifteen years. According to former HEW secretary Joseph Califano, the document revealed smoking to be more dangerous than supposed in the 1964 report. Califano contended that the report "demolished" claims by cigarette manufacturers that there is no proven link between smoking and cancer and chronic diseases. Additional surgeon general reports have further validated these extremely conclusive findings on the harmful effects of smoking, especially in regard to cardiovascular diseases, cancer, and chronic obstructive lung disease.

Among the findings the surgeon general's report reemphasized are these:

1. Smokers, male and female, die from a variety of ailments at a rate two-thirds higher than nonsmokers.
2. The risk goes up as the amount smoked goes up. For example, two-pack-a-day smokers have a death rate twice as high as nonsmokers. . . .
3. Women are dying from lung cancer at a rate three times as high as in 1964.
4. Coronary heart disease from smoking causes more premature deaths than lung cancer and other lung diseases.
5. Pipe and cigar smokers "experience overall mortality rates that are slightly higher than those of nonsmokers, but at rates substantially lower than those of the cigarette smokers."
6. Smokers of low tar and nicotine cigarettes run lower risks of lung cancer and coronary heart disease but "may in fact increase their hazard if they begin smoking more cigarettes or inhaling more deeply."
7. Children or adolescents who smoke may suffer immediate harm in the form of lung damage and respiratory problems.
8. Ninety percent of the people who smoke "have either tried to quit smoking or would probably quit, if only they could find an effective way to do so."[10]

PHYSIOLOGICAL EFFECTS

Nicotine affects the brain and the spinal cord as well as the peripheral nervous system. It can cause increased blood pressure, increased heart rate, reduced skin temperature, release of epinephrine (adrenalin) from the adrenal glands, and increased activity of the gastrointestinal tract. The substance also exerts an antidiuretic action for two to three hours (reducing urine formation), increases tone and motor activity of the bowel (occasionally causing diarrhea), stimulates, then depresses, production of saliva and bronchial secretions, vasoconstricts the blood vessels of the skin, increases amounts of free fatty acids in the bloodstream, increases platelet adhesiveness (a blood-clotting factor), and decreases DNA synthesis of lymphocytes, consequently altering the body and its steady-state mechanisms. Consistent with the effects of other stimulants, nicotine-caused excitation of the brain is followed by a period of postuse depression. Skeletal muscle activity, including the work of the diaphragm, which affects breathing, is reduced because of neuronal-function depression. Nerve fibers coming from the muscles are also affected, leading to a marked reduction in muscle tone that may be involved in the relaxation that accompanies smoking.

Continued smoking increases tolerance to nicotine and can eventually result in a seemingly incessant desire for another cigarette. Certainly, nicotine is one of the strongest dependency-producing psychoactive substances known, and although much of this dependence is psychological, there is significant degree of physical dependence as well. Discontinuation of the drug may result in withdrawal symptoms including restlessness and anxiety, irritability, depression, and dizziness. Though withdrawal is not fatal, it can be extremely uncomfortable, difficult, and prolonged.

Gases

Carbon monoxide (CO), hydrogen cyanide, and nitrous oxides are gases in cigarette smoke that affect the homeostatic condition of the circulatory and respiratory systems. Carbon monoxide is an odorless, colorless, and poisonous gas possessing an affinity for hemoglobin 250 times that of oxygen.[11] It impairs oxygen transportation to body tissues in at least two ways: by competing with oxygen for hemoglobin-binding sites and by increasing the affinity of the remaining hemoglobin for oxygen, thereby strengthening the oxyhemoglobin bond and making it difficult for the tissues to draw oxygen away from the hemoglobin. Body tissues receive oxygen, but not as much as they would under normal circumstances. Carbon monoxide literally drives the oxygen out of the body's red blood cells. As a result, the oxygen-carrying capacity of the blood is impaired and the body lacks sufficient quantities of this necessary element.

Nonsmokers normally have between 0.5 and 2.0 percent COHb (carboxyhemoglobin) in their circulation. Smokers, depending on the brand smoked and the number of cigarettes consumed per day, have COHB levels two to three times greater. Studies on the system effects of the CO burden of each cigarette have shown that COHb levels produced by smoking one cigarette are 0.96 to 1.6 percent after twelve hours of abstinence.

Hydrogen cyanide, a powerful, rapidly acting blood and nerve poison, is the element in cigarette smoke that is most responsible for the impairment of cilia function in the lungs. Removal of this poisonous gas from the smoke allows the cilia to continue to work until overcome by other harmful elements in the smoke.

Nitrous oxides have a deleterious effect on macrophages—the large, vacuum-cleaner-like white cells that live in the fluid that lines the inner surfaces of the lungs and that serve as cleaning mechanisms along with the cilia. Macrophages attack invading particles that are inhaled by digesting them or transporting them to the bronchioles, where they are transferred to the lymphatic system and removed from the lungs. Studies conducted at the University of Pittsburgh showed that when rabbit macrophages were exposed to high concentrations of nitrous dioxide (NO_2), the number of microbes eaten by the macrophages were reduced and the microbe-killing capacity of the defending cells was also lowered.[12]

CHRONIC DISEASE

In the twenty-plus years since the release of the 1964 Surgeon General's Report, the American public has incurred more than $930 billion in cigarette-induced medical costs (see Table 6–1).[13] Elizabeth Whelan of the American Council on Science and Health feels this is a conservative estimate since it is based only on statistics for cigarette-related cancer, heart disease, and chronic lung diseases. The unfortunate thing is the cost of smoking is paid for by all (smokers and nonsmokers). Nonsmokers pay through state-supported public welfare programs that provide benefits to those disabled by smoke-related diseases and to their survivors. They also pay in the form of increased insurance premiums and increased prices for consumer goods as a result of smokers' high rates of absenteeism from work.

The cost of smoking in terms of lost health and depleted economic resources has become astronomical. For example, a middle-aged man who smokes two packs of cigarettes per day will incur an average of more than $56,000 in costs of illness in his lifetime as a direct cause of smoking.[14]

Because of increasing public pressure, Congress has stepped up its warning campaign on packages of cigarettes. Figure 6–1 illustrates how these warnings reflect the growing evidence of the dangers of tobacco cigarettes.[15]

The Federal Trade Commission approved a plan to rotate four new warnings on cigarette packages. Under the system, which started in October of 1985, each brand was assigned a rotation of four warnings, to be changed quarterly depending on the date the cigarettes were manufactured or packaged. The rotations differ from brand to brand. These warnings are the same ones listed in Figure 6–2.[16]

Cardiovascular System

The amount of smoking-induced damage to the cardiovascular system is directly proportional to the number of cigarettes smoked, the age smoking began, and the number of years the user has been smoking. Since nicotine increases both heart rate and blood pressure, smokers respond with

TABLE 6–1   Costs to American Economy for Cigarette–Induced Major Illnesses, 1964–1983

Health-care costs for cigarette-induced cancer	56,200,000,000.00
Productivity lost because of cigarette-induced cancer	186,300,000,000.00
SUBTOTAL: CANCER	$242,500,000,000.00
Health-care costs for cigarette-induced cardiovascular disease	108,300,000,000.00
Productivity lost because of cigarette-induced cardiovascular disease	265,600,000,000.00
SUBTOTAL: CARDIOVASCULAR DISEASE	$373,900,000,000.00
Health-care costs for cigarette-induced chronic lung disease	120,000,000,000.00
Productivity lost because of cigarette-induced chronic lung disease	195,400,000,000.00
SUBTOTAL: CHRONIC LUNG DISEASE	$315,400,000,000.00
TOTAL COST	$931,800,000,000.00

Source: National Interagency Council on Smoking and Health, "American Council on Science and Health Bills Tobacco Industry," *Smoking and Health Reporter.* 1, no. 4 (July 1984): 1. Copyright © 1984 National Interagency Council on Smoking and Health. Used with permission.

FIGURE 6–1   Changes In Tobacco Warnings

Original Warning:

> **Caution: Cigarette Smoking May Be Hazardous to Your Health**

Present Warning:

> **Warning: The Surgeon General Has Determined That Cigarette Smoking is Dangerous to Your Health**

Senate Proposal:

> **WARNING: Cigarette Smoking Causes CANCER, EMPHYSEMA, and HEART DISEASE; May complicate PREGNANCY; and is ADDICTIVE**

sustained increases in blood pressure, which increase the work load of the heart. The chronic hyperactivity of the sympathetic nervous system, caused by nicotine absorption, is also a predisposing factor in heart disease and myocardial infarction.[17]

An increase in coronary-artery blood flow after smoking parallels the rise in systemic blood pressure and ventricular output. In a study of nine patients who smoked regularly and always inhaled freely, a significant rise in arterial pressure five minutes after smoking a cigarette was reported.[18]

Carbon monoxide interferes with circulation by increasing material membrane permeability, creating edema (abnormal accumulation of fluid), and inviting cholesterol deposits. These deposits may eventually lead to arteriosclerosis, considered to be the first stage of many dangerous circulatory conditions. Approximately 90 percent of all patients with symptoms of arteriosclerosis are smokers; very few are nonsmokers.

Another circulatory disease associated with nicotine is Buerger's disease. Patients with this problem have decreased blood flow to the extremities, which in extreme cases require amputation.

In the 1983 Surgeon General's Report, *Health Consequences of Smoking: Cardiovascular Disease,* the key finding was that *cigarette smoking* should be considered the most important known modifiable risk factor for heart disease in the United States. The report stated that up to 30 percent of all coronary deaths are related to smoking.[19] This appears to reaffirm the statistics from the Framington Heart Study, which links cigarette smoking to sudden death due to heart disease. Furthermore, "cigarette smoking is the most significant risk factor for sudden death in men."[20] It is thought that smoking might cause sudden death by increasing the adrenalin and carbon-monoxide levels, making platelets stickier, irritating the myocardium, or raising the blood pressure.

Another significant relationship is that between smoking and coronary bypass operations. For years, physicians have known that smoking causes changes in blood chemistry that facilitate plaque buildup in arteries, which in

FIGURE 6-2   The House of Representatives' Version of Tobacco Warnings

Surgeon General's Warning: Smoking Causes LUNG
CANCER, HEART DISEASE and EMPHYSEMA

Surgeon General's Warning: Quitting Smoking
Now Greatly Reduces Serious Health Risk

Surgeon General's Warning: Smoking by
Pregnant Women May Result in Fetal Injury and Premature Birth

Surgeon General's Warning: Cigarette
Smoke Contains Carbon Monoxide

leads to heart attacks and strokes. But it is only in the past few years that we have seen just how important smoking is as a cause of serious blockage of coronary arteries. A team of physicians have found that 92 percent of the coronary bypass patients under the age of forty were smokers.

Strokes (Apoplexy)

Smokers are more likely than nonsmokers to die from cerebrovascular disease, a condition in which hardening of blood vessels in the brain may lead to a stroke. Both the carbon monoxide and the nicotine in tobacco affect the adhesiveness of platelets—the main clotting factor in blood—in the brain, speeding the formation of a clot.[21] Nicotine also causes blood vessels to constrict, reducing the passageways by which blood reaches the brain. If these arteries become too constricted, the blood supply is greatly diminished or cut off and the smoker suffers a stroke.

Respiratory Diseases

Cigarette cough is so common—it afflicts millions of Americans—that it is accepted as normal rather than as the warning of damage to the lungs that it actually is. Shortness of breath and the nagging smoker's cough are the cumulative effect of toxic chemicals found in tobacco smoke. Tars, nicotine, hydrogen cyanide, and nitrous oxides are associated with the lung diseases of chronic bronchitis and emphysema, known together as chronic obstructive pulmonary disease (COPD).[22]

In the case of smoking-induced bronchitis, cigarette smoke irritates and inflames the air passages (bronchi) leading from the windpipe to the lungs. After prolonged smoking, the cilia become useless and tars build up. This buildup causes a reduction in normal respiration, resulting in regular coughing and regurgitation of phlegm—the body's way of attempting to expel the foreign particles the cilia can no longer eliminate. The only "cure" for this vicious cycle is to quit smoking and give the lungs a chance to resume normal functioning.

Emphysema is a lung disease in which the lungs lose their normal elasticity and retain abnormal amounts of air. Smoking destroys the tiny air sacs in the lungs, where oxygen is absorbed into the body, resulting in a loss of oxygen

absorption and a subsequent loss of breath. Breathing becomes extremely difficult, and people with advanced emphysema may use 80 percent of their strength
just in breathing. The condition is extremely agonizing and usually ends in heart
failure. Since damaged lung tissue can never be replaced, there is no real cure,
but quitting smoking will stop the disease from progressing. Nonsmokers can
also develop emphysema, but such cases are considerably less common.

The overall conclusion of the 1984 Surgeon General's report on smoking is:

> Cigarette smoking is the major cause of chronic obstructive lung disease in the
> United States for both men and women. The contribution of cigarette smoking to
> chronic obstructive lung disease morbidity and mortality far outweighs all other
> factors.[23]

Lung and Other Cancers

According to reports published by the American Cancer Society,
lung cancer accounted for approximately 117,000 deaths in 1983.[24] Lung cancer
is the cause of about 25 percent of all cancer deaths and 5 percent of all deaths in
the United States. Over 80 percent of all cancer deaths are attributed to cigarette
smoking, and *cigarette smoking is the leading cause of cancer mortality in this
country*. The risk of developing cancer is directly related to the length of time the
individual has smoked and the number of cigarettes consumed. The longer and
more heavily a person has smoked, the more likely he or she will develop cancer.
However, upon cessation the risk declines, and if a person remains a nonsmoker
long enough, the risk will eventually be no different from that of a person who
has never smoked. If, for example, a person has smoked twenty cigarettes (one
pack) per day for twenty years and stops smoking for ten years, the risk of
developing lung cancer diminishes almost to that of a nonsmoker.

Tobacco smoking is also strongly associated with cancer of the larynx
(voice box), mouth, esophagus, and bladder.[25] Cigarette smokers have three to
eighteen times the risk of nonsmokers of dying from cancer of the larynx.

One of the grimmest developments of 1985 was that lung cancer became
the leading cause of cancer death in American women. Breast cancer was long in
the forefront, but its survival rate, about two women in three, is far greater than
that of lung cancer, which only one woman in seven survives.

SIDE EFFECTS

Metabolism

Smoking tends to stimulate the adrenalin-releasing effect of nicotine; the cessation of smoking depresses energy consumption and favors fat- and
carbohydrate-deposit formations. Since carbohydrates tend to aggravate the
process of weight gain through the action of insulin, a low-carbohydrate, low-fat
diet such as the Mayo Clinic diet may be useful after quitting.[26]

There is conflicting evidence concerning the release of fatty acids as an effect of nicotine. Ciapoline et al. examined the effects of cigarette smoking on blood-lipid values in ten healthy volunteers between the ages of twenty and forty. The results showed that cigarette smoking caused a prompt rise in free fatty acids and a delayed rise in serum triglycerides.[27] Some data indicate increased serum-cholesterol levels in heavy smokers, whereas other data revealed no correlation.[28]

Tobacco smoke has been implicated in gastrointestinal disturbances. The volume and acidity of continuous gastric secretions are decreased in normal subjects who smoke, and the acidity of the basal gastric secretion often decreases in patients with peptic ulcers who smoke. Schredorf and Ivy have found that smoking tends to increase the motor activity of the colon. Also, smokers have a high propensity for losing lower-esophageal sphincter pressure, resulting in heartburn from gastric reflex.

Cigarette smoking apparently interferes with the body's normal immunological defenses. A study conducted over a two-year period found that 50 percent more heavy smokers were hospitalized for one reason or another than nonsmokers. In another study (Niker 1974), nicotine was added to cultures of human peripheral lymphocytes (infection-fighting cells), causing a significant decrease of the lymphocytes. Even light smoking may have an effect on cellular immunity.[29] Harkey, who performed some of the earliest studies on the antigenicity of nicotine (its ability to elicit a specific immunologic response), could not exclude the possibility that nicotine may act as a hapten, a compound that is not antigenic itself but reacts with an antibody and conveys antigenic specificity when combined with another compound. Silvette et al. reviewed several papers dealing with the immunology of nicotine and concluded that nicotine was antigenic.[30]

Appetite Reduction

Tobacco is frequently used for appetite reduction. Smoking depresses hunger contractions (for fifteen to sixty minutes per cigarette) as well as causing the liver to release glycogen, which results in a small increase in the blood-sugar level. This increase makes the smoker feel satiated and no longer in need of food. If the person smokes incessantly, appetite will continue to diminish and in some cases may disappear.

Nicotine also suppresses taste-bud sensitivity, reducing the taste value in food. When people quit smoking they usually notice an improvement in the taste of the foods they consume, an observation that often results in a weight gain. Increased food consumption may also be a behavioral-oral substitution for the mechanical aspect of smoking. However, following several months of nonsmoking, initial increases in food consumption often level off, with a return to previous dietary habits.

A study conducted by the Minnesota Lipid Research Clinic confirms that there are marked differences in weight between smokers and nonsmokers, regardless of caloric intake and/or physical activity.[31] One explanation of this may be that in smokers there is an increased caloric utilization initiated by the release of adrenalin, or other hormones affecting metabolism.

Fetal Nutrition and Pregnancy

In 1970 one third of all women of childbearing age in the United States smoked,[32] despite the fact that nicotine crosses the human placental barrier. In a study of thirty-seven pregnant women who smoked, nicotine was detected in the amniotic fluid of twenty-two, in quantities up to thirty milligrams per milliliter. Among sixty-seven nonsmokers, no nicotine was found.[33]

Women who smoke during pregnancy tend to give birth to smaller babies, probably because of the increased carboxyhemoglobin levels in their bloodstream.[34] This condition reduces their oxygen level, resulting in less oxygen being available to the fetus. A second probable cause of smaller babies is that nicotine decreases hunger in the pregnant woman who smokes, causing her to eat less and thereby reducing the nutrients available to the developing fetus.

Spontaneous Abortions   Although several investigators have found a significantly higher dose-related incidence of spontaneous abortion among cigarette smokers than among nonsmokers, the lack of control of significant variables does not permit conclusions to be drawn. Ingestion of nicotine, however, has been proved to cause spontaneous abortions in animals.[35]

A recent prenatal program in the United States studied 50,000 pregnant women and children and determined that the risk of miscarriage and infant death increases for women who smoke cigarettes prior to pregnancy (depending on the quantity of cigarettes smoked and the duration of smoking).[36] Findings indicate that smoking before pregnancy may damage the small arteries in the uterus, depriving the fetus of necessary oxygen and nutrients. This damage may be permanent and affect future pregnancies. Furthermore, the risk of sudden infant death syndrome (SIDS) is increased by approximately 50 percent when the mother smokes during pregnancy.

Stillborn and Neonatal Deaths   Investigators in the Ontario Prenatal Mortality Study 1960–61 found a statistically significant relationship between the amount of cigarette smoking and prenatal mortality. Also, women having low socioeconomic status or a history of spontaneous abortion have an increased stillbirth rate if they are also smokers.[37] In 1964, the Public Health Service reported 46,000 stillbirths associated with pregnant women who smoked. The PHS also noted a decrease in deaths if smoking was given up by the fourth month of pregnancy. Butler, in 1969, found a highly significant association between maternal smoking after the fourth month and both late-fetal and neonatal deaths. Infants of smokers had a higher late-fetal mortality rate than infants of nonsmokers. Also, black women smoke fewer cigarettes than white women, but have a higher rate of fetal mortality.[38]

Nicotine in Mothers' Milk   The surgeon general's 1972 and 1973 reports cited findings concerning nicotine in the milk of nursing mothers.[39] For example, Rerlman found nicotine in the milk of all mothers he had tested who smoked. There was a direct relationship between the concentration of nicotine in the milk and the number of cigarettes smoked.[40]

Anomalies   Some research indicates a higher incidence of congenital malformation, such as cleft lip and cleft palate, in infants born to smokers. In a study of 100 mothers (37 smokers and 63 nonsmokers),[41] two fetuses of smokers had Klinefelter's syndrome.* Erickson, Kallen, and Westerholm identified a relationship between smoking and the rate of infant birth malformations.[42] In their study of hospital records concerning such malformations, they found a significant increase in cleft lip or palate in infants born to women who smoked.

Exercise and Physical Performance

A reduction in the oxygen-carrying capacity of the red blood cells—which occurs from smoking—means a reduction in physical capacity. Smoking also causes swelling of the mucous membranes in the trachea and the bronchial tubes, leading to increased airway resistance; extra effort is needed to get air in and out of the lungs. The alveoli (air sacs) in the lungs may also receive a reduced amount of oxygen. During exercise, when the demand on the respiratory system is elevated, the increased respiratory resistance caused by smoking may be noticeable.

During heavy exercise, the oxygen cost of exhaling for chronic smokers is on the average twice as great as that for nonsmokers. This is true even if only a few cigarettes are smoked within one hour prior to exercise. In heavy smokers (people who smoke twenty to thirty cigarettes per day for at least twenty-seven years), the cost is nearly four times that of nonsmokers. If no cigarettes are smoked within twenty-four hours prior to exercise, the oxygen cost is still about 60 percent higher than that for nonsmokers.[43]

Sexual Activity

Smoking impairs sexual performance in two primary ways: (1) the CO intake reduces the blood's oxygen level and impairs the production of the male sex hormone testosterone, and, (2) the nicotine intake constricts the blood vessels, which need to swell to cause sexual excitement and erection in males. A study by Carl Schirren also found severe disturbance of sperm motility in a group of men who smoked. Their sperm counts were low, and the sperm that were present were sluggish, displaying low motility. Schirren reported that if the men stopped smoking entirely, within six to ten weeks a considerable improvement in sperm motility resulted.[44]

The reduced lung capacity smoking causes also affects sexual activity by lowering stamina and thus the ability to prolong the sexual experience. In addition, nicotine discolors the teeth and causes bad breath, reducing the smoker's sexual attractiveness. It is no mere coincidence that patients of sex counselors and doctors report "that after they quit smoking, their sex lives improved."[45]

*A condition in which the sex-chromosome constitution is abnormal, in that a Y chromosome is associated wth more than one X chromosome. A Klinefelter male may appear normal or be very tall, sterile, or mentally retarded.

Other Health Factors

Nicotine and Oral Contraceptives   The Walnut Creek study of the long-term effects of the use of oral contraceptives on health,[46] started in 1969, has provided a good deal of nicotine-related information. The study, involving 17,929 suburban, predominately white women, found that smoking may increase the likelihood of subarachnoid hemorrhage (bleeding between portions of the brain). The risk to cigarette smokers was 5.7 times that to nonsmokers, and the risk to smokers who used oral contraceptives was 22 times that to women who neither smoked nor used oral contraceptives.

A study of the interactions of oral contraceptives and nicotine showed increased urinary levels of epinephrine and norepinephrine.[47] (Norepinephrine is a hormone that stimulates the sympathetic nervous system, which mediates functional activity. Therapeutically it is useful for maintaining blood pressure in acute hypotensive states, central vasomotor depression, and hemorrhage.) In addition, continuous circulatory fluctuations resulting from smoking and oral-contraceptive use are known to increase the risk of myocardial infarction.[48]

Peridontal Disease   Tobacco smokers have much higher rates of periodontal disease, which can cause excessive damage to the gums. "Trench mouth" and loss of teeth from gum damage may also be caused by cigarette smoking.

Medication Effectiveness   The 1979 surgeon general's report on smoking and health reveals that smoking alters the effectiveness of some medications.[49] For example, theophylline, used for treating acute and chronic asthma and bronchitis, and pentazocine, a prescription narcotic antagonist and pain-killer, must be taken in larger doses by smokers than nonsmokers; overdoses are therefore possible if smoking habits vary. It has also been suggested that vaccines are less effective in smokers than in nonsmokers, and responses to diagnostic tests may be affected by smoking. The level of white blood cells, the size of red blood cells, and the time required for blood clotting are also adversely affected by smoking.[50]

Nicotine and Coffee Intake

From a psychological standpoint, smoking may fill a behavioral need for oral stimulation. Studies indicate that smokers may further fulfill this need with additional oral habits, such as greater alcohol and coffee intake. From a physiological standpoint, caffeine and nicotine work together to affect homeostasis. Hickey et al. suggest that tobacco smoking and coffee may be self-selected behavioral regulators of the homeostatic process.[51]

Vitamins

Smoking causes changes in plasma and leukocyte concentrations of Vitamin C and impairs biochemical functions of this vitamin. Vitamin B-12 is metabolized in the detoxification process of cyanide derived from smoking. Some heavy smokers develop amblyopia (an eye disease), which is reversed by either vitamin B-12 supplements or termination of smoking. There is evidence that smoking may also alter the metabolism of lipids, carbohydrates, proteins, and other vitamins such as B-6.[52]

PSYCHOLOGICAL EFFECTS

The Smoking Habit

Smoking involves more than just a physiological addiction to nicotine. Various psychological and social factors work together to cause an individual to start smoking. Unfortunately, the habit is usually initiated with naive intentions, but social forces reinforce the smoking behaviors until the individual develops physical dependence on the drug and then cannot quit without experiencing some type of withdrawal.

As with other forms of nonmedical drug use, the initial experimentation and regular use of tobacco begins in youth. Initiation of the behavior depends on three factors:

1. an opportunity to engage in the behavior
2. a high degree of curiosity about the effects
3. discovery that smoking is a way to express conformity to the behaviors of others or to rebel

Reasons for Smoking and Not Smoking

People begin smoking for many reasons: curiosity, boredom, peer pressure and social acceptance, expression of independence and maturity, parental example, imitation of supposed glamorous social figures, low (or high) academic achievement, response to stress, relief of tension. Smoking often induces feelings of stimulation or tranquility in addition to an increased sense of well-being and improved working efficiency. The habit is relaxing and pleasurable to many and is seen as a means of facilitating communication, a way to role-play, and a way to fill time.

Cigarette smoking received its boost in popularity during World War I, when troops were given free cigarettes by the tobacco companies. In the midst of worry, homesickness, and the nerve-racking experience of warfare, cigarettes acted as a peacemaker to the central nervous system. They numbed the nerve endings and reduced the perception of both pleasurable and unpleasant sensations. Their threat to health was of limited importance since the men could die in battle the next day.

The results of surveys of sex-role convergence and aging effects, smoking initiation, and current smoking and smoking behavior of men and women professionals indicate that men smokers still exceeded women smokers as of 1975 but that presently more women than men are smoking. Women smokers may

FIGURE 6-3   Reasons for Smoking.

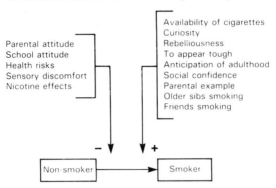

The main psychosocial factors determining the onset of smoking.
On the right are the positive reinforcers or incentives to smoke.
On the left are the factors that discourage smoking.[53]

have taken up the habit to identify with males and achieve liberation from the traditional female stereotype, a supposition supported by the fact that women employed outside the home are more likely to smoke than housewives.

Types of Smokers

There are various types of smoking patterns.

Habitual Smoking   In this pattern, smokers are hardly aware that they have a cigarette in their mouth. For these people, smoking may once have been an important sign of status, but now is simply automatic. The act of smoking enhances the habitual smoker's mood and feelings of competency.

Positive-Effect Smoking   Here smoking serves as a stimulant, producing pleasure, relaxation, or heightened enjoyment, as at the end of a meal. Smokers in this pattern may most enjoy the handling of a cigarette or the sense and sight of the smoke curling out of their mouths. Beginning smokers may fall into this pattern to demonstrate their defiance of their parents.

Negative-Effect Smoking   This is sedative smoking, using the habit to reduce feelings of distress, fear, shame, or disgust, or any combination of these feelings. People in this pattern may not smoke at all under normal circumstances, but may reach for a cigarette when things go badly.

Addictive Smoking (Dependency)   Addicted smokers are always aware they are smoking. They are also aware of not smoking, since the lack of nicotine builds a need and desire for it, and discomfort sets in. The increasing need leads to a growing expectation that a cigarette will reduce the discomfort— and it does give relief, but just for a moment. For dependent smokers, the pleasure of smoking is real, just as the buildup of discomfort when not smoking is real, and sometimes rapid and intolerable.

ALTERNATIVES TO SMOKING AND CONSEQUENT
PROBLEMS _____

During the past twenty-five years, because of the publicizing of the deleterious effects of tars and nicotine, cigarette companies have reduced the amount of these substances in cigarettes and begun large-scale manufacturing of filtered cigarettes. Unfortunate, even though the dependency-producing agent (nicotine) has been reduced, the poisonous gases have remained constant, and in a few cases even increased.[54] It is also unfortunate that the fraction of nicotine removed from the mainstream smoke by a filter is very small. To avoid nicotine's vascular effects, one would have to use a filter that passes no smoke at all.

Since nicotine is the element in cigarettes that produces the smokers' desired effects, smokers draw more deeply and inhale more often when they smoke low-nicotine brands. Consequently, they increase their tar and gas intake. The Snell Laboratories programmed smoking machines to behave like smokers who take faster puffs and inhale deeply. They tested six low-tar, low-nicotine brands and found that in almost every instance the quantity of gas increased, sometimes dramatically. Hence, smoking filtered, low-nicotine brands may produce more of the three poisonous gases than nonfilter brands.[55]

Nicotine gum has been discussed in several studies as a less harmful substitute for smoking. The idea may sound like a vast improvement over smoke inhalation, but most studies list many drawbacks. The main problem is that the gum is absorbed through the throat and lungs. Chewing it may also release three times as much nicotine as a cigarette, but the effects take longer to achieve. This slower effect produced by buccal absorption may, however, produce less dependency in the tobacco chewer. On January 13, 1984, the Food and Drug Administration finally approved the use of nicotine chewing gum as a prescription drug for use in quitting smoking. Merrel Dow Pharmaceuticals was authorized to begin marketing Nicorette (Nicotine Resin Complex) in the United States.[56]

Other efforts are being made to develop methods of delivering a maximum of nicotine to the bloodstream of tobacco dependents with a minimum of smoke to their lungs. This would reduce or eliminate the hazards of lung cancer, although the effects of nicotine on the body would continue. Efforts presently under way include development of a short cigarette with a high nicotine content; a cigarette with noninhalable smoke; smoke-free ways to deliver nicotine to the lungs, as in nicotine inhalers; and methods of ingesting nicotine through the mouth, perhaps in pill form.[57] Obviously, these alternatives are not as desirable as discontinuing the nicotine-consuming act itself or selecting nonchemical alternatives to smoking.

Future research should also concentrate on producing a nicotine substitute that has no adverse effects on the heart or other organs but satisfies the craving for nicotine. Development of this alternative is possible because of the numerous molecules closely related chemically to nicotine, many of which are known to have no effects on heart action.

KICKING THE HABIT ────────────────────────────

Methods

Behavioral Programs   The American Lung Association (ALA), American Cancer Society (ACS), and American Heart Association (AHA) have united in a goal of a smoke-free society by the year 2000. All have initiated programs to maintain the new nonsmoking lifestyle. The ALA has Freedom from Smoking, the ACS offers an I Quit Kit and FRESHSTART, and the AHA has Save a SweetHEART. These programs also attempt to counter the billions of dollars of cigarette advertising produced each year by the tobacco industry.

Company Programs   Companies are now beginning to realize that they can save money in the long run by investing in quit-smoking programs for their employees. Health-insurance premiums for employees are a growing concern for America's major corporations, for they are being dramatically influenced by the growing number of cigarette-induced diseases. The latest studies indicate that all told, it costs our country about three dollars for every pack of cigarettes sold. However, if a single smoking employee were to kick the habit, total savings for the employer would exceed $34,000.[58] Employers now have the information they need to determine the savings they could expect from implementing a smoking-cessation program for employees or their family members. For example, Campbell Soup, American Telephone and Telegraph, Johns-Manville, and Boeing Aircraft employ consultants who help workers quit smoking. It is now clear that *smoking control among employees and their dependents is the single most cost-effective way of containing health-care costs for employers.*

Death in the West   Another effective approach to smoking cessation has been to fully expose the tough-cowboy image. Seven years after it premiered on British television, the controversial antismoking documentary *Death in the West* surfaced in hundreds of cities across the United States.[59] *Death in the West* contrasted the macho image of the Marlboro Man, a rugged cowboy featured in their advertising, with six real-life cowboys who were dying from terminal illness caused by their smoking.

Benefits of Quitting

A 1978 Department of Health, Education and Welfare poll estimated that 17 million Americans tried to quit smoking that year and that 3.5 million succeeded.[60] "Clearly people are getting and responding to the public message . . . that smoking is *slow motion suicide,*" said former HEW secretary Joseph A. Califano in a speech to the National Interagency Council on Smoking and Health. Approximately 30 million people have quit smoking since 1964, and in anywhere from ten to fifteen years these people would be back to the same level of health risk as nonsmokers.[61]

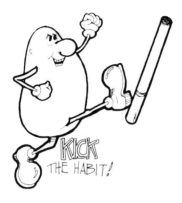

Regardless of the number of years a person has been smoking, chances for longer life and good health are greatly improved once he or she has stopped. Digestive and eating patterns change, absorption of food is greater, appetite is improved, and both the taste of food and the sense of smell are better.

Circulation improves as the blood vessels begin to expand to normal size, returning blood pressure to normal, slowing pulse rate, and increasing heart efficiency; even facial complexion improves. The ex-smoker is less tired, and often rises earlier in the morning and is more alert during the day.

Precancerous cells in the respiratory tract are gradually replaced by new ones. The breathing rate decreases and there is an increase in maximal breathing capacity. A better exchange of oxygen between the lungs and the circulatory system also results. Conditions such as bronchitis improve and coughing disappears. Emphysema patients breathe more easily and many asthma conditions improve considerably.

There are monetary benefits to quitting as well. A heavy smoker can save up to $20,000 in a lifetime by putting cigarettes aside. Insurance premiums can be lowered since insurance companies offer lower rates to nonsmokers, realizing that smoking endangers health and shortens life expectancy and that cigarette smokers are more accident-prone. These various benefits, along with the risks of smoking, are summarized in Table 6–2.

Changing to Other Forms of Tobacco Consumption

Though some people kick the smoking habit through any of a number of treatment programs, including behavior modification, role playing, aversion therapy, and self-monitoring, others simply turn to other forms of tobacco consumption. Pipe and cigar smoking, chewing tobacco, and snuff are increasing in popularity as the hazards of cigarette smoking are brought into the foreground.

Pipe and Cigar Smoking   People who smoke pipes and cigars instead of cigarettes reduce some hazards to their health but increase others. Since most pipe and cigar smoke isn't inhaled, the harmful particles and poison-

TABLE 6–2   Risks of Smoking and Benefits of Quitting

Risks of Smoking	Benefits of Quitting	Relative Risks: Filter-Tipped, Low T/N Brands
Risk: Shortened life expectancy. 25-year-old 2-pack-a-day smokers have life expectancy 8.3 years shorter than nonsmoking contemporaries. Other smoking levels: proportional risk.	Benefit: Reduces risk of premature death cumulatively. After 10-15 years, ex-smokers' risk approaches that of those who've never smoked.	Reduced risk of death from certain diseases (see below) implies increased life expectancy.
Risk: Lung cancer. Smoking cigarettes "major cause in both men and women."	Benefit: Gradual decrease in risk. After 10–15 years, risk approaches that of those who never smoked.	Filter tips reduce risk, but it is still 5 times that of non-smokers. Low-T/N brands reduce male risk by 20 percent, female risk by 40 percent.
Risk: Larynx cancer. In all smokers (including pipe and cigar) it's 2.9 to 17.7 times that of nonsmokers.	Benefit: Gradual reduction of risk after smoking cessation. Reaches normal after 10 years.	Filter tips reduce risk 24 to 49 percent.
Risk: Mouth cancer. Cigarette smokers have 3 to 10 times as many oral cancers as nonsmokers. Pipes, cigars, chewing tobacco also major risk factors. Alcohol seems synergistic carcinogen with smoking.	Benefit: Reducing or eliminating smoking/drinking reduces risk in first few years; risk drops to level of nonsmokers in 10–15 years.	(no identified benefit)
Risk: Cancer of esophagus. Cigarettes, pipes and cigars increase risk of dying of esophageal cancer about 2 to 9 times. Synergistic relationship between smoking and alcohol.	Benefit: Since risks are dose related, reducing or eliminating smoking/drinking should have risk-reducing effect.	(no identified benefit)
Risk: Cancer of bladder. Cigarette smokers have 7 to 10 times risk of bladder cancer as nonsmokers. Also synergistic with certain exposed occupations: dyestuffs, etc.	Benefit: Risk decreases gradually to that of non-smokers over 7 years.	(no identified benefit)
Risk: Cancer of pancreas. Cigarette smokers have 2 to 5 rimes risk of dying of pancreatic cancer as nonsmokers.	Benefit: Since there is evidence of dose-related risk, reducing or eliminating smoking should have risk-reducing effect.	(no identified benefit)

Risks of Smoking	Benefits of Quitting	Relative Risks: Filter-Tipped, Low T/N Brands
Risk: Coronary heart disease. Cigarette smoking is major factor; responsible for 120,000 excess U.S. deaths from coronary heart disease (CHD) each year.	Benefit: Sharply decreases risk after one year. After 10 years ex-smokers' risk is same as that of those who never smoked.	Low-T/N male smokers had 12 percent lower CHD rate, female low-T/N smokers 19 percent lower than high-T/N smokers.
Risks: Chronic bronchitis and pulmonary emphysema. Cigarette smokers have 4–25 times risk of death from these diseases as nonsmokers. Damage seen in lungs of even young smokers.	Benefit: Cough and sputum disappear during first few weeks. Lung function may improve and rate of deterioration slow down.	(no identified benefit)
Risks: Stillbirth and low birthweight. Smoking mothers have more stillbirths and babies of low birthweight—more vulnerable to disease and death.	Benefit: Women who stop smoking before 4th month of pregnancy eliminate risk of stillbirth and low birthweight caused by smoking.	(no identified benefit)
Risks: Children of smoking mothers smaller, underdeveloped physically and socially, seven years after birth.	Benefit: Since children of nonsmoking mothers are bigger and more advanced socially, inference is that not smoking during pregnancy might avoid such underdeveloped children.	(no identified benefit)
Risk: Peptic ulcer. Cigarette smokers get more peptic ulcers and die more often of them; cure is more difficult in smokers.	Benefit: Ex-smokers get ulcers but these are more likely to heal rapidly and completely than those of smokers.	(no identified benefit)
Risk: Allergy and impairment of immune system.	Benefit: Since these are direct, immediate effects of smoking, they are obviously avoidable by not smoking.	(no identified benefit)
Risks: Alters pharmacologic effects of many medicines, diagnostic tests and greatly increases risk of thrombosis with oral contraceptives.	Benefit: Majority of blood components elevated by smoking return to normal after cessation. Non-smokers on Pill have much lower risks of thrombosis.	(no identified benefit)

Source: American Cancer Society, *Dangers of Smoking . . . Benefits of Quitting and Relative Risks of Reduced Exposure* (New York, 1980).

ous gases it contains don't reach lung tissue or pass into the bloodstream. As a result, pipe and cigar smokers' chances of developing coronary heart disease or severe lung diseases are less than those of cigarette smokers. However, when people who smoke pipes and cigars do inhale, as they do with certain brands and sometimes because of the cigarette-inhaling habit, their chances of developing serious heart and lung diseases are even higher than those of cigarette smokers. These chances increase in direct proportion to how deeply they inhale and how often.[62]

Tobacco smoke that is not inhaled still affects the site it touches. Hot smoke lingers inside the mouth and can travel into the throat and windpipe, even into the upper breathing passages. Smoke can be dissolved in saliva and absorbed in the mucous membranes of the mouth, and can be swallowed and enter the digestive tract. The incidence of cancer of the mouth, throat, larynx, and stomach is high—even higher than for cigarette smokers, according to some studies—and pipe smoking, either alone or in combination with other forms of smoking, seems to be a direct cause of cancer of the lip. Also, malignant skin tumors grow more rapidly and in larger numbers in animals whose skin has been painted with cigar tars rather than cigarette tars.[63]

In general, however, smokers who limit themselves to pipes and cigars live longer than cigarette smokers, yet they do not live as long as nonsmokers.[64] There is some evidence, too, that cigarette smokers who cut down on cigarettes and substitute cigars and pipes somewhat decrease their chance of premature death.

Smokeless Tobacco   Since the 1970s there has been a resurgence in the use of all forms of smokeless tobacco in the United States.[65] Today's users are more sophisticated than those of yesterday, and apparently more considerate than those old-timers who were not overly concerned about where they spat. Smokeless tobacco is being heavily promoted through the mass media by well-known sports personalities and entertainers.

DIPPING AND CHEWING   Snuff dipping consists of placing a pinch of powder tobacco (which is sold in cans) between the cheek and gum, whereas chewing tobacco consists of placing a leaf tobacco (which comes in a pouch) or plug (in the form of a brick) in the area near the inner cheek.[66] A "chaw" is a golf-ball-size quid of leaf or plug tobacco. "Chewing clubs," complete with charters, membership cards, and even T-shirts emblazoned with mottos like "Don't Spit On Me," have been spawned in high schools and colleges by this new tobacco craze.

The tobacco industry's advertising campaign is designed to appeal to impressionable young males, especially elementary through college-age students and athletes. It is no accident that macho sports idols provide the basis for the appeal. Besides the ads there are attractive young men and women handing out free samples to try to "get youth started." Use of smokeless tobacco has increased on college campuses, in high schools, and even in elementary schools. There may be as many as 7 million users of smokeless tobacco in the United States.[67]

HARMFUL EFFECTS   Habitual use of chewing tobacco and snuff means you may face health hazards such as:

leukoplakia (leathery white patches inside the mouth that result from direct contact with, and continued irritation by, tobacco juice). Approximately 5 percent of diagnosed cases develop into oral cancer.

less sense of taste and smell. This results in the need to salt and sugar food, both of which are unhealthy if used a lot.

dental problems such as receding gums, greater wear and tear on tooth enamel, and more tooth decay—and, like most tobacco users, more bad breath and discoloration of teeth.

EXPOSURE   Recent research by the Baylor College of Medicine and Texas Lutheran College has shown that use of smokeless tobacco can have significant effects on the heart and blood vessels in both animals and humans. Squires and co-workers found that within twenty minutes of snuff use by subjects younger than twenty years, average heart rate increased from 69 to 88 beats per minute.[68] Average blood pressure readings increased significantly (118/72 to 126/78) during the same period. The researchers concluded that oral tobacco use may pose a health hazard in certain medically compromised individuals, especially those who already have high blood pressure.

Massachusetts will become the first state requiring packages of snuff to carry warnings of its health hazards. Manufacturers will be forced to put labels on cans and packages sold in Massachusetts that say, "Warning: Use of snuff can be addictive and can cause mouth cancer and other mouth disorders."

It should be stressed that at the federal level Rep. Mike Synar, D–Okla, offered a bill requiring warning labels on smokeless tobacco but has met some opposition.

In short, smokeless tobacco is being used as an alternative to smoking tobacco. However, it is not a safe alternative.

Clove Cigarettes   In various parts of the country there has been an increase in the use of clove cigarettes. Quite often these are passed off as safe substitutes for tobacco cigarettes. However, anyone contemplating smoking these cigarettes should first consider the following facts:

1. Clove cigarettes contain 60 percent tobacco and 40 percent ground cloves, clove oil, and other ingredients.

2. On the average, clove cigarettes contain higher levels of tar, nicotine, carbon monoxide, and carbon dioxide than regular commercial cigarettes.

3. Clove oil (eugenol) is on the FDA's list of chemicals that are "generally recognized as safe," but only when it is consumed orally in its unburnt form.

4. Clove oil stimulates the central nervous system and can result in delirium, hallucinations, and seizures.

5. Clove oil affects the cardiovascular system by lowering blood pressure. This causes sweating, weakness, dizziness, and ringing in the ears.

6. Clove oil is an irritant that can burn the body's mucous membranes, resulting in coughing, hoarseness, and difficulty in breathing. It is also an anesthetic, which is why the burning sensation is not apparent.
7. Commercial cigarettes dipped in clove oil are more dangerous than imported clove cigarettes because of the quality of the clove oil.[69]

TOBACCO AND THE NONSMOKER

Effects of Tobacco Smoke on Nonsmokers

The chemicals in tobacco smoke are derived from two sources: mainstream smoke and side-stream smoke. *Mainstream* smoke is inhaled from the burning tobacco during puffing and *side-stream* smoke rises from the cigarette, cigar, or pipe as it burns. The American Lung Association states that side-stream smoke contains concentrations of harmful ingredients greater than those inhaled by the smokers: twice as much tar and nicotine; three to four times as much benzopyrene (a carcinogen); five times as much carbon monoxide; and fifty times as much ammonia; there is also more cadium, a cause of emphysema, hypertension, and chronic bronchitis.[70]

Since each individual has a particular technique when it comes to smoking, different concentrations of substances are found in exhaled mainstream smoke, depending on the tobacco product, the composition of the tobacco, and the degree of inhalation by the smoker. These concentrations, together with the harmful side-stream smoke, put the nonsmoker in a dangerous position when exposed to another person's smoke. Regardless of the controversy surrounding this issue, "passive smoking" or "involuntary smoking" can harm the nonsmoker's health.

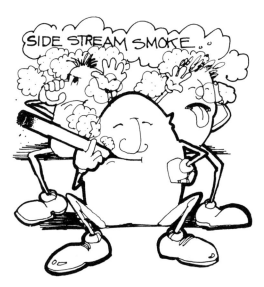

The amount of carbon monoxide smoking puts into the environment is also of major concern to the nonsmoker. The level of this gas varies with (1) the size of the space in which the smoking occurs (dilution of CO); (2) the number and type of tobacco products smoked (CO production); and (3) the amount and effectiveness of ventilation (CO removal). Fifty parts CO per million (ppm) is considered safe according to the American Conference of Government Industrial Hygienists. In experiments conducted by researchers, it was found that only under conditions of unusually heavy smoking and poor ventilation did CO levels exceed this maximum safe limit. However, even with adequate ventilation, the measured CO levels did exceed the maximum ambient level of nine parts per million.[71]

Investigations have been made to determine the amount of carbon monoxide absorbed by the involuntary smoker. This was done by measuring changes in the carboxyhemoglobin levels in nonsmokers exposed to cigarette-smoke-filled environments. Results showed that in a well-ventilated room with a CO level of 4.5 ppm, there was no change in COHb levels of nonsmokers. Without ventilation, the CO level rose to 30 ppm and the COHb level increased from .9 to 2.1 percent in two hours. In another experiment, where the CO level was measured at 38 ppm and ventilation was poor, the COHb level increased from 1.6 to 2.6 percent in nonsmokers.[72]

These increases in COHb levels may not significantly affect a healthy adult, but they can produce deleterious effects in people with angina pectoris or coronary heart disease. In angina pectoris, the volume of blood able to be pumped through the heart muscle decreases under exercise stress. If oxygen-carrying capacity is reduced by the presence of CO in the blood, a person's ability to perform physical activity is shortened. COHb levels necessary to bring on this discomfort are within the levels produced by involuntary smoking. At these same CO levels, CO has been shown to decrease cardiac contractility in persons with coronary heart disease. Also, the heart's functional reserve is reduced.[73]

Cigarette-smoke-filled environments have also been found to cause slight deterioration in some psychomotor performance, especially in attentiveness and cognitive function. Resulting CO levels, however, do not impair one's ability to operate a motor vehicle.[74] Children of parents who smoke are more likely to have respiratory infections, bronchitis, and pneumonia during the first year of life, due in part to their exposure to cigarette smoke.

There are very few instances when the concentration and quantity of cigarette smoke is great enough to cause permanent damage or chronic disease. Exposure to cigarette smoke can result, however, in conjunctival (eye) irritation, dry throat, and the breathing of unpleasant odors. Involuntary inhalation of side-stream smoke from cigars and pipes can also cause the heart to beat faster, the blood pressure to rise, and the CO level in the blood to rise.

Nonsmokers' Rights

Antismokers are campaigning for their rights, and their voices are increasingly affecting public regulations on smoking. Some thirty-three states have passed laws prohibiting smoking in public places, except in designated smoking areas, and are issuing citations for disobedience of the specified laws. Smoking and nonsmoking sections in airplanes, restaurants, and trains are now commonplace. But change will take time.

The National Interagency Council on Smoking and Health has highlighted three additional ways in which nonsmokers'-rights groups appear to be gaining support.

Churches Question Morality of Tobacco Industry   The North Carolina Council of Churches has issued a report questioning the morality of the billion-dollar tobacco industry.[75] Although tobacco employs more than 150,000 North Carolinians, although the state manufactures more than half of all American cigarettes, and although North Carolina farms raise almost 40 percent of the tobacco grown in America, the report questions the morality of making money from an industry whose product poses such health risks. The report was prepared to stimulate discussion of this issue from North Carolina's pulpits.

San Francisco   In a victory for nonsmokers, voters in San Francisco narrowly approved (80,740 to 79,481) an ordinance believed to establish a precedent likely to be followed by other major municipalities. The ordinance prohibits smoking in the private sector workplace as well as in public areas.[76] Moreover, the ordinance was passed in spite of a massive opposition by the tobacco industry, which invested a reported $12.58 per vote (a total of about $1.3 million) to kill the measure. Violators of the new law (employers) may be fined up to $500 a day for noncompliance.

Smokers Support Nonsmokers   A recent national survey has revealed for the first time that a majority of Americans—including both smokers and nonsmokers—now believe "smokers should refrain from smoking in the presence of non-smokers."[77] According to the survey, released by the American Lung Association, an overwhelming 82 percent of nonsmokers and a surprising 55 percent of current smokers agree that smokers should not light up among nonsmokers. A majority of the smokers prefer designated smoking areas in the workplace, in restaurants, and on airplanes, trains, and buses. It appears that the nonsmokers' movement is gaining momentum.

DIVERSIFICATION

When the 1964 surgeon general's report was released, the American tobacco industry was dominated by six large cigarette manufacturers. These corporations had few nontobacco interests. By 1984 the situation was markedly different. The big six had emerged as multinational conglomerates with financial interests reaching from pet food to insurance underwriting, from breweries to security services.[78] Table 6–3 illustrates these dramatic changes away from tobacco production by the tobacco companies.

TABLE 6–3   Tobacco Industry Conglomerates: Status Report on Diversification in the To-bacco Industry, 1984

Tobacco Manufacturer (conglomerate owner or affiliate)	Tobacco Brands	Other Representative Products
Philip Morris Inc.	Marlboro, Merit, Benson & Hedges, Virginia Slims, Parliament	Miller Brewing Company (Miller, Lite, Meister Brau, Lowenbrau, Magnum Malt Liquor), The Seven-Up Company (7-up, Diet 7-up, Like Cola), Mission Viejo Realty Group
R. J. Reynolds Tobacco Company (R. J. Reynolds Industries)	Camel, Winston, Salem, Sterling, Bright, Doral, More, Century, Now, Vantage, Winchester, Work Horse chew, Prince Albert, Carter Hall, Madiera Gold	Kentucky Fried Chicken, Canada Dry, Del Monte, Chun King oriental foods, Hawaiian Punch, Morton Frozen Foods, Patio Mexican foods, Snap-E-Tom, Milk Mate, A-1 Steak Sauce, Escoffier Sauces, Grey Poupon, Ortega Mexican foods, My-T-Fine, Brer Rabbit Molasses, College Inn, Vermont Maid, Heublein, Inc. (Arrow Cordials, Black Velvet, Cuervo, Don Q Rum, Irish Mist, Jose Cuervo, Popov, Smirnoff, The Club Cocktails, Yukon Jack, Inglenook Wines, Napa Valley Wines, Harveys Bristol Creme, Lancer's Vin Rose)
Brown & Williamson Tobacco (div. British American Tobacco Industries; Canadian Affiliate—Imasco)	Kool, Barclay, Belair, Vice-roy, Richland 25's	Marshall Field & Company, Gimbels Department Stores, Saks Fifth Avenue, Kohl's Department Stores, Appleton Papers, Yardley, Imasco (Imperial Tobacco, Hardee's Restaurants, People's Drug, Shoppers Drug Mart, Burger Chef, Embassy Cleaners)
Liggett Group (Liggett & Myers Tobacco) (div. Grand Metropolitan,	Chesterfield, L & M, Lark, Eve, most "generic" cig-arettes sold in the U.S., Pinkerton Tobacco Company (Red Man Chew)	Carlsberg Beer, Alpo Dog Food, Diversified Products (gym equipment), Children's World, Inc., Intercontinental Hotels Corp., International Distil-

Tobacco Manufacturer (conglomerate owner or affiliate)	Tobacco Brands	Other Representative Products
		lers & Vintners (J & B Scotch, Gilbey's Gin, Bombay Gin, Bailey's Original Irish Cream, Grand Marnier, Absolut Vodka)
Lorillard	Newport, Satin, Kent, Triumph, Kent Golden Lights, True, Old Gold, Max, Beech-nut Chewing Tobacco	CNA Financial (Continental Casualty Corporation and its insurance and financial affiliates), General Finance Corporation, Loews Hotels, Loews Theatres, Bulova Watch Company
American Tobacco Company (div. American Brands, Inc.)	Lucky Strike, Pall Mall, Carlton, and Tareyton cigarettes; Half and Half and Bourbon Blend smoking tobaccos; LaCorona, Antonio y Cleopatra, Roi Tan, and Grenadiers cigars	Franklin Life Insurance Company, Southland Life Insurance, Pinkertons, Inc., Master Lock Company, Swingline Office Supplies, James B. Beam Distillery, Sunshine Biscuits, Wilson-Jones Office Forms, Acme Visible Office Supplies, Titleist and Acushnet golf products, Andrew Jergens Company
U.S. Tobacco Company	Skoal, Skoal Bandits, Copenhagen, Borkum Riff, Amphora, Perfecto Garcia	Chateau Ste. Michelle wines, Zig Zag cigarette papers, Cedar King pencils, Dr. Grabow pipes
Culbro, Inc.	General Cigar Co. (Garcia y Vega, White Owl, Robt. Burns, Corina, Wm. Penn, Tiparillo, Tijuana Smalls, London Dock, Kentucky Club), Helme Tobacco Company (Gold River, Mail Pouch, Silver Creek, Redwood, Chattanooga Chew)	Snacktime Company (Golden Pop, Chesty Potato Chips, Pepitos, Snack Time), Imperial Nurseries

Sources: Company annual reports (1982 or 1983) and news releases, based on latest available information. Prepared by William J. Bailey, Masters of Public Health.

William J. Bailey, "Opinion: Opportunity of Threat-Tobacco Industry." *Smoking and Health Reporter.* 1, no. 4 (July 1984) pp. 10–11. © National Interagency Council on Smoking and Health. Used with permission.

SUMMARY

The use of tobacco in the United States goes back to the Indians, who introduced tobacco to Columbus. It was commonly accepted thereafter, until it became associated with various diseases. The 1979 surgeon general's report stated that the smoking of tobacco cigarettes is directly related to an increase in heart problems, lung and other cancers, and respiratory diseases including emphysema. It also interferes with metabolism, increases the number of stillborn and neonatal deaths, appears in the milk of nursing mothers, reduces availability of oxygen during exercise, and is a causative factor in many other health-related problems.

Smokers derive pleasure from the effects of smoking, but once a person is dependent on tobacco it is difficult to stop smoking. Clinics have been organized to help smokers kick the habit, and smoking has been made somewhat safer by the addition of filters and the reduction of nicotine. Alternative uses of tobacco, such as chewing, pipe and cigar smoking, and snuff may help some to give up cigarette smoking, but these forms of tobacco also harm one's health.

Nonsmokers have mobilized a campaign to protect their health from the dangers of involuntary breathing of tobacco smoke. Their efforts have led to smoking and nonsmoking sections in restaurants and airplanes and to the prohibiting of smoking in some public buildings. Sweden was the first country to launch a campaign to become a nation of nonsmokers.

Because of the harmful effects caused by smoking there is an increasing and growing movement away from smoking. Even the tobacco industry senses this movement as evidenced in their increasing diversification away from tobacco products.

NOTES

[1]National Interagency Council on Smoking and Health, "Dramatic Drop in Number of Smokers and Cigarette Production Sends Shock Waves through Tobacco Industry," *Smoking and Health Reporter* 1, no. 3 (April 1984):1.

[2]"Risks in Low Tar Smokers," *Journal* 6, no. 7 (July 1, 1977).

[3]Oakley S. Ray, *Drugs, Society and Human Behavior*, 3rd edition (St. Louis: C. V. Mosby, Co., 1983). Reproduced with permission.

[4]American Cancer Society, *Dangers of Smoking . . . Benefits of Quitting and and Relative Risks of Reduced Exposure* (New York, 1980), pp. 413–29.

[5]Louis S. Goodman and Alfred Gilman, eds., *The Pharmacological Basis of Therapeutics*, 4th ed. (New York: Macmillan, 1970) p. 115.

[6]Ray, *Drugs, Society and Human Behavior*, pp. 100–106.

[7]J. W. Hurst et al., *The Heart, Arteries and Veins* (New York: McGraw-Hill, 1974), pp. 1563–66.

[8]Goodman and Gilman, *The Pharmacological Basis of Therapeutics*.

[9]Department of Health, Education and Welfare, *1979 Surgeon General's Report* (Washington, D.C.: U.S. Department of Health and Human Services. Public Health Service. Rockville, MD). p.29.

[10]Ibid.

[11]Center for Disease Control, *The Health Consequences of Smoking* (Washington, D.C.: Department of Health, Education and Welfare, 1975).

[12]See Walter S. Ross, "Poison Gases in Your Cigarettes: Hydrogen Cyanide and Nitrous Oxides," *Reader's Digest* 109, no. 656 (December 1976):92–98.

[13]National Interagency Council on Smoking and Health, "American Council on Science and Health Bills Tobacco Industry," *Smoking and Health Reporter* 1, no. 4 (July 1984):1–2.

[14]National Interagency Council on Smoking and Health, "New Study Reveals: Smoking Costs and Extra $56,000 in Health Related Expenses over Lifetime," *Smoking and Health Reporter* 1, no. 4 (July 1984):7. Copyright © 1984 National Interagency Council on Smoking and Health. Used with permission.

[15]National Interagency Council on Smoking and Health, "Senate Committee Approves New Cigarette Warning," *Smoking and Health Reporter* 1, no. 1 (October 1983):1. Copyright © 1983 National Interagency Council on Smoking and Health. Used with permission.

[16]Ibid.

[17]American Cancer Society, *Dangers of Smoking.*

[18]G. A. Cellini et al., "Direct Arterial Pressure, Heart Rate, and Electro-Cardiography during Cigarette Smoking of Unrestricted Patients," *American Heart Journal* 89, no. 1 (January 1975):18–25.

[19]1983 Surgeon General's Report, *Health Consequences of Smoking: Cardiovascular Disease,* U.S. Department of Health and Human Services, Public Health Service Office of Smoking (Rockville, MD.) p. 384.

[20]"Medical News: Can You Alter Your Heart Disease Risk?" *Journal of the American Heart Association* 245, no. 19 (May 15, 1981):1904, 1907.

[21]Hurst et al., *The Heart, Arteries and Veins,* pp. 1563–66.

[22]Center for Disease Control, *The Health Consequences of Smoking.*

[23]1984 Surgeon General's Report, *Health Consequences of Smoking: Chronic Obstructive Disease,* U.S. Department of Health and Human Services, Public Health Service Office on Smoking (Rockville, MD.) p. 312.

[24]National Interagency Council on Smoking and Health, "Lung Cancer Facts and Figures," *Smoking and Health Reporter* 1, no. 2 (January 1984):4.

[25]Center for Disease Control, *The Health Consequences of Smoking,* p. 10.

[26]Public Health Service, *The Health Consequences of Smoking* (Washington, D.C.: Department of Health, Education and Welfare, 1967).

[27]Cited in H. Van Vunakis et al., "Nicotine and Cotenine in the Amniotic Fluid of Smokers in the Second Trimester of Pregnancy," *American Journal of Obstetrics and Gynecology* 120, no. 1 (September 1, 1974):62–64.

[28]Hurst et al., *The Heart, Arteries and Veins.*

[29]G. H. Neher, "Nicotine-Induced Depression of Lymphocyte Growth," *Toxicology and Applied Pharmacology* 27, no. 2 (February 1974):253–58.

[30]Luther Terry, "Pushing the Anti-Smoking Crusade in New Directions," *Today's Health* 51, no. 1 (June 1973).

[31]David R. Jacobs and Sara Gottenberg; "Smoking and Weight: The Minnesota Lipid Research Clinic," *American Journal of Public Health* 71, no. 4 (April 1981): 450.

[32]Center for Disease Control, *The Health Consequences of Smoking,* p. 11.

[33]Van Vunakis et al., "Nicotine and Cotenine," p. 11.

[34] American Cancer Society, *Dangers of Smoking,* p. 413. 198

[35]Ibid.

[36]"Smoking and Pregnancy," *Family Health* 2, no. 5 (May 1979):32.

[37]American Cancer Society, *Dangers of Smoking.* p. 414.

[38]Ibid.

[39]Ibid.

[40]Ibid.

[41]Ibid.

[42]A. Erickson, B. Kallen, and P. Westerholm, "Cigarette Smoking as an Etiologic Factor in Cleft Lip and Palate," *American Journal of Obstetrics and Gynecology* 135, no. 3 (October 1, 1979): 348–51.

[43]Donald K. Mathews and Edward L. Fox, *The Physiological Basis of P.E. and Athletics* (Philadelphia: Saunders, 1971), pp. 178–79.

[44]Genell J. Subak-Sharpe, "Is Your Sex Life Going Up in Smoke?" *Today's Health* 52, no. 8 (August 1974): 65.

[45]Ibid.

[46]Diana Petitt and John Wingerd, "Use of Oral Contraceptives, Cigarette Smoking and the Risk of Subarchnoid Hemorrhage," *Lancet* 2, no. 8083 (July 29, 1978):234–35.

[47]F. P. Zuspan and N. Davis, "The Effect of Smoking and Oral Contraceptives on the Urinary Excretion of Epinephrine and Norepinephrine," *American Journal of Obstetrics and Gynecology* 135, no. 8 (December 15, 1979).

[48]Ibid.

[49]HEW, *1979 Surgeon General's Report*, p. 85.

[50]"Drug Effects Can Go Up in Smoke," *FDA Consumer* 13, no. 2 (March 1979):18.

[51]R. Hickey et al., "Coffee Drinking, Smoking, Pollution, and Cardio-Vascular Disease: A Problem of Self Selection," *Lancet* 1, no. 7810 (May 5, 1973):1003.

[52]HEW, *1979 Surgeon General's Report*, p. 68.

[53]M. A. H. Russel, "Tobacco Dependence: Is Nicotine Rewarding or Adversive?" *The Practitioner* 212 (1974):791–800. (London: Morgan Grampian Ltd.) Used with permission.

[54]See Ross, "Poison Gases in Your Cigarettes," pp. 92–98.

[55]Cited in ibid., pp. 92–95.

[56]National Interagency Council on Smoking and Health, "Model Program Launched—Dow Chemical Begins Massive Smoking Cessation Project in Texas," *Smoking and Health Reporter* 1 (July 1984):6. Copyright © 1984 National Interagency Council on Smoking and Health. Used with permission.

[57]Edward M. Brecher et al., *Licit and Illicit Drugs* (Boston: Little, Brown, 1972), pp. 241–44

[58]John R. Seffrin, "Freedom of Choice?" *Smoking and Health Reporter* 1, no. 4 (July 1984):3. Copyright © 1984 National Interagency Council on Smoking and Health. Used with permission.

[59]See National Interagency Council on Smoking and Health, "British Documentary Released Across the United States," *Smoking and Health Reporter*, 1 no. 2, (January 1984):7. Copyright © 1984 National Interagency Council on Smoking and Health. Used with permission.

[60]Cited in National Institute on Education, *Teen-age Smoking Survey* (Washington, D.C.: Department of Health, Education and Welfare, 1978).

[61]"Update Report Blasts Cigarettes," *Science News* 115, no. 3 (January 20, 1979):39.

[62]Department of Health, Education and Welfare, *1979 Surgeon General's Report*, p. 65.

[63]*Pipe and Cigarette Smoking*, Oregon Lung Association, 1977.

[64]Department of Health, Education and Welfare, *Teen-age Smoking Survey*, p. 65.

[65]A. G. Christen and E. D. Glover, "The Case Against Smokeless Tobacco: Five Facts for the Health Professional to Consider," *Journal of the American Dental Association* 101, no. 3 (1980):464–69. Copyright by the American Dental Association. Reprinted by permission.

[66]Ibid.

[67]*The Lung and Short of It* (Eugene, Oregon), Oregon Lung Association, 1985), p. 1.

[68]W. G. Squires et al., "Hemodynamic Effects of Oral Tobacco in Experimental Animals and Young Adults" (abstract presented to the 54th Annual Meeting of the American Heart Association, Dallas, November 16–19, 1981).

[69]*The Lung and Short of It* (Eugene, Oregon), Oregon Lung Association, 1985).

[70]Samuel C. McMorris, "The Smoking Addiction," *British Journal of Addiction,* Spring 1976, pp. 24–36.

[71]Center for Disease Control, *The Health Consequences of Smoking.* Washington, D.C. p. 65.

[72]Ibid.

[73]Ibid.

[74]Ibid.

[75]National Interagency Council on Smoking and Health. "Churches Question 'Morality' of North Carolina Tobacco Industry," *Smoking and Health Reporter* 1, no. 4 (July 1984):7. Copyright © 1984 National Interagency Council on Smoking and Health. Used with permission.

[76]Michael Lespaire, "San Franciscans Vote to Require Non-Smoking Work Areas," *Smoking and Health Reporter* 1, no. 2 (January 1984):5. Copyright © 1984 National Interagency Council on Smoking and Health. Used with permission.

[77]National Interagency Council on Smoking and Health, "Even Smokers Agree That They Shouldn't Smoke in the Presence of Non-Smokers," *Smoking and Health Reporter* 1, no. 4 (July 1984):10–11. Copyright © 1984 National Interagency Council on Smoking and Health. Used with permission.

[78]William J. Bailey, "Opportunity or Threat: Tobacco Industry, *Smoking and Health Reporter* 1, no. 4 (July 1984): 10–11.

7

DEPRESSANTS AND THE BODY

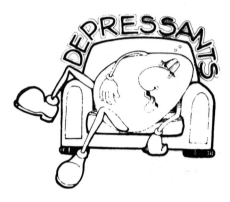

INTRODUCTION

Depressants are drugs that decrease awareness of and response to incoming sensory stimuli.[1] Three major depressants—sedative-hypnotics, minor and major tranquilizers, and deliriants (volatile substances)—are probed in this chapter.

SEDATIVE-HYPNOTICS

Classification

Drugs classified as sedative-hypnotics may differ chemically but produce similar effects.[2] Their action is chiefly one of CNS depression, though the precise mechanism of their action is not known. Both barbiturates and nonbarbiturate drugs are included in this class, as well as a wide variety of organic and synthetic compounds.

Physical Effects

Hypnotics are used to bring on sleep; sedatives are usually used to induce a milder degree of CNS depression, such as anxiety relief. In most instances, the same substances can be used for both sedation and hypnosis, depending on the dose. Large doses depress the cerebral cortex, the respiratory system, and the cardiovascular system.

Sedative-hypnotics impair judgment and motor coordination. Side effects can include nausea, vomiting, headache, drowsiness, gastric upset, rashes, and hangover. Excitement, blurred vision, facial numbness, an aftertaste, and fever can also occur. And if an individual is hypersensitive to a drug in this class, more serious reactions are possible. A further hazard is that the difference between therapeutic and lethal dose levels is often very minimal.

Sedative-hypnotics can produce both psychological and physiological dependence. Symptoms of withdrawal from long-term use are far more severe than they are for alcohol, and require close medical supervision. In therapeutic use, the dangers of dependence and sudden withdrawal are greater than those from direct toxic side effects.[3]

Barbiturates

The basic ingredient of the barbiturate family of drugs is barbituric acid. Various members of the family include phenobarbital, pentobarbital, amobarbital, and secobarbital.

Classification   Barbiturates are classified by duration of action: they are either ultrashort (thirty minutes to three hours), short (three to six hours), intermediate (six to twelve hours), or long-acting (twelve to twenty-four hours). Ultrashort barbiturates produce anesthesia within one minute of intravenous administration. The most commonly used of these drugs is thiopental.

Among the short-acting barbiturates are pentobarbital, secobarbital, and amobarbital. It takes from fifteen to forty minutes for these drugs to go into effect.

Butabarbital is the most commonly used intermediate barbiturate. Its onset time is generally thirty to forty-five minutes.

Long-acting barbiturates have onset times of up to one hour. This category of barbiturates includes barbital and phenobarbital.

History   Barbiturates were among the first drugs of the twentieth century designed to produce relaxation and sleep. Discovery of their hazardous effects, including physiological dependence, brought about a search for substitutes. Numerous compounds were developed, but many of them, including Valium and Librium, were also found to have hazardous effects, such as severe physiological dependence. Barbiturates are now rarely used for medical purposes.

Physical Effects   Barbiturates affect the user in many ways, ranging from subtle changes in mood and sedation to sleep and coma. Typical effects are a reduction in attention span, less awareness of external stimuli, and a decrease in the ability to perform intellectual tasks. Barbiturates also decrease the amount of sleep spent in dreaming (rapid-eye-movement, or REM sleep). Children and elderly users, however, may experience excitement rather than sedation.

Continued barbiturate use often results in tolerance and may eventually result in physical dependence. Pregnant women who ingest large doses of barbiturates throughout pregnancy (or during the last three months) run the risk of congenital dependency in their infants.[4] During chronic barbiturate intoxication, nausea, dizziness, confusion, and an impaired mental state occur. Allergic reactions, though rare, are also possible, resulting in swelling of the face, dermatitis, skin lesions, fever, delirium, convulsions, and degenerative changes in the liver.[5] When administered to expectant mothers, barbiturates may cause fetal oxygen deficiency, which may result in birth defects, brain damage, or death. When taken with alcohol, barbiturates exert a powerful synergistic effect, which may lead to accidental overdose or a planned suicide.

Withdrawal from barbiturates is far more severe than withdrawal from alcohol or heroin, and can be life-threatening without medical supervision. Initial withdrawal symptoms include sweating, insomnia, vomiting, tremors, paranoia, and a short temper. Excessive dreaming and nightmares can occur, and hallucinations and seizures have been reported in extreme cases.

Medical Use   The medical uses of barbiturates are limited today to the treatment of insomnia and some convulsive disorders, and, to a lesser extent, as an antianxiety agent. This is because of the large number of nonbarbiturate sedatives and tranquilizers currently available. There is some evidence, however, that thiopental, a barbiturate-analgesic, may prevent brain damage when given immediately following the loss of oxygen.[6] Harvey Shapiro, an anesthesiologist at the University of California, also found that thiopental reduced brain swelling during operations, as well as lessening cerebral pressure and improving blood circulation.[7]

Barbiturate Abuse   There are several nonmedical uses of barbiturates that can be classified as barbiturate abuse. The first is for maintenance of an anxiety-free state of chronic intoxication.

The second is for stimulation, to amplify altered moods. Such episodic intoxication is found most commonly in young adults or teenagers, often at parties.

Barbiturates are also taken to counteract the effects of amphetamines, or to ease withdrawal from heroin.[8] The heroin dependent may also supplement his or her heroin doses with barbiturates when the supply is low, or unknowingly,

administer heroin cut with barbiturates. Although this pattern of use characterizes a relatively small number of individuals, it is by far the most hazardous,
because tolerance can develop and because lethal doses may accidentally be
taken.

Barbiturates are sometimes taken in combination with alcohol. Recently,
however, people have become aware of the hazards (coma and death) of this,
and mixing of these drugs seems to be declining.

Methaqualone

The primary medical uses of methaqualone are to relieve nervous
tension and anxiety and to promote sleep. Various brand names for methaqualone preparations in the United States include Sopor, Optimal, Parest, Somnafac, Quaalude, and Bi-Phetamine T.[9]

History One of the major reasons for methaqualone's rapid
growth in popularity was that its sedation usually did not result in the classic
barbiturate-like hangover. Further, its use did not disturb dream-stage sleep. In
1965, the W. H. Rorer pharmaceutical house first introduced Quaalude[R] as a
major improvement over barbiturates. By the late 1960s Quaaludes were "the"
drug on many college campuses.[10] Students discovered that in combination with
alcohol, methaqualone produces a sense of well-being and a higher pain threshold. It was also thought of as a "love drug" because it depressed inhibitions and
led to sexual desire. Because it was approved by the FDA, it was not thought to
be as harmful as barbiturates. However, serious problems of overdose and dependence developed in various sections of America.[11] In 1974, 88 persons died
of overdose. By 1977, the death rate was down to 61, but Quaalude-related
emergency-room visits jumped from 1671 in 1974 to 5500 in 1977.[12]

In the 1980s, "stress clinics" where patients obtained superficial examinations from licensed doctors and a prescription for methaqualone sprang up
around the country, and the incidences of overdose and abuse began to rise
again. In 1981 overseas production began to be reduced, and in 1983 Lemmon
Pharmaceutical Company, the major manufacturer of methaqualone, announced it would stop making the pills and would destroy stockpiles of the drug
to reduce its abuse.[13]

Psychological and Physiological Effects When doses of 75
milligrams of methaqualone are taken, dreamy moods are induced and inhibitions are lowered. However, if doses of 150 to 300 milligrams are taken, a sense
of numbness and sleep result. Headache, hangover, menstrual disturbance,
tongue changes, dry mouth, cracking at the angles of the mouth, nosebleeds,
depersonalization, dizziness, skin eruptions, pain in the extremities, diarrhea,
and anorexia can also occur.[14] Other effects may include anxiety, nausea, and
restlessness.

During its early use, methaqualone was thought to be nonaddictive, unlike
barbiturates. Eventually, however, physicians and clinicians became aware that

tolerance and physiological dependence develops with continued use.[15] Withdrawal symptoms include irritability, vomiting, headaches, seizures, cramps, tremors, sleeplessness, mania, convulsions, and death. A fetus can become physiologically dependent if its mother takes methaqualone.

A serious danger with methaqualone is the potential for accidental overdose. It is easy to misjudge the potency of the dosage; the user may forget the quantity of pills already taken, because methaqualone affects memory; or the user may underestimate the risk in taking additional pills, because the drug affects judgment.

MINOR TRANQUILIZERS

Classification

The word *tranquilizer* describes a number of drugs with differing chemical structures. The three major chemical families of minor tranquilizers are meprobamate and its analogues (Soma, Miltown, Equanil); benzodiazepines (Librium, Valium); and dephenylmetanes (Suavitil, Softran).

History

Introduced in 1955 as the first minor tranquilizer, meprobamate (Miltown) was originally prescribed for the treatment of mild to moderate anxiety and mild psychoneurotic or psychosomatic complaints. The drug previously used to treat these problems, barbituric acid, was being used less often because of its adverse effects, including physical dependence. The new minor tranquilizer allowed for a wider variation of dose to achieve the desired results. In a world seeking immediate relief from tension and anxiety, this drug and the others in its class found rapid acceptance.

Acceptance soon turned to widespread use—related, some feel, to overprescribing by physicians. Such overprescription can occur because most medical schools offer only a limited curriculum in pharmacology and because drugs are continually introduced to physicians after they graduate from medical school. Also, massive promotional drives and advertising campaigns in medical journals by pharmaceutical houses have encouraged physicians to prescribe these drugs. Furthermore, our pill-oriented society has made many consumers feel cheated if a visit to their physician does not result in a prescription. Some researchers estimate that as much as 50 percent of minor-tranquilizer prescriptions are unnecessary.[16]

Though all segments and professions in society now use tranquilizers as a coping device (Valium is sometimes referred to as the "executive Excedrin"), tranquilizers simply postpone finding solutions to the problems they are taken to cure. It is hoped that this knowledge, along with knowledge of the drugs' negative effects, will bring about a decline in their use.

Physical Effects

Tranquilizers reduce neuromuscular activity, thereby reducing environmental awareness and facilitating relaxation. Motor coordination, speech patterns, attention span, and libido (sex drive) are all affected. Feelings of aggression are reduced and feelings of sociability occasionally increase. With increasing dosages, drowsiness progresses toward sleep.

Minor tranquilizers have a number of known side effects. These include apathy, illogical fears, low blood pressure, fainting, chills, rashes, upset stomach, disorientation, blurred vision, bladder, menstrual, and ovulary irregularities, and sleep disturbances; if taken with alcohol, toxic and sometimes fatal reactions can occur. The euphoria the drugs produce also promotes psychological dependence. With repeated use, tolerance, as well as cross-tolerance (tolerance for one drug extending to tolerance for another), develops. However, the lethal dose level does not rise. Dose escalation brings one closer to death more quickly than with other drugs. Withdrawal symptoms following chronic administration of large doses of the minor tranquilizers are similar to the symptoms of withdrawal from alcohol and barbiturates: anxiety, muscle twitches, insomnia, headache, fever, nausea, vomiting, abdominal cramps, sweating, and convulsions; death is possible.

The more recently developed minor tranquilizers—benzodiazepine derivatives—are considered safer than older forms. Their dose–response curves are flat (except for diazepam), which means that increased dosage does not always produce increased effect. Hence, benzodiazepine derivatives used in therapeutic doses rarely act strongly on respiration and normally do not result in psychological depression that could lead to suicide.

Future tranquilizers may be even safer than present drugs because of the discovery of inosine and hypoxanthine, chemical compounds found (and probably manufactured) in the brain that act in the same manner as benzodiazepines. These cerebral purines are of relatively high concentration and structurally similar to Valium and may help in the development of drugs that are free of side effects.

Valium (Diazepam)

Derived from the Latin word meaning "to be strong and well," Valium is an antianxiety agent and a muscle relaxant and produces antiepileptic effects without sedation. It is used to treat anxiety and muscle spasms, as a preanesthetic for heart patients, in the early stages of labor, and to control cerebral palsy, convulsive attacks, and low-back pain. Unfortunately, very little is known about how Valium works.[17]

History Developed in 1961 by Leo Sternbach, a chemist for Roche Laboratories, Valium was the most prescribed drug in the world. In 1978, over 45 million prescriptions were written for Valium; in 1980, it was estimated that 10 to 15 percent of all Americans took Valium sometime during the year.[18]

According to the Drug Abuse Warning Network (DAWN), Valium is the most abused medicine in this country.[19] Approximately 30 percent of Valium prescriptions are for anxiety and insomnia, 15 to 18 percent for muscle spasms, 2 to 3 percent for epilepsy and cerebral palsy, and 45 percent for anxiety-related psychosomatic or organic illness (such as ulcers).

Many tranquilizer users are upper- or upper-middle-class and/or white-collar workers, retired persons, or unemployed.[20] The National Institute of Mental Health and the National Institute on Drug Abuse estimate that women users outnumber men by 2.5 to 1.[21] Changing social roles, more leisure time, employment pressures, poor self-image and insecurity, problems in child rearing, and the so-called empty-nest syndrome are among the oft-cited reasons why women become dependent on tranquilizers.[22] Furthermore, there is speculation that women use tranquilizers more than men because they see their physicians more often than men. And because women are generally more able to discuss their frustrations and their physical and emotional pain, their physician's treatment often includes the prescription of tranquilizers to ease the discomfort.

Valium is a popular street drug as well as a prescription drug. The Philadelphia Veteran's Administration Drug Dependence Treatment and Research Center has noted an increase in the use, misuse, and abuse of Valium among opiate dependents. Valium is also used by heroin dependents, particularly those undergoing methadone treatment, as it supplements the CNS-depressing effects of methadone while adding its own antianxiety properties. Combined with alcohol, Valium was the third highest cause of drug-related death in 1978.[23]

Physical Effects   Valium may cause the user to become drowsy and less alert. The drug also causes respiratory depression, a decrease in memory and motor functions, and occasional decreases in arterial pressure. Valium should be used cautiously by those with liver and kidney impairments and should not be used by women who are pregnant or nursing. In July 1970, the FDA ordered that manufacturers of tranquilizers issue warnings to physicians that these drugs should be avoided by women during the first trimester of pregnancy. Subsequent studies associated Valium and the incidence of cleft palate and lips in babies.[24] Children of mothers who used Valium in the first trimester had four times greater incidence of this congenital defect. Furthermore, babies born to Valium users tend to be hypoactive, exhibiting abnormally low muscle tension for the first twenty-four hours following delivery.[25]

A number of side effects are also associated with Valium use. These include lethargy, skin rashes, menstrual and ovulatory irregularities, blood abnormalities, conjunctivitis (pink eye), drowsiness, insomnia, fatigue, changes in emotional reactions, irritability, overexcitement, hostility and confusion, headaches, double vision, constipation, hypertension, stammering, changes in libido, nausea, slurred speech, perspiration, and thirst.[26]

Synergism   Valium alone thus has significant bodily effects and in combination with other drugs it can be even more dangerous. It has been found, for example, that when Valium is combined with ethanol (alcohol), the

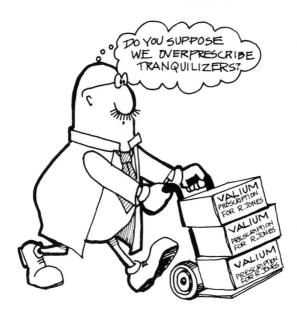

plasma levels of Valium increased, probably because Valium is more soluble in ethanol than in water, thus increasing the permeability of Valium in the blood supply.[27] It has also been noted that "acceleration by ethanol of the absorption of diazepam (Valium[R]) is important and provides a more complete explanation of the marked sedation that can follow this combination of drugs. . . . Overdose with diazepam alone is remarkably safe, but combined with alcohol can produce central nervous system depression and death."[28]

Dependence and Withdrawal   A study conducted by the Ford Foundation in 1970 found Valium's dependence-producing level to be 80 to 120 milligrams a day for three months.[29] Physical dependence can also result from a level as low as 30 milligrams a day, however, if the drug is taken over a longer period of time.[30] Since the drug can produce dependence, withdrawal becomes a hazard of prolonged Valium use. Almost as severe as barbiturate withdrawal, Valium withdrawal begins within forty-eight hours of discontinuation and is characterized by violent shaking and possible grand mal seizures.[31] Symptoms are not alleviated by the administration of other minor tranquilizers. In extreme cases, sudden withdrawal may cause coma or death.[32]

Today, emotional disturbances are given as the most common reason for medical prescription of Valium. The drug is used to help patients cope with anxiety or depression. Valium is prescribed by 97 percent of all general practitioners and internists. The average daily use of Valium is fifteen milligrams a day. It has been noted that because Valium creates a feeling of relaxation, euphoria, well-being, and uninhibitedness, users gradually increase their dosage above the prescribed amount.[33] When this happens, users form a psychological dependence on the drug.

Since Valium is taken as a temporary problem solver, the patient is once again confronted with problems when it wears off. To alleviate this feeling, some patients increase the amount of Valium taken, consequently increasing their tolerance and leading themselves toward physiological dependence. In a study by Maletzky and Klotter, forty-two of fifty subjects were found to have adjusted their own doses of Valium because of the drug's immediate positive effects.[34] Twenty-four of those who had become physically dependent tried to quit: twenty-two were unsuccessful. Dependence develops in patients who become chronic users and is more prevalent among long-time users who take high doses. High doses also induce sleep and may produce an appearance of drunkenness, ataxia (gross motor impairment), excitement, or uninhibitedness.[35] When a Valium dependent decides to quit, withdrawal symptoms may be delayed for as long as forty-eight hours, depending on the half-life of the metabolites. The symptoms are convulsions, tremors, cramps, and sweating. It is advisable to withdraw from Valium slowly to allow the body to readjust to reduced levels of the drug and to minimize withdrawal symptoms. David E. Smith, director of the Haight-Ashbury Clinic in San Francisco, recommends a periodic therapeutic holiday at a reduced or zero level for long-time Valium users so that they can avoid becoming physically and psychologically dependent on the drug.[36]

Valium occupies the spotlight of controversy because researchers failed to recognize its apparent addiction capabilities when it was first being used years ago. Valium has a high rate of abuse because it is so easy to increase the dosage and become dependent and because it rarely proves fatal.

The FDA cites evidence that "Valium is overprescribed and abused and that it can cause psychological and physical dependence."[37] As physicians and the general public have become more aware of Valium's potential for abuse, its sales have diminished. Between 1975 and 1980, Valium sales were cut in half and the number of prescriptions dropped from 61.3 million to 33.6 million.[38] Physicians are being more careful and conservative about prescribing the drug, fearing it may do more harm than good. But when used in moderation and under a physician's supervision, Valium is considered one of the safest depressant drugs and can be extremely helpful.

Librium (Chlordiazepoxide)

The only major chemical difference between Librium and Valium is that Valium is not as soluble in water. Librium is a brand name, Chlorodiazepoxide is the chemical name. Librium is used as much as Valium, as an antianxiety agent, for muscle relaxation, and in various drug-withdrawal treatments. It has been used in the treatment of geriatric patients to reduce the chances of overexertion and in emotional crises. It has also been used to treat emotionally disturbed children.

Physical Effects   Librium has longer-lasting physiological effects than Valium, and a greater potential for dependence when used in excessive amounts. The drug produces mild drowsiness, fatigue, and a reduced ability to coordinate voluntary muscle movement. In some instances, it may cause skin rash, nausea, mild headache, and either an increased or decreased sex drive. Librium may depress blood pressure as well as pulse rate, lower body metabolism, and increase appetite. In large doses, it can produce a partial or complete suspension of respiration.

Librium's euphoric effects may lead some patients to psychological dependence, and tolerance can occur in only a few weeks of use. Physical dependence may ultimately occur, producing symptoms of hyperexcitability, insomnia, vomiting, tremors, muscle twitching, anxiety, and depression. As with Valium, withdrawal from Librium should be medically supervised.

MAJOR TRANQUILIZERS (ANTIPSYCHOTICS) _____

Classification

Antipsychotics, or "major tranquilizers," are grouped on the basis of their most widespread medical use: treatment and management of certain acute psychological disorders, notably schizophrenic and other severe conditions.[39] There are four recognized groups of antipsychotics: the Rauwolfia alkaloids, the phenothiazines, the thioxanthines, and the butyrophenones. Although these groups are chemically dissimilar and their modes of action different, they all act on the central nervous system to block, inhibit, or retard signals along nerve pathways.

The physiological theory of schizophrenia, for which phenothiazine use is indicated, holds that auditory and visual hallucinations are caused by inadequate sorting of relevant and irrelevant stimuli within the brain. Confusing the relevant (pertinent) and irrelevant (or possibly unreal) stimuli might lead to a highly disoriented state. The structures involved in brain arousal and the evaluation and filtering of relevant stimuli include the reticular formation and its ascending reticular activating system (ARAS).

Situated along the brain stem (the part of the spinal cord that leads to the cerebellum and cerebral cortex), the ARAS samples all sensory impulses coming into the brain, and then alerts the cerebrum to receive information. Barbiturates and other sedative-hypnotics directly suppress ARAS neuronal activity. However, phenothiazines appear to depress the *input* reaching the ARAS, thus limiting the amount of information transmitted to the ARAS, and therefore, from the ARAS to the cerebrum. While the patient is awake (that is, when the ARAS is not depressed) there is decreased sensory input into the ARAS.

Current Use

The growing use of antipsychotic preparations in the behavior management of chronic forms of psychosis, senility, and violent behavior has led some experts to credit these drugs with reducing the number of patients requiring hospitalization or institutionalization. Major tranquilizers make certain uncontrollable individuals less harmful to themselves and others. In some cases, chemotherapy along with antipsychotics facilitates external intervention with patients suffering from acute perceptual distortions.

Physical Effects

Though the CNS-depressant action of the various antipsychotics varies with the particular drug, dose, duration of application, and individual metabolic factors, mild doses generally produce a marked decrease in the intensity of neural activity in the brain. Thus, the impact of emotions is reduced, and awareness of internal and external events is minimized. Antipsychotics will bring on sedation accompanied by significantly reduced motor activity and muscle tone, and will lower blood pressure, pulse rate, and body temperature as well.

Antipsychotics, like all drugs, produce contraindications (adverse reactions) in a certain percentage of individuals. These reactions can involve any of the bodily systems, producing anemia, weight gain, dry mouth, altered liver, kidney, or bladder functions, swollen tongue, and emotional dependence. Hypersensitivity reactions may include diarrhea, nausea, vomiting, and fever. Major tranquilizers are also able to cross the placental barrier and reportedly produce prolonged side effects and birth defects in the newborn.

Long-term therapy with antipsychotics may lead to a condition called tardive dyskinesia. This drug-induced nervous disorder is manifested in involuntary movements of the jaws, lips, and tongue. The condition is more common in the middle-aged, or elderly, and once developed, the pattern of uncontrollable chewing, puckering of lips, and repetitive tongue protrusions may become irreversible.[40]

The lethal levels of antipsychotics depend on the specific preparation, individual metabolic factors, tolerance, chemical hypersensitivity, and occurrence of multi-drug use. When antipsychotics interact with alcohol, antihistamines, or opiates, the combined depressant effects are greater than the sum of the effects of the substances taken singly.

DELIRIANTS (VOLATILE SUBSTANCES)

Classification

The variety of volatile substances currently being inhaled as psychoactive drugs may be broken into three classes: the volatile hydrocarbon solvents, aerosols, and anesthetics. The volatile hydrocarbon solvents are primarily used as commercial solvents. Their power as solvents, plus their tendency to evaporate quickly, make them desirable for use in materials where quick drying is required or convenient,[41] such as in plastic-model cement and typewriting correction fluid. Some of the more highly refined petroleum products, such as gasoline and lighter fluid, are also included in this group.[42]

The psychoactive ingredients of aerosols are not found in the substance forced out of pressurized cans but are actually the propellants that provide the pressure. These propellants are most often chlorinated or fluorinated hydrocarbons,[43] and can be found in pressurized cans of deodorants, vegetable-oil spray, and hair sprays.

The anesthetics are considered more exotic than the solvents and aerosols, since they are generally less easy for the general public to obtain. One of the anesthetics often inhaled is chloroform. Although only limited research has been performed on these compounds, they seem to closely resemble various CNS depressants in their effects.

History

Before their medical applications were known, anesthetics such as nitrous oxide (laughing gas) and ether were frequently used for recreational purposes. Some deliriants have also been used during historical periods of stress (war, scarcity, depression) as a substitute for drugs that were more socially acceptable but unavailable. Presently deliriants are used in cleaning compounds, spray cans, airplane-model glue, and many industrial products.

One of the most striking features of volatile substances is their availability. For example, one survey found it was possible to purchase 38 different products containing volatile solvents from a single service station/hardware store.[44] Also, there are at least 300 products currently offered in aerosol form.[45] The lack of regulations on the sale of these products and their general availability contribute to their abuse among adolescents. This abuse has led to the limiting of model-cement sales in some states to certain age categories and to the addition of certain chemical agents with unpleasant side effects to volatile substances. It is hoped that these side effects will be severe enough to discourage inhalation of these substances.

Physical Effects

Volatile substances are rapidly transported across the blood-brain barrier. In low doses, they produce arousal and euphoria typical of CNS depressants. Several inhalations produce intoxication characterized by alterations in judgment, hyperactivity, and some lack of behavioral control. With increased doses, activity is further reduced and sedation becomes pronounced. High doses can produce increased hilarity, dizziness, a floating sensation, and hallucinations.

Solvents have caused temporary changes in kidney, liver, and bone-marrow functions and have affected responses to certain psychological tests.[46] Other deliriant compounds are caustic enough to produce mouth ulcers and severe stomach distress. Appetite reduction may also be caused, leading to nutritional disorders. Inert-gas propellants in aerosols can cause asphyxiation or freeze the vocal cords when inhaled.

Some users of volatile substances report side effects that include confusion, headache, lack of coordination, and watery eyes. Large doses often cause nausea, vomiting, or runny nose. Heavy sedation caused by these drugs can be characterized by stupor, respiratory depression, and unconsciousness, and may lead to death. Continuous rebreathing of a deliriant from a plastic bag or other container will also induce unconsciousnes, and death can result from the accidental overdose or from suffocation by the container.

Psychological Effects

For many, the psychological effects of inhaling volatile substances are very pronounced. These effects include impaired judgment, confusion, hyperactivity, lack of behavioral control, retarded motor-coordination skills, fright, and tenseness. Acute psychosis has also been observed, though it is of temporary duration.[47]

SUMMARY

Despite the number of medical problems that are effectively met by proper and judicious use of barbiturates, abuse of barbiturates remains one of America's hidden drug problems. To combat this problem, physicians have begun diagnosing and treating underlying disorders before relying on barbiturate use.

Methaqualone is a CNS depressant that was to replace barbiturates in reducing tension and anxiety and promoting sleep. Originally it was thought to be free of the dangers of dependency, but with use it was soon discovered that this was not so. The drug produces harmful side effects and when combined with other CNS depressants such as alcohol can lead to death.

Tranquilizers are the number-one prescription drug in the United States, with minor tranquilizers, including Valium and Librium, the most frequently prescribed. Minor tranquilizers reduce stress, anxiety, and tension as well as aiding in muscle relaxation and working as a mild analgesic. However, many physicians are presently reassessing their prescribing of tranquilizers, and it is hoped that people will learn to cope rather than rely on these drugs. The side effects of minor tranquilizers, the potential hazard when they are combined with alcohol or other depressants, and the very real possibility of psychological and physical dependence make these drugs dangerous.

Major tranquilizers have been effective in the treatment and management of severe and chronic psychological disorders in that they reduce potential self-harm and allow clinicians to make therapeutic contact. Despite their tremendous medical potential, however, they can cause harmful side effects.

Volatile substances are CNS depressants and are found in three forms: volatile hydrocarbon substances, aerosols, and anesthetics. Abuse of volatile hydrocarbon substances includes glue sniffing and inhaling typing correction fluid and gasoline fumes; aerosol abuse includes inhaling propellants that have been used in deodorants and hair sprays; and anesthetic abuse includes inhaling more exotic solvents such as chloroform. Deliriants' psychophysiological effects include euphoria, confusion, and increased hilarity, and lead to sleep or coma. Research indicates that regular use leads to changes in kidney and liver functions and a reduction of appetite. The effect on the brain is still uncertain.

NOTES

[1]"Sedatives and Hypnotics: Alcohol and Drug Fact Sheet," *Drug Information Center (DIC)* (Eugene: University of Oregon, 1979).

[2]Ibid.

[3]Ibid.

[4]Pauline Postotnick, "Pregnancy and Drugs," *FDA Consumer* 12, no.8 (October 1978):7–10.

[5]"Barbiturates: Alcohol and Drug Fact Sheet," *Drug Information Center (DIC)* (Eugene: University of Oregon, 1979).

[6]Owen Davis, "Saving the Brain When Accident or Stroke Halts Oxygen," *Science Digest* 84, no. 3 (September 1978):39–42.

[7]Cited in M. Clark and B. Castel, "Saving Coma Victims," *Newsweek* 48 (May 22, 1978):20–22.

[8]"Barbiturates."

[9]"Methaqualone: Alcohol and Drug Fact Sheet," *Drug Information Center (DIC)* (Eugene: University of Oregon, 1980).

[10] Phillip Nobile, "Quaaludes' Abuse Creates Subtle Dangers," *Science Digest* 84, no. 6 (December 1978):53–55. Copyright © 1978 by Phillip Nobile. Reprinted by permission of The Harold Matson Company, Inc.

[11]"Methaqualone: A Dr. Jekyll and Mr. Hyde?" *Pharm Chem Newsletter* 2, no. 1 (1973):4.

[12]Nobile, "Quaaludes' Abuse."

[13]"Quaaludes 'Dead,' Drug Agents Claim," *Register Guard* (Eugene, Oregon), August 19, 1984, p. 17D.

[14]James R. Gamage and E. Lief Zerkin, "Inhalation of Volatile Substances," *National Clearinghouse for Drug Abuse Information* 25, no. 1 (October 1973):7.

[15]Ibid.

[16]John Pekkanen, "The Impact of Promotion on Physicians' Prescribing Patterns," *Journal of Drug Issues* 6, no. 1 (Winter 1976):14.

[17]Susan Edmiston, "The Medicine Everybody Loves," *Family Health* 10, no. 1 (January 1978):25–28.

[18]"Overcoping with Valium," *FDA Consumer* 13, no. 10 (December 1979–January 1980):21–23.

[19]Edmiston, "The Medicine Everybody Loves," p. 52.

[20]Charlotte S. Catz, "Diazepam in Breast Milk," *Drug Therapy* 3, no. 1 (January 1973):19.

[21]Penelope McMillan, "Women and Tranquilizers: A Special Report," *Ladies Home Journal* 93, no. 1 (November 1976):167.

[22]Annabel Hecht, "Tranquilizers: Use, Abuse, and Dependency: FDA Requirements," *FDA Consumer* 12, no. 8 (October 1978):20–33.

[23]"Overcoping with Valium," pp. 21–23.

[24]Mark Safra and Godfrey P. Oakley, Jr., "Association between Cleft Lip with or without Cleft Palate and Prenatal Exposure to Diazepam," *Lancet* 2 (September 13, 1975); and Betty Smith, "Tranquilizer Hazards," *Drug Survival News* 7, no. 2 (October 1978):5.

[25]R. E. Kron et al., "Neonatal Narcotic Abstinence: Effects of Pharmacotherapeutic Agents and Maternal Drug Usage on Nutritive Sucking Behavior," *Journal of Pediatrics* 88, no. 4 (April 1976).

[26]Elmar G. Lutz, "Allergic Conjunctivitis Due to Diazepam," *American Journal of Psychiatry* 132, no. 5 (May 1975):548.

[27]S. L. Hayes et al., "Ethanol and Oral Diazepam Absorption," *Drugs* 14, no. 1 (July 1977):68.

[28]Ibid., p. 69.

[29]Cited in Lutz, "Allergic Conjunctivitis," p. 166.

[30]Wendy Bant, "Diazepam Withdrawal Symptoms," *British Medical Journal* 4, no. 5991 (November 1, 1975):44.

[31]Gilbert Cant, "Valiumania," *New York Times Magazine,* February 1, 1976, p. 44.

[32]Sara J. White and Karen Williamson, "What to Watch for with Minor Tranquilizers," *RN* 42, no. 11 (November 1979):57–59.

[33]Robert M. Julien, *A Primer of Drug Action* (San Francisco: W. H. Freeman & Company Publishers, 1981), pp. 53–54, 122–23.

[34]Cited in "Anxiety and Pain over Valium and Darvon," *Science News* 115, 85, (1979):31.

[35]Kenneth L. Melmon and Howard F. Morvelli, "Basic Principles in Therapeutics," *Clinical Pharmacology* (1979):85.

[36]Cited in "Overcoping with Valium," pp. 1–4.

[37]"Overcoping with Valium," p. 22.

[38]Erich Goode, *Drugs in American Society* (New York: Knopf, 1984), pp. 88–89, 168. Copyright © 1984 Alfred A. Knopf, Inc. Used with permission.

[39]"Antipsychotics: Alcohol and Drug Fact Sheet," *Drug Information Center (DIC)* (Eugene: University of Oregon, 1979).

[40]M. D. Long, *The Essential Guide to Prescription Drugs,* 4th ed. (New York: Harper and Row, Pub., 1985), p. 923.

[41]*The Non-Medical Use of Drugs.* Final Report of the Commission of Inquiry (Ottawa: Crown, 1973), p. 439.

[42]James Gamage and E. Lief Zerkin, "The Deliberate Inhalation of Volatile Substances," *National Clearinghouse for Drug Abuse Information* 30, no. 1 (1974):4.

[43]Ibid.

[44]*The Non-Medical Use of Drugs,* p. 4.

[45]Gamage and Zerkin, "The Deliberate Inhalation of Volatile Substances," p. 4.

[46]"Volatile Substances: Alcohol and Drug Fact Sheet," *Drug Information Center (DIC)* (Eugene: University of Oregon, 1980).

[47]*The Non-Medical Use of Drugs,* p. 443.

ALCOHOL
america's number one drug problem

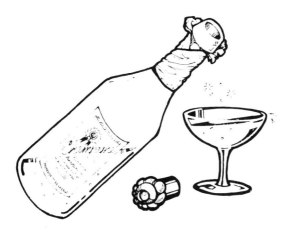

INTRODUCTION _____

You have asked me how I feel about whiskey. Well, here's how I stand on the question. If, when you say whiskey, you mean that devil's brew, the poison spirit, the bloody monster that defiles innocence, dethrones reason, destroys the home and creates misery, poverty, yes, literally takes the bread from the mouths of little children, if you mean the evil drink that topples the Christian man from the pinnacle of righteous, gracious living and causes him to descend to the pit of degradation, despair, shame, and helplessness, then I am certainly against it with all my heart.

But, if when you say whiskey, you mean the oil of conversation, the philosophic wine, the ale consumed when good fellows get together, that puts a song in their hearts and laughter on their lips, the warm glow of contentment in their eyes; if you mean Christmas cheer, if you mean the stimulating drink that puts the spring in an old man's footsteps on a frosty morning, if you mean the drink whose sale puts untold millions of dollars into our treasury which are used to provide tender care for our little crippled children, our blind, our deaf, our dumb, our pitiful aged and infirm, to build highways and hospitals and schools, then certainly I am in favor of it. This is my stand and I will not compromise.[1]

In view of such feelings toward alcohol, it is not surprising that the drug is one of the most widely used and abused by people of all ages and backgrounds in our society. There are approximately 90 to 100 million regular users of alcohol, and 9 to 12 million classified as alcoholics. Alcohol leads to more problems for individuals, families, and society as a whole than any other drug in the United States.

Alcohol is classified as a CNS depressant that produces analgesia. Several alcohols (ethyl, n-butyl, and amyl) are produced by the fermentation process, in which certain yeasts convert the carbon, hydrogen, and oxygen of sugar and water into ethyl alcohol and carbon dioxide. Most natural fermentation will lead to about 14 percent alcohol. Distillation, a process in which alcohol is added to an already fermented beverage, produces a higher alcoholic content, often more than 50 percent by volume. Ethyl alcohol (100 percent ethanol) is also known as absolute alcohol. *Proof* refers to the percentage of pure alcohol in a beverage. The percentage of alcohol is always half the proof (100 percent alcohol would be 200 proof). A common tale on the origin of the term *proof alcohol* dates back to early America, when alcohol was used to help ignite gunpowder. Unless the alcohol concentration in the powder was at least 50 percent, the gunpowder would not ignite. Table 8–1 indicates the approximate percentage of alcohol in various beverages.

Consumption of alcohol worldwide is increasing as more and more countries become industrialized. The alcohol industry is becoming more concentrated as distilleries and breweries fast become multinational companies. This trend is leading to the production of all kinds of alcohol. What this means is not that beer-drinking countries are giving up their beer and wine-drinking countries their wine, but that all are adding beverages over and above these preferred drinks.[2]

CONSUMPTION OF ALCOHOL IN THE UNITED STATES

It is clear that Americans are drinking more beer than wine or distilled spirits. Per-capita consumption for Americans fourteen and older is nearly thirty gallons of beer each year. This is equivalent to 320 twelve-ounce cans of beer. Americans consume nearly as much ethanol from beer (49 percent) as from wine (12 percent) and distilled spirits (39 percent) combined.[3]

Youth

The proportions of tenth, eleventh, and twelfth graders who have ever consumed alcohol has stabilized at a fairly high level: 87 percent of those surveyed reported having had a drink at some time in their lives.[4] Approxi-

TABLE 8-1   Approximate Percentage of Alcohol in Various Alcoholic Beverages

Alcoholic Beverage	Percentage of Alcohol by Volume
Table Wines (still, white, sparkling, red, and rosé)	10–22
Aperitifs, dessert wines, flavored wines	17–20
Beer	3–6
Ale	6–8
Hard cider	5–10
Whiskey	42–52
Brandy	40–50
Rum	34–46
Gin	37–50
Vodka	37
Liqueurs	30–65

mately 15 percent of adolescent drinkers surveyed reported drinking at least once a week and consuming five or more drinks per drinking occasion. Thirty-one percent of tenth, eleventh, and twelfth graders surveyed reported being drunk at least six times a year, and 2 percent reported experiencing adverse consequences from consumption two or more times a year. Among American high school students, 93 percent have tried drinking, and 71 percent drink at least once a month. Of these latter, about 6 percent drink daily.[5] Only marijuana and smoking surpass alcohol in daily use. In total consumption, alcohol remains the drug consumed in the greatest quantity.

Adults

In 1979, self-reported consumption for U.S. adults did not show drastic changes from previous years. Approximately one third reported moderate (24 percent) drinking or 3–5 drinks per week.[6] Although two thirds of the adult population drinks, about half of all alcoholic beverages sold are consumed by only 16 million (or about 11 percent) of those eighteen and older.

The Elderly

The excessive use of alcohol and resulting addiction is a significant problem not only for young people and adults but also for many elderly people. There has been a general belief that as people age, they cut back on their drinking because of declining health. However, it is estimated that from 2 to 10 percent of the aged are alcoholics, with generally higher rates for widowers and lawbreakers.[7]

HISTORY

According to paleontologists, the ingredients necessary to synthesize alcohol (sugar, water, yeast, and heat) were present on earth at least 200 million years ago. Evidence of the drug's use dates back to 6400 B.C.; both intoxicating beverages (wines and stronger drinks) as well as their effects were well known to the Egyptians, ancient Hebrews, Greeks, and Romans.[8]

The date of the discovery of distillation remains a mystery. The Arabians were apparently distilling alcohol by A.D. 900, however, and in the mid 1600s a Dutch physician distilled alcohol by using juniper berries in an effort to produce a diuretic. The diuretic, known as *jenever,* was later called gin.[9]

Alcohol in colonial America consisted mainly of beer, wine, hard cider, and rum. Political and social problems concerning alcohol in the United States led to the "Whiskey Rebellion" in Pennsylvania in 1794 and the temperance movement, which culminated in 1920 with the passage of the Eighteenth Amendment and its prohibition of the manufacture and sale of any alcoholic beverage. Prohibition endured for thirteen years but still did not eliminate the problems associated with alcohol.

WHY DO PEOPLE DRINK?

There are many reasons why people drink. Reasons often offered by junior-high students include

1. acceptance by peers
2. the smart thing to do
3. a way to forget troubles
4. habit
5. advertising
6. movies
7. examples set by older people
8. taste
9. rebellion against authority

These reasons can apply to people of every age who drink. Moderate drinking is thought to aid in socialization and the reducing of tension.

Advertising

When alcohol is advertised to consumers, it is often depicted as a way to gain greater health, sexier lives, rugged individualism, and social sophistication. Its sphere of influence is shown to encompass recreation, work, and business; it's promoted as a casual yet indispensible part of social life. Through advertising, alcohol, like hundreds of thousands of other products, has become a part of our national buying pattern.

Alcohol in its various forms is being produced in larger quantities and is readily available for purchase. The alcohol industry is a major advertiser that heavily promotes its product. A progressively more concentrated group of giant conglomerates are promoting alcohol products through mass advertising, which is a tax-deductible business expense. The alcohol industry's budget for its advertising is many times greater than all the funds spent publicly and privately each

TABLE 8–2   Top Fifteen Magazines in Distilled–Spirits Advertising

Rank	Magazine	Total Adv. (millions)	Liquor Adv. (millions)	Percentage of Liquor Adv.
1	*Newsweek*	$98.9	$12.3	12
2	*Time*	91.0	9.8	8
3	*Sports Illustrated*	71.3	7.7	11
4	*Playboy*	32.7	6.8	21
5	*U.S. News & World Report*	41.0	4.2	10
6	*TV Guide*	45.1	3.4	2
7	*Penthouse*	15.3	3.0	20
8	*New Yorker*	25.8	2.9	11
9	*People*	19.8	2.8	14
10	*New York*	11.3	2.4	21
11	*Cosmopolitan*	21.6	2.1	10
12	*Business Week*	62.3	1.6	2
13	*Psychology Today*	7.8	1.4	18
14	*Ebony*	13.3	1.3	10
15	*Gourmet*	4.1	1.2	28
TOTAL	All Members	$1480.5	$81.0	5

Source: Meyer Kalzper, Ralph Byback, and Marc Hertzman, "Alcohol Beverage Advertisement and Consumption," *Journal of Drug Issues* 8, no. 4 (Fall 1978): Table 1, p. 350.

year on alcohol-prevention campaigns. A recent annual tabulation showed that the distilled-spirits industry spent $160 million on advertising, the beer industry more than $100 million, and the wine makers more than $50 million.[10] The top fifteen magazines in terms of value of distilled-spirits advertising are listed in Table 8–2.

Peer Acceptance, Search for Adulthood, and Rebellion

It seems extremely important for young people to feel accepted by their peers. It is also important to them to be thought of as adult, or in control of their own lives. These two points, in combination, are reasons for teenage drinking. Many teenagers drink to take on the role of adults, and many others drink to be accepted by that group. Young people seem to regard drinking as a badge of adulthood, of virility. They also see it as a way to rebel against adults or society in general when they feel thwarted by them.

Studies show that most adults drink for recreation and enjoyment. Alcohol makes one feel good. Small amounts of alcohol cause a euphoric, relaxed feeling. After a couple of drinks everything looks better and problems seem less devastating. Drinking helps people to feel more comfortable and less inhibited during social gatherings, thus making it easier to get to know others and enjoy themselves.

Small amounts of alcohol can truly enhance many situations. It's when alcohol gets to be *the* situation that the problems begin to occur. Alcoholics and potential alcoholics increase their dependence on alcohol to constantly make situations easier and more enjoyable. Instead of having a few drinks at the party, they will have a few drinks just to feel like going to the party.

Changing Sex Roles

Changing sex roles have affected the numbers of women with alcohol problems. Women who have left the home and entered the traditionally male working world are encouraged by advertising to consume greater quantities of alcohol. Their involvment in more extensive social and business situations exposes them to heavy drinking, and the increased stress they undergo in new roles may also lead to alcoholism. Women now make up about fifty percent of all alcoholics.

Gender and Culture

Self-reported consumption of alcohol by males in 1979, as before, was different from that by females, particularly in the abstainer and heavier-drinking categories.[11] Twenty-five percent of males reported abstaining, versus 40 percent of females. In the heavier-drinking category, males (14 percent) outnumbered females (4 percent). In the lighter-drinking category, females (38 percent) outnumbered males (29 percent). Self-reported moderate drinking was greater for males (31 percent) than for females (18 percent).

According to researchers at Washington University National Alcohol Research Center in St. Louis, "the differences in drinking frequency between men and women are probably the result of cultural rather than genetic factors."[12] In other words, women often abstain from drinking or drink less than men because drinking is considered less appropriate behavior for women. Changes in women's drinking patterns in the future will probably reflect changes in these attitudes. At present more men turn to alcohol and more women turn to tranquilizers as a drug of choice.

Sex

Alcohol consumption before sex is very popular because it can reduce inhibitions and often induces a sense of increased arousal. What alcohol does is make sex more fun to think about, but that's the extent of it.[13] As Shakespeare recognized, "Drink sir . . . provokes desire, but it takes away the performance." Recent research has agreed with this statement: tests have revealed that more alcohol causes less physical arousal, regardless of what the person thinks. Another study showed that alcohol caused testosterone levels in males to drop to as much as five times less than normal.

A recent study of the effects of alcohol on women's sexual behavior determined that drinking seemed to enhance feelings of womanliness.[14] The study noted, however, that alcohol hindered their subjects' ability to gain satisfying interactions with men. The study also found that heavy-drinking women were generally more sexually active than nondrinkers or light drinkers. These women were also found to have had sex more frequently at an early age and were currently more sexually active than their lighter- or nondrinking counterparts. Citing their inability to develop satisfying relationships, the study indicated that heavy-drinking women were unable to receive sexual fulfillment much of the time and tended to have a lower regard for feminine ideals.

PHYSIOLOGICAL EFFECTS

"Alcohol is a depressant that acts as an anesthetic on the CNS. It is absorbed unchanged in the stomach and small intestine and is disseminated by the blood to all parts of the body, including the brain."[15] Though people may feel stimulated and less inhibited after drinking an alcoholic beverage, their central nervous system is actually being depressed. Problem drinkers and alcoholics should be greatly concerned about these effects, since the mortality rate for alcoholics is about 2.5 times that for the normal population.[16]

Circulatory System and Blood

Pulse rate and total blood flow are increased by the consumption of alcohol. "In moderate quantities, alcoholic beverages slightly increase the heart rate, slightly dilate blood vessels in arms, legs, and skin, moderately lower blood pressure, stimulate appetite, increase production of gastric secretion, and markedly stimulate urine output."[17] Levels of lipoproteins (substances in the blood consisting of various fats and proteins) are also affected: high-density lipoproteins increase and low-density lipoproteins decrease. This may be why recent reports indicate that daily consumption of small to moderate amounts of alcohol can prevent drinkers from heart disease.[18] Chronic excessive use, however, causes lesions in the muscular tissue of the heart and can lead to congestive heart failure.

Recent studies by the National Heart, Lung, and Blood Institute reveal that moderate drinking (one to two drinks a day) and exercise are linked to higher levels of blood protein which in turn appears to help protect against coronary heart disease (CHD).[19] Research findings suggest that moderate drinking increases the level of high-density lipoproteins (HDL). These proteins, it is felt, may clear away cholesterol deposits from the walls of coronary arteries. Previous research indicated that low-density lipoproteins (LDL) carry cholesterol, which leads to fatty deposits in blood vessels and increased coronary risk. By contrast, HDL appears to remove cholesterol from the body. Recent studies, including the Framingham Heart Study, have shown that persons with high levels of HDL were less likely to suffer heart attacks.

However, caution should be used in increasing alcohol consumption, since it has long been known that in healthy humans alcohol doses equivalent to two to five ordinary drinks (30 to 75 millileters) slightly increase heart rate, blood pressure (systolic more than distolic), and cardiac output.[20] In other words, regular consumption of large amounts of alcohol, regardless of race or sex, is associated with a substantially higher prevalence of high blood pressure. Furthermore, as W. P. Castell, director of the Framingham Heart Study, has stated, some "people are born with a biological makeup that can enhance the additive qualities of alcohol."[21] He pointed out that "it could be very dangerous to tell some people that two drinks a day will be good for them when their makeup will not allow them to stop at two. Thus, what starts out as prudent advice may turn into advice that could lead to cardiac death from alcohol myopathy (toxic disorder of the heart muscle), rather than to an extension of life by lower coronary atherosclerosis (fatty deposits)."[22]

When people begin drinking, they become relaxed and euphoric; they may say and do things they would not do under normal circumstances. When their blood alcohol content reaches .05 to .10 percent, however, a depressant action begins to interfere with ability to function. Most states hold .10 blood alcohol content to be the point of legal intoxication—the point at which people can no longer safely operate an automobile.

At .10 to .20, the onset of additional CNS depression makes it more obvious that a person is intoxicated. The individual may not be able to walk a straight line, close his or her eyes, touch fingers together, or perform other simple motor activities. At .20 to .30, a drinker is highly intoxicated. At this point, control is lost and the drinker may change from being the life of the party to being strongly sedated. When blood alcohol reaches .40 to .50, the drinker becomes unconscious. At .50 to .60, death may occur.

Blackout may occur with almost any level of alcohol in the body, though usually it is experienced at higher levels of intoxication and after chronic alcohol intake. Blackout is a temporary form of amnesia. While the individual is drinking, he or she is conscious, ambulatory, and appears in control. On the following day, however, much of the time spent drinking is completely forgotten. Blackouts are thought to be an early warning signal in the progression toward alcoholism.

The percentage of alcohol in the blood can be estimated by the number of drinks consumed in relation to body weight. Table 8–3 shows the number of drinks a person needs to reach a blood alcohol level, or concentration, of .08 in one hour. Pacing alcohol consumption over a longer period will help to prevent intoxication, as will having food in the stomach, since food helps slow absorption.

Prolonged use of substantial amounts of alcohol has been found in a large proportion of patients with unexplained cardiomyopathy, a heart-muscle disease, who make up 2 to 3 percent of those hospitalized for heart disease. But abstinence from alcohol produces a good recovery rate in early stages of the disease and can lead to marked recovery even in advanced stages.[23] Also, brief drinking sprees by apparently healthy individuals can result in premature heartbeats or a total loss of rhythmic beating in the heart's upper chambers—the "holiday heart syndrome." Whereas most population studies suggest that moderate drinkers suffer fewer major coronary events, studies of problem drinkers and alcoholics show the opposite.

Table 8–3   Number of Drinks in a One-hour Period Needed to Reach Approximately a .08% BAC

Weight Kg.	Lbs.	Number of drinks						
45	100	1	2					Legal
54	120	1	2	3				Oregon
63	140	1	2	3				BAC Limit for
72	160	1	2	3	4			Driving:
81	180	1	2	3	4			.08%
90	200	1	2	3	4	5		
99	220	1	2	3	4	5	6	
108	240	1	2	3	4	5	6	

One drink = 1.05 oz. of 80-proof liquor = 5 oz. of 12% wine = 12 oz. of 5% beer.

Nervous System

Chronic alcoholism has been shown to cause brain damage in a number of individuals. In fact, many studies have suggested that at least 50 percent of people who have been drinking heavily for years will develop some sort of brain disorder by the time they are forty.[24] Such alcohol-related brain damage may at least partially reverse itself once a person stops using alcohol. One study reported that parts of destroyed brain cells actually begin to grow back after alcohol use has been discontinued.

Alcohol's first CNS-depressing action is exerted on the cerebrum, the part of the brain responsible for inhibitions, judgments, and reasoning. When this area is sedated, thought processes become jumbled and disorganized. The finer grades of discrimination, memory, concentration, and insight are also dulled and finally submerged. When the cerebrum is affected, the cerebral cortex is also restricted. Motor processes become disrupted, and quick changes in mood and outbursts can occur.

The cerebellum, the part of the brain that controls the senses, is affected next. Vision dims, the field of vision eventually narrows; sound becomes distorted and hearing levels are lowered. Gradually the remaining senses—smell, taste, and touch—are also impaired.

The last part of the brain to be affected is the medulla, the vital brain center that monitors respiration. When alcohol sedates the medulla, respiration may be impaired and breathing may eventually cease.

The potentially damaging effects of alcoholism on the brain are of increasing concern. Light and moderate social drinkers appear to experience a loss of some intellectual abilities, even when sober, as a result of drinking. The degree of impairment appears directly related to the amount the social drinker usually consumes each time he or she drinks; frequency of drinking does not appear important.[25] A survey of Detroit workers indicated that although impairment appears to diminish as consumption does, in a dose–response manner, it is still measurable at very low alcoholic levels. And although drinkers may not be clinically impaired, their subtle loss in cognitive powers could significantly interfere with everyday functioning, particularly intellectual activities. Long-time social drinkers, especially those who notice that liquor affects their memory, may wonder if alcohol is having some sinister cumulative effect on their ability to remember. According to Elizabeth Loftus, the evidence suggests that years of partygoing take no inevitable toll. However, it seems that as far as memory is concerned, it would be better to have one drink every day than to save up until Saturday and splurge with seven drinks.[26] Even though the same amount of alcohol is ingested in both cases, the effects on the brain are apparently different. *The amount of alcohol consumed in one setting is critical.* As research continues, additional insight should be gained into the effects of moderate drinking on the brain.

Brain atrophy has been reported in anywhere from 50 to 100 percent of alcoholics.[27] New evidence suggests that heavy social drinking may also result in brain atrophy. The notion that brain damage from chronic alcohol abuse is irreversible is being reexamined. Several studies have shown partial reversal of brain atrophy and neuropsychological impairment in the abstinent alcoholic. Researchers have suggested that the brain damage often accompanying chronic alcohol abuse is not caused solely by malnutrition. That is, those areas of the brain that are particularly vulnerable to ethanol damage—the hippocampus (part of the cerebral cortex) and the cerebellum—are affected by some as yet unclear aspect of chronic alcohol abuse distinct from malnutrition. Although the precise destructive action of alcoholism remains a mystery, members of the research team have formulated several hypotheses. They suggest that ethanol— or its metabolite acetaldehyde—could be indirectly toxic by inhibiting protein synthesis in the brain. Or it could be that alcohol serves to obstruct the flow of blood to areas of the brain that mediate functioning.

Liver

Cirrhosis of the liver is one of the more serious physiological problems related to alcohol. Statistical evidence linking cirrhosis and alcohol consumption include the following:

1. cirrhosis is seven times as common in heavy drinkers as in nondrinkers.
2. there is a high association of the extremes of high intake (1.5 gallons per capita) and low intake (.5 gallons per capita).
3. there is a positive relationship between increases in intake, amount, and duration on the one hand, and cirrhosis on the other.[28]

Some scientists think that proper nutrition will provide effective protection against cirrhosis. Others have indicated that alcohol itself appears to be toxic to the liver, and that physicians should caution alcoholic patients not to rely on a nutritious diet as a safeguard and continue alcohol abuse.[29] After the ingestion of relatively small amounts of alcohol, the accumulation of fat in the liver can be detected. Cirrhosis is the sixth leading cause of death of adults in the United States, and it is estimated that alcohol is directly toxic to the liver when nutritional factors were controlled.[30]

Acetaldehyde, the intermediate by-product of alcohol metabolism, appears to be one of the major villains in the onset of alcoholic drinking, and the trouble probably begins in the liver. Researchers have found that the same amount of alcohol given to alcoholics and nonalcoholics produced much higher blood acetaldehyde levels in alcoholics. It is thought that this is due in part to a malfunctioning of the liver's enzymes. Also, the rate of breakdown of acetaldehyde into acetate is performed at about half the normal rate, apparently because of the accumulation of acetaldehyde.

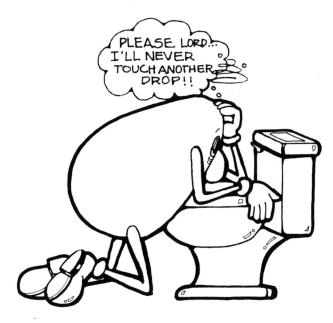

Digestive System

Moderate alcohol use may help the digestive system since it causes an increased flow of saliva and gastric juices. It may also help by alleviating distressing moods that are interfering with digestion. Alcohol may also harm digestion, however, by irritating and inflaming the linings of the oral cavity, esophagus, and stomach. The pyloric sphincter, a muscle valve that separates the stomach from the small intestine, will contract and cause vomiting when sufficiently irritated by alcohol.

Kidneys

When alcohol is consumed, blood vessels in the kidneys dilate, causing increased urine production.[31] Increased urine production is also caused when alcohol affects the brain centers responsible for maintaining body water. Excessive use of alcohol can cause permanent kidney damage.

Body Temperature

Ingestion of alcohol induces a false feeling of warmth because it increases blood flow to the skin and stomach. Actually, the increased blood flow may cause increased sweating, resulting in rapid heat loss and the lowering of the body temperature. Large amounts of alcohol will depress the hypothalamus, the mechanism that controls body temperature, also resulting in a decrease in body temperature. Thus, drinking alcoholic beverages to keep warm in cold environments not only doesn't work but may actually facilitate hypothermia (subnormal body temperature).

Fetal Alcohol Syndrome

In 1973, the term *fetal alcohol syndrome* (FAS), was coined to designate the pattern of growth retardation, physical defects, and mental retardation found in infants born to women who drank heavily and extensively during pregnancy.[32] The Department of Health, Education and Welfare has estimated that in 1978, 1500 children were affected by fetal alcohol syndrome.

How much alcohol can cause FAS? The degree of damage to the fetus is relatively proportional to the level of alcohol consumed by the mother. Drinking less than one ounce of absolute alcohol per day appears to lower the apparent risk of birth defects, but a completely safe level of alcohol consumption, short of no consumption, has not yet been determined. The National Institute on Alcohol Abuse and Alcoholism recommends that not more than two mixed drinks or their equivalent in beer or wine be consumed daily during pregnancy.[33] The National Council on Alcoholism has recommended complete abstinence throughout pregnancy.[34] For the regular or moderate social drinker (two drinks a day, with no drinking problem), the risk of having a child with one or more FAS abnormalities approaches 19 percent. The risk of FAS or various combinations of the symptoms in children of problem-drinking or alcoholic women may be 40 percent or more. If heavy drinking occurs during the first three months of pregnancy, there is an increased incidence of FAS abnormalities; if drinking continues beyond the first three months, the size, weight, and nutritional status of the child are also likely to be affected.[35]

Cancer

Heavy alcohol consumption has been related to increased risk of cancer at various sites, especially the mouth, pharynx, larynx, and esophagus. Cancer risk is further increased for heavy drinkers who also use tobacco.[36]

Testosterone Level

Numerous studies have shown that acute or chronic ingestion of alcohol results in lowered testosterone in the serum of males of all species. This reduction may cause impotency, loss of libido, breast enlargement, loss of facial hair, and testicular atrophy in many male alcoholics.[37]

EFFECTS OF DRINKING ON THE INDIVIDUAL AND SOCIETY

A recent national survey emphasized the *social* rather than physical effects of drinking.[38] Adverse social effects include economic costs, interpersonal problems (a spouse, friend, or relative either threatened to break off the relationship or actually did so), problems with the police (being questioned, warned, or arrested for drinking or drunkenness), and automobile or other accidents involving personal injury or property damage.

Economic Costs

Pinpointing the economic costs that alcoholism and alcohol use impose upon society is hindered by a lack of definitive measurements. The approximate $43 billion that has been given as an estimate has been criticized by some as inflated and by others as conservative. The former argue that none of the costs in the six categories listed in Table 8–4 may be attributed unconditionally to alcohol misuse. The cost of alcohol may run as high as 120 billion a year.

TABLE 8–4   Economic Costs of Alcohol Misuse and Alcoholism in the United States, 1975[39]

Item	Cost (in Billions)
Lost production	19.64
Health and medical	12.74
Motor-vehicle accidents	5.14
Violent crime	2.86
Social responses*	1.94
Fire losses	0.43
TOTAL	42.75

*Drunkenness, child abuse, noise making, generally disorderly

Job-Related Problems

Alcohol consumption even in minimal amounts tends to increase the rate of accidents at work. It is estimated that about 10 to 30 percent of occupational accidents may have been preceded by alcohol intake. Even in modest amounts, alcohol affects the reflexes and judgment of people in situations where there is a risk of accidents (driving or operating machines, working at heights, and so on) or those in a position of executive responsibility.[40]

There is evidence, especially from developed countries, that persons engaged in certain occupations are at particularly high risk of developing alcohol problems. Unfavorable psychological factors affecting conditions of work (such as isolation, monotony, low pay, pressure to increase output, and lack of career opportunities) may contribute to poor morale, stressful situations, and psychological disturbance. These in turn may encourage alcohol use and lead to a new set of problems.

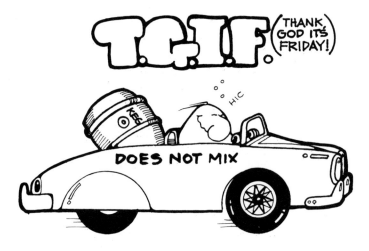

Motor-Vehicle Accidents

The third largest economic cost of drinking is that of alcohol-related motor-vehicle accidents. The drinking driver is a menace to everyone on the road. Alcohol impairs vision, coordination, judgment, sensation of speed, and depth perception, making the driver careless or uninhibited. Of the 50,000 people killed in traffic accidents each year, half are killed by drinking drivers; millions more are injured. The risk of motor-vehicle accidents tends to increase in proportion to the blood alcohol concentration of the driver.

In addition to motor-vehicle accidents, research has shown that alcohol is involved in about half of nonvehicle accidents. It is implicated, for example, in up to 50 percent of adult deaths from fires, and 50 to 68 percent of drownings.[41]

Crime

Alcohol is closely associated with certain forms of crime. Individuals under the influence of alcohol resort more frequently to physical assaults, domestic violence, disorderly conduct, and rape. More specifically, in the case of homicide, a blood alcohol level of above .10 has been found in 67 percent of the offenders who were determined to be drinking at the time of the crime. For aggravated assault, it has been estimated that alcohol was present in 80 percent of the offenders.[42] The combined cost of violent crimes and the social responses to alcohol problems is near $5 billion per year.

The Family

The family can be totally disrupted by a substance-abusing member(s). The whole family can eventually become a source of neurosis. The use of alcohol may increase financial or occupational problems (if money is spent on alcohol that should have been spent on food, clothing, or medical expenses). Children of alcoholics are a high-risk group for whom early intervention strategies are being developed and implemented. It is estimated that there are some 12 million such children in the United States, but that only 5 percent are receiving help.[43]

It should be emphasized that the family is also a powerful treatment milieu. Families can be a great source of strength in the recovery process and are becoming increasingly involved in the process of intervention in alcoholism.

Suicide

The risk of suicide among alcoholics is about thirty times greater than it is in the general population. Among Native Americans, five of the top ten causes of death are alcohol-related: accidents, cirrhosis, alcoholism, suicide, and homicide. Among ethnic groups, Native Americans appear to have the highest prevalance of drinking problems.[44] According to figures released by the Indian Health Service, suicide rates among Indians below thirty-five are 2.4 to 3.3 times as great as among all United States citizens in the same age groups.

Calvin Frederick, chief of the Disaster Assistance and Mental Health Section of the National Institute of Mental Health states,

> They don't feel they have anywhere to go. They're caught between a desire to move out of their own sphere into a more modern society and a desire to maintain the traditions of their old lives. Yet the realities of today make it impossible to continue their old way of life. They wind up frustrated. They drink heavily, become depressed, and become self destructive.[45]

The self-destruction takes the form of accidents, murders, and suicides.

ALCOHOLISM

What is Alcoholism?

There are some who believe alcoholism is a disease, and some who do not. One definition of alcoholism states that it is "a chronic disease, or disorder of behavior, characterized by the repeated drinking of alcoholic beverages to an extent that exceeds customary dietary use or ordinary compliance with the social drinking customs of the community, and which interferes with the drinker's health, interpersonal relations or economic functioning."[46] The American Medical Association (AMA) had earlier come to a similar conclusion, and in 1956 it formally acknowledged that alcoholism was to be included in the treatment realm of medical science. Furthermore, both the AMA and the American Bar Association have declared that alcoholics are entitled to the same rights and privileges under the law and the same medical treatment granted to persons with other diseases. The National Institute on Alcohol Abuse and Alcoholism views alcoholism as a treatable dysfunction from which as many as two thirds of those affected can recover (though they cannot return to drinking). Many states now allow chronic alcoholism to be a defense against drunkenness charges and refer chronic drunk drivers to appropriate treatment resources rather than sending them to jail.

Those who believe alcoholism is not a disease frequently cite the lack of a clear etiology (history and causes) of alcoholism as the reason for their disbelief. Claude Steiner, author of *Games Alcoholics Play,* is one of the most critical opponents of the disease concept. Steiner rejects the concept largely out of his interpretation of the term *disease,* which he feels is reserved for a condition in which there is a specific biochemical, microorganismal, or viral alteration. He and others also feel that the disease concept aims only at abstinence rather than control and prevention through education. Still others feel that:

> Alcoholism is a disease, it is the only disease that is bought and sold, and it is the only disease that is contracted by the will of man, it is the only disease that requires a license to propagate it, it is the only disease that requires outlets to spread it.
> If Alcoholism is a disease . . . it is the only disease that produces revenue for the government and it is the only disease that is habit forming, it is the only disease that provokes crime, it is the only disease that brings violent death on the highways, it is the only disease that is spread by advertising, and it is the only disease without a germ or virus cause. It just might be that it's not a disease at all.[47]

Many people still consider alcoholism to be untreatable, and consider the person with alcohol problems to be intractable and unwilling to be helped.

When discussing alcoholism, chemical dependency, and/or physiological addiction to alcohol, we need to keep the three phenomena of tolerance, withdrawal, and compulsive use in the forefront. Alcohol use is the response to drinking more and more because of the tolerance and withdrawal relationship. The same effects—illness, irritability, and sickness are associated with the absence of alcohol in the system. *Compulsive use* is a result of high tolerance and the desire to avoid withdrawal. It is the absolute need to keep the system saturated or medicated with the necessary quantity of alcohol.

Alcoholism is a chronic disease. In many cases it is present years prior to eventual diagnosis. It is a progressive disorder: left untreated, it intensifies. It is a disease, interestingly enough, that seems to continue despite sobriety; alcoholics who decides to resume their drinking behavior do not start at the beginning but continue where they would have been even had they not stopped drinking. Even in the absence of alcohol use, a number of characteristics of the disease seem to continue developing.

In a very genuine sense alcoholism, like many other chemical-dependency states, is incurable. There is no total eradication of the disorder. If one is to be free from the ravages of the disease, absolute and prolonged sobriety is the only alternative. Over the years, a number of clinicians in the medical and psychological arenas have struggled with this realization. More and more people, however, are coming to understand that sobriety is the only alternative to alcoholism and the death that inevitably results from it.

Alcoholism has a pathogenesis, in that any stage in the disintegration one can look back to the origins of the pathology and see the systematic deterioration occurring. Interestingly enough, the warning signals of the disease are very common among alcoholics, and the course of the deterioration has a very large number of similarities. This is not to say that once you've seen one alcoholic you've seen them all. However, to some degree this is true.

The biochemistry of the disease can be explained in fairly simple terms. The ethanol molecule, when ingested, is quickly metabolized in the blood system, primarily by the liver. The initial stages of metabolism by hepatic protein enzymes results in alcohol being transformed into acetaldehyde, which is closely related to the famous pickling agent formaldehyde. Because of its poisonous nature it is quickly transformed into acidic acid (vinegar) and then into carbon dioxide and water, which are eliminated through breathing and urination. This process occurs when normal drinkers consume alcohol. However, the metabolism of an alcoholic is dramatically different in one sense. Though most of the alcohol is transformed and eliminated in that fashion, approximately 1 percent of it is diverted to an alternative fate. It is this fate that results in biochemical dependency. This very small percentage of residual alcohol combines with the neurotransmitter dopamine to form an addictive alkaloid called tetrahydraisoquardrelone (THIQ). This substance is closely related to the opium family and morphine. Furthermore, THIQ combines with other neurotransmitters in the central nervous system to form other similarly addictive alcoholoids. It is now felt that for the most part these substances are not truly metabolized and eliminated from the central nervous system; they remain within the system to act, it appears, much in the same fashion as heroin. Hence, "once an alcoholic, always an alcoholic," for reasons similar to those causing opiate dependency. This explains why after twenty years of sobriety one may return to the use of alcohol.

Though the jury is still out on this theory, it also appears that several other supplemental factors are occurring simultaneously in a number of alcoholics. One of these is that the livers of many alcoholics have an insufficiency of ADH (alcoholdehydrogenase), which lowers their ability to metabolize alcohol at a sufficient rate. Hence, the active ingredient remains in the system longer in an alcoholic than in normal drinkers. One can hypothesize that this prolonged presence in the system allows more diversion of the alcohol to the "dopamine connection."

Furthermore it appears that a person can not only contract a carrier-type and pass it on through birth but can also become a transmitter even though there may be no prior history of alcoholism in the family. People from nonalcoholic family systems who eventually drink to the point of developing the disorder can transfer the disorder should they have children. Again, though the research is still being evaluated, it appears that these theories will eventually be proved true.

There is also a psychological component to this biochemical model that further predisposes one to alcoholism. The behavioral theory of learning has two major aspects: instrumental or operant conditioning and classical conditioning. The first includes the stimulus–response–reward relationship, in which a precipitating factor causes the individual to respond by consuming alcohol; the reward consists of the desired effects. One of the best examples is the five o'clock happy hour on Friday afternoon following a hard day (week) of work. People meet at their favorite watering hole to respond to that hard period of work by consuming alcohol for the desired effect of conviviality, good cheer, and relaxation. Most people drink in partial response to this behavioral principle. The stimuli may be varied, the response is to drink, and the rewards may also vary with the individual. The classical-conditioning aspect consists of anticipation of the reward prior to the consumption of alcohol. The anticipated feeling of relaxation furthers the reinforcement offered by that upcoming drinking episode.

Research psychiatrist Stanley Gitlow suggests that there is a progression to alcoholism. He points to the belief that alcoholics appear to suffer from stimulus augmentation. That is, their perceptions appear to be acute and their appetites (and a need for relief from them) are greater than those of nonalcoholics. He notes that his own clients exhibit a defective identification with the same-sex parent. More often than not in alcoholic family systems, sons are emotionally and physically estranged from their fathers and daughters from their mothers. Consequently, children growing up in these systems learn to distance themselves from people. This involves isolating themselves and eventually being unable to relate easily to others on an emotional basis. This is markedly different from families where alcoholism is not present and where normal bonding and nurturing occur.

Appetite needs are normally met by a dampening mechanism that comes from satisfactory interpersonal relations. But when a boy or a girl cannot relate effectively to the parent of the same sex, the normal mechanism for dampening down particular need is unavailable. Because of this alcohol offers a medicinal effect when consumed. Individuals in an alcohol-using society discover sooner or later that alcohol either allows them to relate to others or relieves them of the sense of need to do so. Either way, alcohol use is perceived by the alcoholic to be a solution. It is not an accident that Alcoholics Anonymous is as successful as it is because of the emotional bonding occurring within its group structure.

There are a number of stages in the disease of alcoholism, and they include the following:

1. *The well individual.* The use of alcohol has not yet damaged the individual's physical, social, or economic capacities. There is no reason for concern regarding his or her use of alcohol.

2. *The episodic-excessive drinker.* The frequency of drinking has begun to increase to the point where the individual is visibly intoxicated up to twelve times per year. Initial signs of health impairment do not necessarily include evidence of addiction. However, there may be secondary damage related to alcohol—trauma (a shock-like effect on the system) or accident—and primary damage related to alcohol (reversible). Other symptoms may include transient nutritional deficiencies that reverse with the cessation of drinking and proper nutritional treatment. There may be some economic costs as well from the standpoint of an employer expressing fear or concern over the individual's ability to function on the job.

3. *The habitual-excessive drinker.* The frequency of drinking continues to intensify to intoxication episodes equaling or surpassing thirteen times per year. Damage to health continues as in stage 2. Interpersonal and social relationships now begin to show signs of deterioration as the individual loses long-time friends, is separated or divorced, and so on. Social relationships now *necessarily* involve alcohol use and other heavy users. Economic costs progress to the loss of employment because of alcohol abuse. The individual may be temporarily employed in a special setting, one in which the employer has a specific interest in treating alcoholism and is inclined to tie job security to a treatment plan promoting recovery.

4. *Alcohol addiction; physiological changes.* The frequency of drinking has progressed to the point of inability to abstain even one day. Health continues to deteriorate: there is additional documentation of withdrawal symptomatology, including delirium tremens, hallucinations, shakes, sweats, whips-and-jangles seizures, and so on. Interpersonal and social relationships continue to deteriorate, as does the individual's capacity for financial self-support.

5. *Alcohol addiction; irreversible damage.* The frequency of drinking continues as in stage 4, with further evidence of permanent physiological deterioration. There are a variety of areas in which the body can be dramatically harmed, including hepatic, gastrointestinal, cardiovascular, and central and peripheral nervous systems. Furthermore, a variety of psychiatric concerns can develop, such as Korsicoff's syndrome and Wernicky's disorder. In this late stage of deterioration one can lose control of the bladder and bowels as well. These are only a few examples of the excessive medical deterioration that will develop in the late stages of alcoholism.

6. *Death.*

These stages of alcoholism include a variety of specific cognitive-behavioral indicators by which the disease can be diagnosed. Many of these indicators appear among virtually all alcoholics. Some of the indicators are as follows:

1. *Symptomatic drinking.* The drinker begins to use alcohol to satisfy conditions of his or her inner environment, for personal rather than social reasons. The social setting becomes an excuse, rather than the reason, for drinking.

2. *Increased tolerance.* The individual can drink more with less apparent effects. The psychophysiological systems adapt to the presence of the ethanol molecule so effectively that larger quantities of alcohol are tolerated.

3.   *Blackouts (alcoholic amnesia).* The individual has no recall of events during these periods, which can last from several minutes to several hours or days. During the blackouts the individual may not appear to be intoxicated and may carry on conversations or elicit a variety of other behavioral functions, such as driving a car with apparent control. However, at a later date the individual cannot remember any of the events taking place. Typical of this is the incident in which the individual wakes up the morning after a drinking bout not knowing how she got home or where she parked her car.

4.   *Sneaking drinks.* Because of his rising tolerance to alcohol and dependence on its anxiety-relieving properties, the individual needs to drink more in order to gain satisfaction from the experience. A need arises to find ways to consume more alcohol than his companions without revealing himself. The individual may drink before going to a party or bring along a concealed supply to be consumed away from companions. This is often quite confusing to his social-drinking friends who may see him becoming intoxicated while apparently consuming the same quantity as other guests. This is the same individual who is embarrassed when observed drinking in a secluded area.

5.   *Preoccupation with drinking.* Drinking has now become an increasingly important role in the individual's life and seems to dominate her thinking.

6.   *Gulping drinks.* The individual is becoming more and more concerned with the biochemical effects of alcohol and is less concerned with the social setting and conviviality.

7.   *Avoidance of references to drinking.* Sensing the change in his drinking behavior and probably experiencing some related guilt, the individual tends to avoid discussions of his drinking behavior. When such discussions are unavoidable, he understates the amount and frequency of his drinking. This is a hallmark characteristic of alcoholism.

8.   *Increased frequency of blackouts.* The fear and discomfort created by the frequency of blackouts is overshadowed by the individual's need to secure the medicinal effects of alcohol.

9.   *Loss of control.* Gradually, and often imperceptively to the individual, she exercises less and less control of her ability to control the amount, intending 1 or 2 and having 10–15. This loss of control often identifies itself in the form of a series of "benders." The individual may be able to abstain for relatively long periods of time, but with the first ingestment of a small quantity of alcohol a demand is set that ceases only when advanced intoxication makes further intake impossible—in other words, drinking to the point of passing out. Once drinking has begun, only situational or circumstantial factors stop it, such as running out of alcohol or money or becoming physically unable to continue drinking. Intervention on the part of concerned others will also stop drinking in this instance. The individual may seek to sustain a certain amount of alcohol in her system twenty-four hours a day.

10.   *Creation of an alibi system.* With loss of control the patient begins to develop a system of excuses. The individual believes these rationalizations and feels that his drinking is a result rather than a cause of the problems.

11.   *Reproof by family.* If the alcoholic is married, drinking will affect the family, materially and emotionally, and he will react with pleading, cajoling, threats, and a variety of other forms of emotional bribery in an effort to stop the alcoholic's drinking. Eventually the family rejects the alcoholic.

12.   *Extravagance.* The alcoholic will often become extravagant, "buying the house a drink." She may also make a variety of other money-spending displays, long-distance phone calls and unnecessary or costly purchases. Quite often these are done while she is intoxicated.

13.   *Aggression.* As the illness progresses the individual may reveal deep-seated but repressed hostility through aggressive behavior. He will often strike out at those closest to him—family members and close friends. The individual may also unconsciously

use this aggressive behavior as a means of seeking rejection to confirm his own feelings of inadequacy and to once again give himself an excuse for continued drinking.

14. *Persistent remorse.* Following periods of heavy drinking the alcoholic is plagued by persistent feelings of deep guilt and remorse, and on some level she is aware of the effect of her drinking on her own life as well as those of family members. This particular characteristic often involves the individual making sincere promises to herself and others to modify her drinking behavior. These attempts are usually unsuccessful.

15. *Water wagon.* The individual resolves to take control of himself in a very drastic fashion by stopping drinking altogether. Usually, however, he relapses and resumes his drinking patterns.

16. *Changes in drinking pattern.* After unsuccessful attempts to go on the wagon, the alcoholic will try other forms of controlling her drinking—switching types of beverages, drinking only at certain times or only in certain places, and so on.

17. *Loss of friends.* By now the use of alcohol has become so problematic that the individual begins to lose even his best friends. At this point, because of the rejection of people he has known over a period of time, the individual is forced to drink with people he may at one point have considered his inferiors. However, these are people with whom he shares a common denominator—alcohol dependency.

18. *Vocational difficulties.* The impact of the person's alcoholism interferes with her ability to secure and maintain gainful employment. Typically, she drinks on the job, is absent because of hangovers, is late for work, and is less productive and more hazardous in her behavior. Frequent job changes and firings occur.

19. *Changing family habits.* The individual's family pattern changes in response to his unpredictable behavior. The family begins to withdraw from social and community activities, and the children's performance in school, for instance, begins to drastically deteriorate while they also isolate themselves from their peers. Hostility, guilt, and aggression strain the family atmosphere to the breaking point.

20. *Medical complications.* Many alcoholics experience physical difficulties due in part to their generally poor nutrition and the presence of extremely high amounts of alcohol and acetaldehyde in their system. A variety of medical disorders can occur.

21. *Resentment.* The individual becomes increasingly resentful of her growing isolation from the community, her family, and her friendship group. A certain amount of paranoia and suspiciousness culminates in feelings of persecution.

22. *The geographic cure.* With his world falling around him and having failed to abstain or modify his drinking behavior, the alcoholic may attempt to control his drinking by seeking a completely new environment. This means packing the bags and moving; it may or may not include the family.

23. *Protecting the supply.* The illness has reached such a point that alcohol is the only salvation. It is the only means of escaping from or dealing with a world that is increasingly frustrating and painful. The thought of being caught without the ability to drink becomes frightening. At this point the individual will foresake almost everything else to safeguard the means of supplying alcohol.

24. *Morning drinking.* The medicinal value of alcohol has now become so necessary that the individual starts drinking from the moment she gets up. This drinking continues throughout the day and into the evening, when the individual literally drinks herself to sleep. Morning drinking is often done in response to severe hangovers as well.

25. *The moment of truth.* At this point the alcoholic has reached rock bottom. He is at the crossroads in his life, death faces him squarely. He has reached his moment of truth and is finally forced to make a decision between life and death. The sad reality is that thirty-five of thirty-six alcoholics not in treatment (not choosing prolonged sobriety) die!

Causes of Alcoholism

Although research indicates a significant relationship between hereditary (genetic) factors and alcoholism, results from such research remain inconclusive. Since alcoholism occurs in the children of total abstainers, social environment may also be a factor. Physiological factors, such as nutritional deficiencies and/or lowered blood chloride levels, may additionally contribute to alcoholism. Acetaldehyde synthesis and metabolism from alcohol consumption may be the key to explaining biochemical alcohol dependency. Further research in all these areas is crucial.

Several studies focusing on genetic factors in alcoholism among twins indicate a genetic factor in drinking behavior. However, the evidence for a genetic determinant remains inconsistent. Studies done with adoptees, separated at an early age from their biological parents, indicate that sons and daughters of alcoholics are four times as likely to become alcoholics as are sons and daughters of nonalcoholics, whether raised by alcoholic parents or nonalcoholic parents.[48] In a study of familial incidence of alcoholism, "rates of alcoholism [were found to be] substantially higher in relatives of alcoholics than in relatives of non-alcoholics."[49] Among the conclusions from that study are these:

> almost one-third of any sample of alcoholics will have at least one parent who was an alcoholic; if one member of a family is an alcoholic, 82 percent of the time there is at least one other alcoholic in the family; while data support the widely held view that alcoholism can be a familial disease, it is important to realize that [this] is not sufficient to allow the finding of a hereditary or environmental etiology of alcoholism.[50]

There are some who feel that an "alcoholic personality" is a cause of alcoholism. According to this theory, individuals who find tension relief through alcohol may in time become behaviorally conditioned by the positive reinforcement. Unfortunately, research in this area is often contradictory and nonspecific. Researchers have found, however, significant relationships between a person's self-concept and alcoholism.[51] Alcoholics often have dependent personalities and lack a good self-image.

Women and Alcohol

In recent years there has been a marked increase in the number of reported female alcoholics, and some researchers estimate that nearly half of the country's 10 million alcoholics are female.[52] Although there is no typical alcoholic woman, nor are the exact causes of alcoholism known, there appear to be social and emotional problems that distinguish women alcoholics from men. In addition, female alcoholics seem to share certain physical characteristics and notable behavior patterns. For example, women alcoholics who have been the subjects of studies have said they felt warm, loving, considerate, and expressive when drinking.

For years there has been a double standard of acceptable behavior for women, one that does not include drinking. For example, the heavy-drinking man is often accepted but a heavy-drinking woman is often criticized.[53] In some social settings, drinking by women may be associated with sophistication and maturity. But in general, it has been stigmatized as immoral and a betrayal of a woman's "proper role" of wife and mother. It is becoming increasingly difficult for the modern woman to conform to society's expectations, to achieve the "superwoman" goal of playing the roles of career woman, wife, mother, lover, etc., while maintaining a sense of family.[54]

There are some indications that women's new lifestyle is changing their drinking habits and placing them in different drinking situations. A study of suburban and urban populations of women alcoholics showed that the suburban housewife is the most secretive in her drinking and the professional woman the least secretive.[55] The National Institute on Alcohol Abuse and Alcoholism (NI-AAA) reports that eight of ten working women, ages twenty-one to thirty-four, drink and that the average age has dropped during the 1970s from forty to thirty. In fact, almost two of three women now being treated for alcoholism are under thirty-five.[56] Also, there is a higher rate of alcoholism among employed women than among homemakers; married working women are especially prone.[57]

The guilt expressed by female alcoholics in treatment predominates most counseling sessions.[58] Their drinking is often covered and protected by spouse and family, which often delays them from seeking treatment. The husband is often embarrassed by his wife's drinking and feels it may reflect poorly on his masculinity, so he tries to hide the problem. Interestingly, a husband is more likely to leave a wife with alcohol problems than a wife is to leave an alcohol-abusing husband.[59]

There are some common physical and psychological characteristics among women alcoholics. Research has shown that problem drinking and alcoholism may progress faster in women than in men. One reason for this may be that men have approximately 10 percent more water in their bodies than women. Since alcohol is distributed throughout the body in proportion to the water content of body tissues, alcohol tends to be more diluted in the bodies of men than in those of women. Research suggests that women may become more intoxicated than men on the same amount of alcohol even when both have the same body weight. Women have less body fluid and more body fat, whereas men have more muscle tissue than fatty tissue. Therefore, since alcohol does not diffuse as rapidly in body fat as it does in water, the concentration of alcohol in a woman's blood will be higher than the concentration in a man's blood even when they consume the same amount of alcohol.[60] Studies also show that women who are about to experience their menstrual period become more intoxicated than other women. In other words, a woman's changing sex-hormone levels may be related to the effect alcohol has on her.

Treatment and Rehabilitation Services

Though myths, stigmas, and misunderstandings make it difficult for the alcohol-dependent person to obtain the help he or she needs, a wide variety of facilities, programs, and agencies do exist to treat alcoholism. The philosophies and methods of these programs differ, but the ultimate goal of each is to either stop or control the intake of alcohol. Generally available services include alcoholism-information programs, general hospitals, mental-health facilities, and rehabilitation clinics. Halfway houses, outpatient clinics, community human-service organizations, and volunteer-run organizations such as Alcoholics Anonymous (AA) are also located in many areas.

Volunteer-Run Organizations   Alcoholics Anonymous is probably the best-known alcoholism-treatment organization run by volunteers. Unlike other organizations, AA does not participate in political or public policy action related to either the causes of or the problems associated with alcoholism. Its activities are devoted only to maintaining and encouraging abstinence by alcoholics.

The National Council on Alcoholism (NCA) is another organization run exclusively by volunteers. It provides national leadership in public alcoholism education, advocates increased government involvement in alcoholism treatment, and provides knowledgeable consultants. The NCA also works at the community level by offering information and referral services to problem drinkers and their families.

The Center of Alcohol Studies at Rutgers University is a third group staffed by volunteers. The center provides information and documentation services for the entire alcoholism field, sponsors numerous summer-school symposiums for training professional staffs of state alcoholism programs, and participates in continuing research, documentation, publishing activities, and the establishment of alcoholism programs. The center publishes the *Quarterly Journal of Studies on Alcohol,* one of the leading research journals in its field.

General Hospitals   Until recently, general hospitals offered little or no treatment for alcohol dependents. The American Hospital Association now has a national plan, however, to promote alcoholism programs in all general hospitals and to extend such programs into community treatment systems for alcoholics.[61] Hospital admission policies have also been changed in order to admit alcoholics into general wards with the diagnosis of alcoholism. Specialized wards in certain hospitals have been made available to the nonprofessional community to provide and conduct alcoholism programs.

Intermediate Care (Halfway Houses)   After trying and failing many times to move the alcoholic from the therapeutic milieu back into community life, alcoholic rehabilitation workers saw the need for some form of intermediate care. The result of this need was the halfway house, where information about alcoholism could be disseminated, shelter and security provided, and residents eased back into a life of sobriety and community living. Halfway houses are sometimes given governmental support, but are usually run by nonprofit community groups interested in alcoholism treatment and recovery. Professionals may be available for medical or psychological treatment.

Treatment Approaches

Drug Treatment For many years, various drugs have been used to treat alcoholic patients. Recently, however, clinical examinations and controlled double-blind studies have shown that these drugs are not as effective as they had been thought to be.[62] The early success of most of the drugs appears to have been due to the patient's eagerness to be cured, rather than to the drugs' ability to cure. Some of these drugs, however, including disulfiram (antabuse), tranquilizers, antidepressants, and lithium are still utilized in treating alcohol dependency, but they are only one component of a total treatment program.

DISULFIRAM (ANTABUSE) Alcohol ingestion causes an increased acetaldehyde concentration in the blood. Antabuse appears to inhibit liver enzymes that are needed to oxidize acetaldehyde, producing symptoms that serve as a deterrent to further alcohol drinking.[63]

Antabuse has a slow absorption rate, and may take from three to twelve hours to become effective. Tolerance and dependency do not develop, but the interaction of the drug with alcohol may produce numerous adverse effects, such as a rise in blood pressure, deep flushing, a sensation of warmth, decreased respiratory efficiency and oxygen debt, accelerated heart rate, severe dizziness, nausea, and vomiting. A rapid fall in blood pressure, unconsciousness, and death are also extreme possibilities. Antabuse should therefore be administered only after a complete physical examination and under close medical supervision.

Despite widespread use of Antabuse, some clients can have serious adverse reactions to the drug, including strong psychotic reactions. In fact, the widespread practice of court-mandated Antabuse therapy for repeat alcohol offenders may not be producing the intended effects, since the best treatment rates with Antabuse are seen when clients voluntarily admit themselves to an Antabuse program.[64]

TRANQUILIZERS AND ANTIDEPRESSANTS Tranquilizers and antidepressants are an inexpensive way to treat large numbers of patients. The goal of such treatment is to reduce patient anxiety and concomitantly the need for alcohol.[65] Efforts to determine these drugs' effectiveness have been relatively few. However, the results of a double-blind study of ten different psychopharmacologic agents indicated that none of the drugs was superior to a placebo in producing *significant* abstinence.

LITHIUM Lithium, a soft metal belonging to the alkali group, has recently been used in the treatment of alcoholism. Researchers at Memorial University in Newfoundland report that 36 percent of patients undergoing lithium treatment were still abstaining from alcohol after six months of treatment.[66]

Detoxification Detoxification, the process by which a substance foreign to the body is changed to a compound or compounds more easily excretable, is the necessary first step in the successful rehabilitation of an alcohol dependent. Most detoxification programs do not require expensive or elaborate medical facilities, but many alcoholics entering such programs need specific medical attention.

Self-Help Programs   There are several groups whose supportive interaction helps members to remain sober. As we have noted, the most well-known of these groups is Alcoholics Anonymous, co-founded in 1935 by two alcoholics who were searching for a self-help approach to alcoholism.

AA membership does not require dues, only the admission of being an alcoholic and the desire to stay sober while helping other alcoholics do the same. AA depends primarily on a spiritual approach and unselfish devotion to other recovering alcoholic members.[67] Rehabilitation includes discussion of day-to-day problems.

There are three other groups related to AA: Al-Anon, Al-a-teen, and Al-a-tot. Al-Anon was founded around 1940 when wives of AA members found that they too had problems—coping with alcoholic husbands (early AA groups were invariably *all men*) and finding ways in which they could help their husbands fight alcoholism.[68] Supportive discussion is the key to Al-Anon's effort, and with the increasing number of female alcoholics the group now has male members as well.

Al-a-teen came into being in 1957 because many children of alcoholics felt uneasy trying to relate to older people in Al-Anon groups. These children were often embarrassed and distrustful, and were more willing to seek and accept advice from their contemporaries. Al-a-tot was founded for similar reasons to help preteenage children of alcoholics. Both groups are supported and sponsored by Al-Anon.

The question often arises, "Can alcoholics become social drinkers?" In the majority of cases the answer is no. According to AA philosophy, a return to normal or social drinking is impossible because of the alcoholic's biophysiological makeup. AA remains steadfast in its belief that alcoholism is a progressively irreversible disease characterized by the inevitable loss of control over alcohol use. Some recent studies, however, conclude that some alcoholics can return to social drinking, but these cases seem to be the exception, not the rule.

Crisis Intervention   Treating alcoholism is a long process that involves not only the alcoholic but also his family. There are many methods of treatment, but the first step in any process of detoxification is for the alcoholic to admit he has a problem and make a commitment to do something about it. Often this comes about because of a crisis in the alcoholic's life that is a direct result of alcohol abuse. For example, he might have received a drunk-driving ticket, had an automobile accident when he was drunk, lost his spouse when she couldn't deal with the problem any longer, or hurt himself or someone else while under the influence. Once the person admits to having a problem, *then* he can be treated.

Sometimes this takes "tough love" on the part of family members or friends. This means that the alcoholic is not protected or sheltered but instead is confronted with the facts. Specific written documentation of what has happened when the alcoholic drinks must be presented to the alcoholic in a nonemotional, nonthreatening manner. Such an approach will help lead to early intervention. In a nutshell, this is the approach called crisis intervention.

Sometimes, though, the family and friends of the alcoholic are referred to as *co-alcoholics*, because without realizing it they help the alcoholic to continue living her life with the problem. For example, they might constantly bail her out of jail, make excuses for her, or even give her the money to buy her alcohol. They need help just like the alcoholic does. Intervention, if carefully worked out early, can do a great deal to stop alcoholism in its early stages.

Group Therapy   Regardless of the medical treatment needed, the alcohol dependent will usually participate in a counseling or psychotherapy program to help deal with immediate problems and to recognize factors underlying drinking patterns. Such treatment seems to be most effective when employed by a group of men and women similarly affected.

Psychodrama, a method of learning through role playing, is a treatment method often used in group therapy. Its primary goals are to improve the individual's failing self-image[69] and to improve sociopsychological behavioral patterns. Psychodrama has proved effective because of its ability to deal with the variety of problems, personalities, and situations confronting the alcoholic.

FAMILY THERAPY   Family therapy is an outcropping of group therapy. In this form of treatment, relatives, including adults, teenagers, and younger children, take an active and responsible part in the rehabilitation of the alcohol dependent. The method allows families to receive help together and helps nonalcoholic family members to accept and appreciate their own feelings while assisting in the alcohol dependent's recovery. There are indications that family therapy offers the most effective psychological approach to recovery for many alcoholics (especially those with strong, supportive families).

Abstinence   Since midcentury abstinence-oriented ideology has dominated the strategies and procedures used to treat alcoholism. This ideology holds that the alcoholic is unable to regulate his or her rate of alcohol intake, that this loss of control is inevitable and irreversible, and that any return to normal or socially accepted levels of consumption is impossible.[70]

THE MOVEMENT AGAINST DRUNK DRIVING _____

Mothers against Drunk Drivers

MADD is a grass-roots movement whose members are concerned citizens, men and women, victims and nonvictims. Its goals are first to keep the issue of drunk driving alive by making people aware of the problem and second to mobilize the public to help individuals modify their drinking habits so they choose to make drunkenness and drunk driving socially unacceptable.

MADD was started by Candy Lightner, whose daughter Cari was struck and killed by a drunk driver near her home in Fair Oaks, California. The driver that hit Mrs. Lightner's daughter had a prior arrest for hit-and-run driving and drunk driving and had been released from custody on bail only two days before killing Cari. The driver was sentenced to two years in prison but was made to serve only sixteen months in a work camp. Angry and frustrated, Candy Lightner protested a judicial system that allowed someone with an extensive history of drunk driving to continue to drive. She finally decided to develop a powerful nationwide group to do something about it.

In addition to the goals mentioned above, MADD is engaged in educating citizens on how they can be individually responsible, organizing community efforts to fight drunk driving, reforming laws relating to drunk driving, and conducting programs for victims of drunk-drivers. MADD has been very successful in reducing the legal blood alcohol content in various states and has initiated several effective programs to limit drinking and driving.

Students against Driving Drunk

SADD was started in September 1981, as part of a mandatory health-education program for sophomores at Wayland High School near Boston, Massachusetts. The program was developed under the leadership of Robert Anastas, who has made curriculum materials for others desiring to start a SADD program. The students organized for the following reasons: to help save their own lives and the lives of others; to educate students on the problem of drinking and driving; to develop peer counseling among students about alcohol use; and to increase public awareness and prevention of alcohol abuse everywhere.

The students realized that drunk driving began to appear as a death threat to them personally and to their generation. Since they felt it was their problem, they wanted to provide leadership in preventing deaths and injuries. The program is gaining popularity and spreading throughout the country. One attractive feature of the program is the teenager–parent contract:

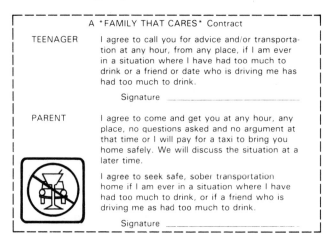

A *FAMILY THAT CARES* Contract

TEENAGER   I agree to call you for advice and/or transportation at any hour, from any place, if I am ever in a situation where I have had too much to drink or a friend or date who is driving me has had too much to drink.

Signature _____

PARENT   I agree to come and get you at any hour, any place, no questions asked and no argument at that time or I will pay for a taxi to bring you home safely. We will discuss the situation at a later time.

I agree to seek safe, sober transportation home if I am ever in a situation where I have had too much to drink, or if a friend who is driving me as had too much to drink.

Signature _____

This type of approach keeps communication open between parents and teenagers.

RESPONSIBLE DRINKING ——————————————————

It should be stressed that the vast majority of social drinkers imbibe for pleasure and other beneficial effects. Some feel the time has come to inform those who choose to drink to do so in a responsible manner—in moderation. It is estimated that there are over 100 million regular alcohol users in the United States and approximately 10 million or more alcoholics. A considerable amount of energy has gone into encouraging abstinence, and enormous sums of money have been spent on the problem of alcoholism. However, what is being done for the over 90 million social drinkers to keep them from losing control?

It appears that the social drinker will receive greater attention in the future. A few suggestions are being offered. One suggestion is to limit alcohol consumption to one drink per hour. One drink is defined as 12 ounces of beer, *or* 4 ounces of wine *or* 1.5 ounces of eighty proof distilled liquor. Going beyond this amount can lead to problems. Another suggestion is not to mix alcohol with other drugs because of possible synergistic effects.

The following guidelines can help you prevent drunkenness if you are hosting a social gathering:

Don't serve alcohol only. Many people will behave responsibly when other beverages are available.

Serve food first. The more food in the stomach, the slower the rate of alcohol absorption. However, avoid serving salty snacks: they just make people more thirsty.

Don't serve alcohol to someone who already appears intoxicated.

Don't allow an intoxicated person to drive.

When necessary, advise guests that they should drink responsibly at your social functions.[71]

SUMMARY ——————————————————

Alcohol-related problems far exceed problems related to any other psychoactive drug found in the United States. The psychological effects of drinking affect almost every sector of society; the physiological effects range from loss of coordination to death. Prolonged drinking may lead to cirrhosis of the liver, brain impairment, heart problems, and fetal alcohol syndrome.

There has been a national recognition of the problems associated with irresponsible drinking. Groups such as Mothers Against Drunk Driving (MADD) and Students Against Driving Drunk (SADD) have been able to create a national awareness about not drinking and driving. States are lowering the limits for legal intoxication and many drivers are volunteering to remain sober while others drink.

Individuals are more aware of driving in a responsible manner. Also, through increased education and television programs the general public is better informed about what to do if a person's drinking is getting out of control. It is no longer necessary to hit rock bottom before getting help for alcoholism. Many individuals go for crisis intervention approaches prior to having serious drinking problems.

Though the debate still continues over whether alcoholism is a disease, hospitals, intermediate care facilities (halfway houses), and drug-treatment and detoxification programs all work to help the alcoholic. In addition, self-help groups, group therapy, and family counseling provide support systems for medical care.

NOTES

[1]Wayne Polen, Garen Len, and Gail Vive, *Alcoholism: A Treatment Manual* (New York: Gardner Press, 1979), p. 14.

[2]"Worldwide Consumption Continues to Climb," *U.S. Journal of Drug and Alcohol Dependence* 5, no. 2 (March 1981): 19.

[3]*Alcohol and Health,* Fourth Special Report to the U.S. Congress from the Secretary of Health and Human Services (Rockville, Md.: National Institute on Alcohol Abuse and Alcoholism, 1981).

[4]*NIAAA Information and Feature Service* No. 82, New York: National Clearinghouse for Alcohol Information, (Rockville, Md. April 1, 1981):4.

[5]National Institute on Drug Abuse, *Student Drug Use in America: 1975–81* (Rockville, Md.: National Clearinghouse for Alcohol Information, 1981).

[6]*NIAAA Information and Feature Service No. 82, (*April, 1, 1981), p. 4.

[7]Oscar J. Kaplan, *Psychology of Aging* (New York: Academic Press, 1979) pp. 212–13.

[8]Richard H. Blum et al., *Society and Drugs* (San Francisco: Jossey-Bass, 1970).

[9]Ibid.

[10]Meyer Kalzper, Ralph Ryback, and Marc Hertzman, "Alcohol Beverage Advertisement and Consumption," *Journal of Drug Issues* 8, no. 4 (Fall 1978): 339–53.

[11]*Alcohol and Health,* p. 4.

[12]*NIAAA Information and Feature Service* No. 81 (March 1981).

[13]"Drugs and Alcohol: The Aphrodisiacs That Aren't," *Executive Fitness Newsletter* 2, no. 17 (August 23, 1980):1–2.

[14]Richard A. Zucker, Victor A. Battistach, and Ginette B. Langer, "Sexual Behavior, Sex-Role Adaptation to Drinking in Young Women," *Journal of Studies on Alcohol* 42, no. 5 (May 1981):457–65.

[15]David A. Works, *New Hope, New Responsibilities* (Washington, D.C.: Department of Transportation, 1974), p. 7.

[16]*NIAAA Information and Feature Service,* No. 84 (June 1, 1981):6.

[17]National Institute of Mental Health, *Alcohol and Alcoholism* (Chevy Chase, Md., 1970), p.22.

[18]See, for example, Charles H. Hennekens et al., "Effects of Beer, Wine, and Liquor in Coronary Deaths," *Journal of the American Medical Association* 242, no. 18 (November 2, 1979).

[19]*Alcohol and Health,* p. 30.

[20]W. P. Castell, "Editorial," *Journal of the American Heart Association* 242, no. 18 (1985):2000.

[21]Ibid.

[22]Ibid. p. 4.

[23]Ibid.

[24]"Alcohol Brain Damage: Circle the Wagons," *Science News* 116 (October 20, 1979):262.

[25]"Alcohol and Brain Damage," p. 262.

[26]Elizabeth F. Loftus, "Did I Really Say That Last Night? Alcohol, Marijuana, and Memory," *Psychology Today* 13, no. 10 (1980):48. Reprinted with permission from *Psychology Today.* Copyright © 1980 American Psychological Association (APA).

[27]"Alcohol-Related Brain Damage Subject of Research," *NIAAA Information and Feature Service,* no. 81 (April 1, 1981):4.

[28]N. Spritz, "Review of Literature Linking Alcohol Consumption with Liver Disease and Atherosclerotic Disease," *American Journal of Clinical Nutrition* 32, no. 12 (December 1979).

[29]"Liver Hurts Livers, Regardless of Diet," *Journal of the American Medical Association* 228, no. 4 (April 22, 1974).

[30]Fifth Special Report to the U.S. Congress on Alcohol and Health from the Secretary of Health and Human Services. December 1983, DHHS Publication No. (ADM) 84-1291. Printed in 1984, p. 8.

[31]N. Kessel and H. Walton, *Alcoholism* (London: MacGibbon & Kee, 1965), p. 25.

[32]See K. L. Jones et al., "Pattern of Malformation in Offspring of Chronic Alcoholic Mothers," *Lancet* 1, no. 7815 (June 9, 1973):1267–71.

[33]S. Cohen, "The Fetal Alcohol Syndrome: Alcohol as a Teratogen," *Drug Abuse and Alcoholism Newsletter* 7, no. 4 (May 1978).

[34]"Fervent Support for FAS Concerns," *U.S. Journal of Drug and Alcohol Dependence* 1, no. 11 (December 1977):70.

[35]L. B. Robe, "Alcoholic Drinking During Pregnancy," in *Just So It's Healthy* (Minneapolis: Comp. Care Publications, 1977).

[36]*NIAAA, Information and Feature Service,* No. 32, April, 1981, p. 4.

[37]Jones et al., "Pattern of Malformation," p. 1267.

[38]*Alcohol and Health,* p. 25.

[39]*NIAAA, Information and Feature Service,* No. 82, April 1, 1981 p. 5.

[40]Ibid., pp 4–5.

[41]Ibid., p. 5.

[42]"Counting the Cost," *Bottom Line* 3, no. 4 (August 1980):10–14.

[43]*NIAAA, Information and Feature Service,* No. 82, April 1, 1981, p. 5.

[44]Ibid., p. 4.

[45]Quoted in ibid., p. 3.

[46]Department of Health, Education and Welfare, *Alcohol and Alcoholism* (Rockville, Md., 1981).

[47]Claude Steiner, *Games Alcoholics Play.*

[48]David Rutstein, Richard Veech, and D. Phil, "Genetic Factors and Alcoholism," *New England Journal of Medicine* 298, no. 20 (May 18, 1978):1140–41.

[49]Nancy Cotton, "The Familial Incidence of Alcoholism," *Journal of Studies on Alcohol* 40, no. 1 (January 1979):89–112.

[50]Ibid.

[51]Albert J. Yakichuk, "A Study of the Self-Concept Evaluations of Alcoholics and Nonalcoholics," *Journal of Drug Education* 8, no. 1 (1978):41–47.

[52]"The New Alcoholics," *Glamour Magazine,* March 1983.

[53]J. Langone. *Women Who Drink* (Reading, Mass.: Addison-Wesley, 1980), p. 2.

[54]Ibid.

[55]E. N. Corrigan, *Alcoholic Women in Treatment* (New York: Oxford University Press, 1980).

[56]"A Special Redbook Report," *Redbook,* June 1982, p. 77.

[57]"The New Alcoholics," p. 18.

[58]"Female Alcoholics: Are They Different?" *Focus on Family,* November/December 1984, p. 16.

[59]Ibid.

[60]*Here's to Your Health: Alcohol Facts about Women* (Washington D.C.: U.S. Government Printing Office, Department of Health and Human Services, 1981), p. 2.

[61]*Alcohol and Health,* Special Report to the U.S. Congress by the Secretary of Health, Education and Welfare (Rockville, Md., Department of Health, Education and Welfare, U.S. Government Printing Office, 1974).

[62]Ibid.

[63]John Guarnaschelli, Edward Zapanto, and Frederick Pitts, "Intercranial Hemorrhage Associated with the Disulfiram-Alcohol Reaction," *Bulletin of the Los Angeles Neurological Societies* 37 (January 1972):19–23.

[64]"Antabuse: A Special Report," *Amethyst Multnomah County Alcohol and Drug Scene* 3 no. 7 (September 1979).

[65]E. J. Larkin, *The Treatment of Alcoholism: Theory, Practice and Evaluation* (Toronto: Addiction Research Foundation of Ontario, 1974), p. 19.

[66]"Lithium Treatment for Alcoholics," *Science News* 114, no. 16 (October 14, 1978).

[67]National Institute on Alcohol Abuse and Alcohlism, *Treating Alcoholism* (Washington, D.C.: Department of Health, Education and Welfare, 1974). p. 10.

[68]Morris E. Chafetz and Harold W. Demono, *Alcoholism and Society* (New York: Oxford University Press, 1962), p. 167.

[69]Ruth Fox, *Alcoholism: Behavioral Research, Therapeutic Approaches* (New York: Springer, 1967), p. 218.

[70]E. M. Jellineck, *The Disease Concept of Alcoholism* (Chicago: Hillhouse Press, 1960), p. 1.

[71]Drug Information Center, *Using Alcohol Responsibly* (Eugene: University of Oregon, 1983).

9

OPIATES

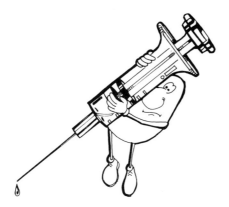

NONSYNTHETIC OPIATES

Opiates, sometimes called narcotics, are drugs derived from opium (the thickened juice of the opium poppy) that are used to induce sleep and relieve pain. Opium has been in existence since at least 4000 B.C., when it was known as "the plant of joy."[1] Raw opium was highly regarded by the early physicians Hippocrates in Greece and Galen in Rome, and spread into Europe and China during the first century A.D.

In 1805, the major active constituent of opium, an alkaloid, was isolated and named morphine after the Greek god of dreams, Morpheus. Codeine, another alkaloid, was isolated approximately thirty years later. Heroin, a semi-synthetic drug produced by synthesizing acetic anhydride (a common industrial acid) and morphine, was produced in 1874. With the use of these drugs and the invention of the hypodermic needle, opiates were employed freely and approved of for general use. In 1906, the American Medical Association even believed heroin to be nonaddictive, though this error was discovered some time later.

Many reasons are given for the widespread use of opium, but according to Norman Taylor, a noted botanist,the main reasons are that it is cheap to produce, readily available, and the greatest chemical flight from reality known.[2] Opium's unlicensed cultivation is forbidden in most countries, but it is grown nonetheless in Turkey, Asia Minor, Macedonia, Yugoslavia, Bulgaria, Iran, China, and India, and transported for distribution. Raw opium can be prepared for smoking by dissolving, boiling, roasting, or fermenting. Americans seldom use opium in its raw state, however, but use its derivatives, morphine and heroin.

Smoking or eating opium produces dullness or stupor, and, in larger doses it may produce sleep, coma, or even death. Tolerance and physical dependence will result with repeated use, as will psychological dependence. Once dependence has set in, opium users often don't continue to take the drug to seek a high but rather to remain free from withdrawal symptomatology.

Morphine

Morphine is about ten times stronger than opium and takes effect much more rapidly. It can be pure white, off-white, or light brown and can be purchased as a cube, capsule, tablet, or powder, or in solution. Intravenous injection gets the medication into the bloodstream for immediate transportation, but use of hypodermic syringes must be carefully regulated so that drugs are injected in the proper dosage and so that dirty needles which lead to such conditions as hepatitis, blood poisoning, and endocarditis (inflammation of the membranes lining the heart), are avoided.

Morphine acts as a primary and continuous depressant on respiratory action in the brain stem.[3] It decreases the amount of oxygen and carbon dioxide that is exchanged, depresses the coughing center, and stimulates the vomiting center.[4] Some researchers also believe that free morphine leaves the blood and concentrates in tissues such as the kidneys, liver, and lungs.[5]

Individuals intoxicated by morphine have pinpoint pupils that do not react to light. If they inject the drug frequently, vein membrane walls break down, eventually forming scar tissue referred to as *tracks*. Although the blue discoloration caused by the needle may disappear, the tracks will remain permanently.

Heroin

When first synthesized in 1874, heroin was thought to be a cure for morphine addiction. It was soon discovered, however, that heroin is two times as likely to produce dependency as morphine, and that it is ten times stronger than morphine. It is usually found as a white, odorless, crystalline powder that dissolves in water.

Since heroin is a CNS depressant, drowsiness follows injection, the pupils constrict, respiration and pulse are slowed, and, after large doses, coma or death may occur. The danger of dependency seems to be greater than for other opiate agents because tolerance develops more rapidly (about twice as fast as with morphine).

Chronic use of heroin by pregnant women may result in a variety of obstetrical complications.[6] Heroin dependency may cause poor nutrition and inadequate hygiene, and may involve other drugs, which can contribute their own complications. Babies born to chronic users also run the risk of congenital heroin dependence and may need special care for several weeks following delivery, though withdrawal symptoms may not show. Many of these infants have low birth weights, but this has not been attributed to heroin use alone.

Since the beginning of the 1980s, researchers have tried to find more about what heroin does to pregnant women and the developing fetus. "There are an estimated 100,000 women of childbearing age in the United States and they give birth to almost 10,000 babies each year."[7] Some of the effects of addiction can be passed on to a fetus, leading to retardation, behavioral abnormalities, and delayed development of the muscular and nervous systems. Even methadone and other heroin substitutes can cause these problems. Symptoms will occur in about 75 percent of newborns of heroin-dependent mothers. Methadone-dependent mothers will almost always have infants that go through withdrawal symptoms. Another major reason for problems with newborns is that heroin-dependent mothers rarely have proper prenatal care.[8]

Withdrawal Symptoms   Symptoms of withdrawal from heroin can be violent and long-lasting.

About 12 or 24 hours after the last dose, the addict may fall into a tossing, restless sleep known as the "yen," which may last several hours but from which he awakens more restless and more miserable than before. As the syndrome progresses, . . . dilated pupils, anorexia (loss of appetite), gooseflesh, restlessness, irritability, and tremor [set in] . . . at 48 to 72 hours . . . the patient exhibits increasing irritability, insomnia, marked anorexia, violent yawning, severe sneezing, lacrimation, and coryza (inflammation of nasal mucous membrane with profuse nasal mucous discharge). Weakness and vomiting are common, as are intestinal spasm and diarrhea. Heart and blood pressure are elevated. Marked chilliness, alternating with flushing (skin reddening) and excessive sweating is characteristic. Pilomotor activity (contraction of skin's smooth muscle causing hairs to stand erect) resulting in waves of gooseflesh (curtis anserina) is prominent, and skin resembles that of a plucked turkey. This feature is the basis of the expression "cold turkey" to signify abrupt withdrawal without treatment. Abdominal cramps and pains in the bones and muscles of the back and extremities are also characteristic, as are the muscle spasms and kicking movements that may be the basis for the expression "kicking the habit. . . ."

The failure to take food and fluids, combined with vomiting, sweating and diarrhea, results in marked weight loss, dehydration, . . . and disturbance in acid-base balance. Occasionally there is cardiovascular collapse. . . .

. . . In addition, there seem to be subtle behavioral manifestations of protracted abstinence that include an incapacity to tolerate stress, a poor self-image, and overconcern about discomfort.[9]

Nonphysical Dependence   According to Stewart, de Witt, and Eikelboom, recent behavioral and neuropharmacological findings suggest that opiates (and stimulants) act on common neurochemical systems of the brain to generate appetitive states that maintain drug behavior.[10] It has become clear, they say, through comparative study of drug self-administration by humans and by laboratory mammals that there is a particular affinity of the regulation of appetites by the brain for depressant drugs such as heroin and morphine. Their study of the reactions of animals to these drugs is not only directly relevant to our understanding of drug abuse, but may provide us with important information about the control of appetitive behavior and about the neural substrate of the motivational systems of the brain.[11]

It has been demonstrated that physical dependence is not necessary for opiates to be sought and taken. Yet the prevailing view has been that continued self-administration of opiates is a function of the need to reduce or avoid withdrawal. Stewart and colleagues quote other studies that show that the initial acquisition of opiates that are self-administered can occur rapidly in an animal having no previous drug experience, and that opiate use can be maintained over long periods at doses too low to bring on withdrawal or deprivation.

Likewise, the conditions surrounding relapse to drug taking by individuals who have been drug-free for long periods suggest that avoidance of withdrawal or desire to reduce need does not provide an adequate account of drug-taking behavior. Reexposure to the environment previously asociated with drug taking leads to relapse in a large percentage of experienced but drug-free individuals, even after prolonged abstinence.

Maddox and Desmond studied the effect of opioid use on 248 addicts in San Antonio for three years. They found that moving away from the environment of regular use led to abstinence, but upon return to San Antonio, 81 percent of the addicts relapsed within one month.[12] Three reasons they suggest for abstinence through relocation are reduced availability, separation from conditioned stimuli, and separation from models. In short, physical dependence may not be the only reason people crave drugs.

Heroin-Related Deaths   For opiate dependents who do not kick the habit, opiate poisoning (overdose) can occur. Numerous deaths have been attributed to overdoses, though some researchers in the field suggest that many of these deaths were *not* a result of too much heroin. For example, Edward Brecher states that

> "virtually all the victims whose deaths are falsely labeled as due to heroin overdose . . . are addicts who have already developed a tolerance for opiates and even enormous amounts of morphine or heroin do not kill addicts. . . . A conscientious search of the United States medical literature throughout recent decades has failed to turn up a single scientific paper reporting that heroin overdose, as established by these or any other reasonable methods of determining overdose, is in fact a cause of death among American heroin addicts."[13]

When an individual dies in the absence of a physician who can determine the cause of death, it becomes the duty of the local coroner or medical examiner to determine it. Following the autopsy, no coroner wants to find himself faced with inquiries from the press, police, and anxious family members without knowing the cause of death. Milton Halpern, a physician, states that

> in some fatal acute cases, the rapidity and type of reaction do not suggest overdose alone but rather an overwhelming shocklike process due to sensitivity to the injected material. The toxicologic examination of the tissues in such fatalities, where the reaction was so rapid that the syringe and needle were still in the vein of the victim when the body was found, demonstrated only the presence of alkaloid, not overdosage. In other acute deaths, in which the circumstances and autopsy findings were positive, the toxicologist could not even find any evidence of alkaloid in the tissues or body fluids. Thus, there does not appear to be any quantitative correlation between the acute fulminating lethal effect and the amount of heroin taken.[14]

Others interested in drug abuse have identified the sugar and quinine adulterants often added to heroin as the true culprits of overdose-attributed deaths. Michael M. Baden, one-time deputy chief medical examiner of New York City, states that

> the majority of [heroin] deaths are due to an acute reaction to the intravenous injection of the heroin-quinine-sugar mixture. This type of death is often referred to as an "overdose" which is a misnomer. Death is not due to a pharmacological overdose in the vast majority of cases.[15]

Further speculation about heroin-related deaths centers in the area of synergism. On many occasions, heroin is used with other CNS depressants, such as alcohol and barbiturates, and combining such drugs may amplify their chemical effects, causing death. Administering an opiate to an already depressed central nervous system may simply be too severe.

Three of the most publicized overdose deaths of the 1970s were those of rock performers Jimi Hendrix, Janis Joplin, and Jim Morrison (of the Doors). In particular, Janis Joplin "drank like an F. Scott Fitzgerald Legend."[16] On October 19, 1970, shortly after her death, *Time* reported,

> The quart bottle of Southern Comfort that she held aloft onstage was at once a symbol of her load and a way of lightening it. As she emptied the bottle, she grew happier, more radiant, and more freaked out. . . . Last week, on a day that superficially at least seemed to be less lonely than most, Janis Joplin died on the lowest and saddest of notes. Returning from her Hollywood room after a late-night recording session and some hard drinking with friends at a nearby bar, she apparently filled a hypodermic needle with heroin and shot into her left arm. The injection killed her.[17]

. . . Not to mention the Southern Comfort. However, her death was attributed strictly to overdose.

Medical Uses   On the legitimate-use side, a five-year study was conducted by the Sloan-Kettering Cancer Center in New York on the efficacy of various analgesics. Heroin was included in this study since there has been growing support for making heroin available to terminally ill cancer patients experiencing intractable pain (pain so intense that patients are aware of nothing else). Present medication provided to such patients is either given in dosages too small to help or must be continually increased because tolerance is reached. Available studies suggest that heroin would aid terminal patients with intractable pain, but legislators and others are afraid legalization will increase street use.

Proponents of heroin use for terminally ill patients with intractable pain feel that such use is safe and invaluable. Surprisingly, the use of heroin in this way alone does not lead to addiction even when it is administered regularly.[18] In the United States, various groups have actively sought to reintroduce heroin into the medical community. The following two acts, among others, show that their voices are being heard:

1. The Compassionate Pain Relief Act (H.R. 5290) would give physicians the freedom and responsibility to provide heroin to patients who need it. H.R. 5290 also states specifically that heroin would be available only to cancer patients whose pain is not relieved by conventional analgesics.
2. The Waxman Bill (as amended and approved in March 1984 by the Committee on Energy and Commerce) would allow distribution of heroin according to prescriptions written by physicians registered under section 302 of the Controlled Substances Act, and then only through hospitals, pharmacies, or hospices.[19]

A growing number of people, especially in Great Britain, where heroin is legal, feel that the lawful availability of heroin poses no greater security threat than similar drugs do. The Heroin Movement created in 1974 by the National Committee for the Treatment of Intractable Pain has helped foster in the United States initial efforts in pain research, terminal care, and studies on the comfort of patients.[20] Pain control is discussed openly on rounds: nurses and doctors are beginning to be concerned now not about addiction but about giving enough of the right narcotic to the suffering patient. American medicine appears to be giving serious consideration to placing heroin on the prescribed drug list.

Great Britain has been administering heroin and morphine to terminally ill patients with intractable pain for a number of years. Both drugs are prescribed in English hospices and treatment centers. Hospices, in fact, often prefer heroin to morphine because it has fewer side effects (less nausea and vomiting, reduced constipation potential, reduced anorexia) and is highly soluble in water, making it a substantially stronger analgesic.

Codeine

Codeine, derived from morphine, is less effective than morphine in inducing sleep and alleviating pain. It is widely used in cough medicines through which it appears to exert analgesic and antitussive (cough-reduction) effects on the central nervous system. It is also found in pills for treating various types of mild to moderately severe pain. Little is known, however, about the location and nature of codeine's effects.

In therapeutic doses, the side effects of codeine are seldom serious, but may include such gastrointestinal reactions as nausea, vomiting, constipation, and dizziness. The drug possesses a certain potential for dependence, but the incidence of codeine drug abuse does not remotely approach that of morphine or heroin. The lethal dose of codeine is not known with certainty.[21]

SYNTHETIC OPIATES

Methadone

Methadone is a synthetic narcotic classified as a CNS depressant whose effects are similar to those of morphine, though they develop more slowly and persist longer.[22] First synthesized during World War II, the drug is currently approved for uses in reduction of severe pain and in detoxification and maintenance treatment for opiate dependents. Methadone is a white crystalline powder that is soluble in alcohol and water and may be injected or drunk.

Because methadone maintenance and detoxification programs have become widespread in the past five years, more methadone has been available on the illicit market and "drug-program abuse" is frequent. Diversion of medication, missed medication, lost medication, medicine supplementation, multiple registrations of patients, and other forms of program abuse exist throughout the country.

Physical Effects   When taken into the body, methadone produces a loss of appetite, constriction of pupils, sweating, reduced respiration, elevated blood sugar levels, constipation, the release of antidiuretic hormones, drowsiness, and impotence. It has less hypnotic action than morphine but is very dependency-producing. Methadone is absorbed rapidly after administration—within ten minutes it can be found in significant concentrations in plasma. Like other opiate analgesics, it quickly leaves the blood and localizes in the lungs, liver, kidneys, and spleen. Concentration levels in the brain reach their peak one to two hours following administration. The drug readily crosses the placental barrier and enters into fetal circulation, and may produce a methadone-dependent infant.

Withdrawal   Studies have been made of infants born to mothers taking methadone; these cases have been compared with those of infants born to mothers who used heroin during pregnancy.[23] Withdrawal symptoms exhibited by the methadone group were approximately the same, though a bit less pronounced, than those exhibited by heroin-dependent infants. Other studies concur in finding milder withdrawal symptoms in methadone-dependent babies, but one study[24] found that longer treatment was needed for those infants.

Overdose   Acute methadone poisoning may result from clinical overdosage, accidental overdose, or deliberate overdose (suicide attempts). By the time the patient reaches medical assistance, he or she may be asleep or stuporous or, if a large overdose has been taken, may lapse into a deep coma from which there is no arousal.

Propoxyphene Hydrochloride (Darvon)

Propoxyphene hydrochloride (best known under its trade name of Darvon), a white crystalline powder that is water-soluble and usually combined with aspirin or acetaminophen, was first synthesized in 1953. It was considered a medical breakthrough because it had the potency of codeine but not its side effects or potential for abuse or dependency. Unfortunately, this initial optimism was short-lived, since research later proved that Darvon was structurally related to methadone.[25] Darvon is generally taken to relieve mild pain.

Physical Effects   Many of the people who become dependent on Darvon were first introduced to the drug when it was prescribed by their physician for specific pain relief. Users then went on to use the drug for every physical discomfort they encountered, without further consulting their doctor. Many found the euphoria Darvon produces a pleasant relief from the problems of day-to-day life. The drug can eventually lead to psychological dependence.

For most individuals, recommended doses do not cause clinically significant changes of respiration, blood pressure, or pulse rate. Research indicates, however, that Darvon may impair cognition and motor-skill coordination. Adverse reactions can include dizziness, headache, sedation, insomnia, skin rashes, and gastrointestinal disturbances (including nausea, vomiting, abdominal pain, and constipation).

Continuous ingestion of large doses of Darvon will produce physical dependence. As tolerance develops, the dosage must be increased approximately every six weeks to obtain the desired effects. The drug can be easily abused, since it is not thought of as one of the strongest synthetic opiates, and the claim is now being made that Darvon is one of the deadliest prescription drugs in the United States.

Accidental or intentional overdose of Darvon has symptomatology similar to that of opiate overdose and includes convulsions, coma, respiratory depression, and severe cardiovascular depression. In 1978, over 600 deaths were attributed to Darvon.[26]

DRUG ABUSE–RELATED LEGISLATION

National Addiction Rehabilitation Administration (NARA)

Passed by Congress in 1966, the National Addiction Rehabilitation Administration marked a major shift in this country's policy on opiate dependence. For the first time since the Harrison Act became effective in 1914, the problem of opiate dependence was looked at from a medical rather than a legal-criminal point of view.[27] That is, the passage of NARA marked a national acceptance of the dependence as an illness rather than an act punishable by imprisonment.

Lexington, Kentucky, and Fort Worth, Texas Programs   The major effect of the act was the establishment, under the auspices of the National Institute of Mental Health (NIMH) and the Department of Justice, of medical treatment programs at Lexington, Kentucky, and Fort Worth, Texas. If opiate dependents qualified for treatment at one of these centers, they could be sent there instead of to prison if they had committed drug-related offenses:

> (1) The user could be committed for treatment rather than criminal prosecution of a drug-related crime. If the offense was non-violent in nature, the Surgeon General of the Public Health Service took responsibility for examination, treatment, and rehabilitation. (2) If the user was already convicted of a crime, [he] could be committed to the Attorney General for treatment. The treatment period was not to exceed 10 years or the maximum sentence period for [the] crime. (3) The user could voluntarily submit himself to the Attorney General for treatment. This form of civil commitment could be implemented even if criminal charges for an offense didn't exist.[28]

The Lexington facility comprised two treatment centers. One was operated in conjunction with the Department of Psychiatry at the University of Kentucky Medical Center. This program consisted of an outpatient center within the university hospital and provided crisis intervention, individual psychotherapy, referral, education and family counseling, vocational training, job placement, and legal intervention.

> The other center, the NIMH's Clinical Research Center (CRC), is a comprehensive residential in-patient facility. Services include detoxification, therapeutic community setting, group and individual therapy, encounter groups, sensitivity and self-awareness groups, vocational training, supervised work assignments, social services referral, job placement, legal intervention, medical-health care, and recreational therapy.[29]

The treatment program at the latter was not unlike one at an average large inpatient psychiatric facility. The admitting procedure included a complete history of drug use, a family history, education and vocational history, psychological testing, and physical examination. A physician then made a diagnosis and instituted specific treatment based on the patient's data. If the patient was physically dependent on opiates at the time of admission, he or she was placed in a detoxification ward. The treatment procedure included the administration of 60 to 100 milligrams per day of methadone, followed by incremental reductions of approximately 10 milligrams per day.

Follow-up studies tracking 1912 Lexington "graduates" one to four years after their release showed that only 6.6 percent of them had abstained from further drug use through this period. A second study involving 453 former patients spot-checked at six months, two years, and five years following release found a total of only 12 who had abstained through the five-year period.[30] "Almost all [became] re-addicted and re-imprisoned early in the [next] decade and for most the process [has been] repeated over and over again."[31]

Further Legislation

As laws dealing with narcotics failed, new legislation repeatedly increased the severity of the penalty for drug-related offenses. In 1909, three federal laws specified only a two-year imprisonment for narcotics use. In 1917, the Harrison Act increased this period to five years. Ten years became the typical penalty in 1922, and some states provided for sentences of twenty, forty, and up to ninety-nine years. During the 1950s, the death penalty and life imprisonment were added to federal statutes as well as to some state codes.

This mandatory sentencing, however, failed to close down illicit drug trafficking. Subsequent federal and state legislation was then enacted, depriving convicted narcotics users of the right to parole or time off for good behavior. But these actions too were ineffective and drug dealing continued to grow. What the laws did bring about was the imprisonment of people addicted to drugs but who engaged in no criminal activity as well as those engaged in drug-related crime.

Many deplored what they felt was the injustice of laws stipulating mandatory sentencing for drug addiction. In 1969 Stanley Yolles, director of the National Institute of Mental Health, testified to that effect before the House Select Committee on Crime. Dr. Yolles stated that:

> This type of law has no place in a system devised to control an illness. It has no place being used for individuals who are addicted to drugs. This type of law angers us as doctors, because it should not be applied to people who are sick. It destroys hope on the part of the person sentenced—hope of help, hope of starting a fresh life. It's totally contradictory to the whole concept of medicine. A prison experience is often psychologically shattering. The young person is exposed to severe assaults. He may for the first time learn criminal ways. Such mandatory sentences destroy the prospects of rehabilitation.[32]

The Supreme Court eventually ruled that punishment for simply being drug-dependent was cruel and unusual. But the federal government and several state were still able to incarcerate opiate dependents by sending them to "rehabilitation centers" under an imprisonment procedure called civil commitment. One of the largest civil-commitment programs was launched by the state of California. Many convicted drug users in California were sent to the California Rehabilitation Center. There they were detained up to seven years, spending part of their time confined within the center and the remaining time as outpatients after being paroled.[33] Vocational rehabilitation and educational advancement through high school were offered, but five times a month, for at least the first six months, users had to submit to urinalysis, at both planned and spontaneous times, to test for use of drugs. Following parole, a halfway house helped

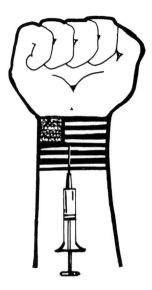

ex-residents to readjust to community life. A resident became eligible for final discharge after three drug-free years as an out-patient, but of the 5300 persons admitted between 1961 and 1965, only 27 were finally discharged.[34]

DETOXIFICATION

The increasing number of individuals requiring treatment for legal and illegal opiate abuse has provoked new, often innovative, personal-treatment programs. These range from "talk therapy" to "chemotherapeutic" treatment (methadone maintenance).

The most widely used method of opiate detoxification was developed by staff members of the U.S. Public Health Service Hospital at Lexington, Kentucky. The initial concern in this process is to determine if polydrug dependence is evident, since withdrawal from barbiturates is potentially more dangerous than withdrawal from opiates. Polydrug use must be determined early on because opiate detoxification symptoms may mask barbiturate withdrawal symptoms.[35]

A moderately long acting barbiturate can be administered to test for dependency. If an individual is significantly dependent on barbiturates, the various signs of intoxication will not appear. If signs do not appear, the extent of dependency must be determined. The client should then be stablized on a determined amount of pentobarbital while he or she undergoes gradual withdrawal from the opiate. When that has been accomplished, withdrawal from the barbiturate may begin, with administered doses reduced by 100 milligrams per day.[36]

Methadone is the widely used opiate detoxicant because it is easily absorbed and is able to "block" heroin's euphoria. When opiate use has ended, withdrawal symptoms of yawning, perspiration, lacrimation, rhinorrhea, and "yen" sleep have begun to intensify, and pupil dilation, gooseflesh, tremors, hot and cold flashes, aching bones and muscles, and anorexia have set in, methadone treatment begins. (Doctors must also be sure that patients do not fake symptoms to secure a prescriptive dose.) Doses of methadone are administered in 10-to-40-milligram amounts for two to three days, and then reduced by 20 percent a day. This schedule may be extended for those unable to tolerate it (though it should not exceed twenty-one days) but an even shorter detoxification program should be encouraged.

General Effects

Detoxification and withdrawal are not enjoyable experiences. Their severity, however, is often overstated, and with proper medical treatment they *can* be relatively painless. On the street, drug dependents already suffering from malnutrition and an array of drug-related illnesses may go through withdrawal with hallucinations, convulsions, weight loss, nausea, vomiting, diarrhea, temperature flashes, muscle cramps, and pain. Because they expect the worst, the worst may happen. Under clinical care, however, discomfort can be controlled, drug-related medical problems can be treated, and medical personnel can help to reduce anxiety by conveying a sense of ease and optimism. When detoxification has been carried out, good nutrition and hygiene instruction can be provided and plans can be made for continued treatment and follow-up.

THERAPEUTIC APPROACHES

Whereas some opiate dependents try to break their habit with chemicals such as methadone, others prefer to try a chemical-free approach. Most of these programs involve groups of individuals in noninstitutional treatment centers; the goal of the programs is positive psychological change, resulting from group pressure and reinforcement.

Small-Group Support

A number of groups whose aim is to help drug dependents work on their problems have sprung up across the country. In these groups, members feel that commonly shared goals, values, and beliefs, plus a sense of personal responsibility and the chance to participate in one's own treatment, will help to bring about the end to drug addiction. Jerome Frank, professor of psychiatry at Johns Hopkins Medical School, agrees that group pressures, kept in proper perspective, *can* be very beneficial to the individual:

> An important over-all beneficial effect of group methods with inpatients, as well as outpatients, is to restore to patients a sense of individuality and of some control over their destinies. The expectations that they are capable of self-control and of assuming some degree of responsibility for themselves and others, which is implicit

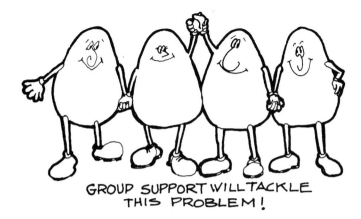

GROUP SUPPORT WILL TACKLE
THIS PROBLEM!

in all forms of group therapy, bolsters their self-respect, stimulates their hopes and in general, helps to restore their morale.[37]

Group pressures and influences are frequently utilized in small-group encounter sessions. In these meetings, between eight and twelve persons meet for a predesignated amount of time to handle individual and interpersonal difficulties. Through these meetings, participants hope to begin seeing themselves as responsible for their own actions. Meetings often become quite intense, with participants pouring out emotions, frustrations, and tears. Physical violence is not tolerated, and although no topic is immune from discussion, the emphasis is on present and personal behavior.[38]

Therapeutic Communities

The idea of group pressure as a drug-free way to achieve opiate independence is carried a step further in the therapeutic community. Here, in such communities as Daytop, Odyssey House, Phoenix House, Liberty Park Village, and Synanon, members (who join voluntarily) must submit to organization rules, relinquish all personal assets, and be responsible for assigned tasks. Members reinforce each other as they attempt to gain control over their actions and become responsible.

The success of these programs as a way of treating opiate dependency has not been substantial. By the mid 1960s, leaders of the Synanon community were ready to admit that they were not achieving the results they had hoped for. With few exceptions, Synanon "graduated" no drug-abstinent individuals. Members thought to be cured promptly relapsed when they left the security of the community.

A major reason for the failure of therapeutic communities seems to be that they are too self-contained and isolated, too unlike the "real" world. Day and night, members are reinforced and supported; their own egos become subservient to the group, and drug-using desires are completely repressed. When members choose to leave, they are faced with pressures and temptations their community had selectively eliminated. Returning to a "normal" environment can cause a relapse into narcotic-seeking behavior.

The future of therapeutic communities remains unclear. Some may become ongoing treatment facilities where recovered users would permanently live and work. Others may offer postdependence-syndrome assistance, since techniques they have developed seem effective. Therapeutic communities are an alternative to the institutional approach. But although they do offer good treatment, by no means are they a cure.[39]

Personal Responsibility and Commitment

Traditional drug treatment in the United States has been oriented toward heroin and similar narcotics.[40] However, alcohol and cocaine programs are increasing in number and in their new approaches to treatment. It's important to find an appropriate kind of help based on personal resources (family, friends, work, internal motivation) and deep involvement, regardless of the drugs being used. Therapy groups, education, and individualized recovery plans and follow-up care are important elements to success.[41] But treatment alone does not get a person off drugs. Personal responsibility and commitment do. Treatment can only help. A change in behavior is a three-step process: (1) motivation to act, (2) maximization of success, and (3) maintenance of new behavior.

METHADONE MAINTENANCE _____

Introduction

When first presented as a new form of opiate-dependency treatment, methadone maintenance was predicted to produce positive results. Since then, however, a number of problems have dimmed that optimism, including the discovery that methadone is even more capable of causing dependence than heroin. Despite the method's shortcomings, methadone maintenance remains the most often used technique for the treatment of opiate dependency.

Marie Nyswander and Vincent P. Dole first proposed the idea of methadone maintenance in 1964. During a study of metabolic processes involving drug dependents undergoing methadone detoxification, Nyswander and Dole noticed a definite attitude change in patients when methadone was administered past the usual ten-day detoxification period. Said Dr. Dole, "The interesting thing about methadone maintenance is that it permits people to become whatever they potentially are, whereas dependents, under the pressure of drug abuse and drug seeking, look very much the same. When [drug dependents are] freed from this dependency, they differentiate and become part of the spectrum of humanity."[42]

Nyswander and Dole found that therapeutic dose levels of methadone were able to assuage opiate desire without producing disabling sedation. Because of cross-tolerance, methadone is also able to block an opiate's euphoric affects. Methadone can produce its own euphoria, however, when taken in large doses, and large doses of heroin can also break methadone's euphoria block. Treatment should include only gradual methadone dose increases. Dose levels can be stabilized over a period of time.

Despite the method's seeming success, patients in actuality simply trade one form of dependence for another. Additionally, research quickly revealed that discontinuance of methadone treatment was generally followed by relapse to drug-using behavior—a craving for heroin, not methadone. But the rationale behind the method's use still makes it a plausible treatment:

> In absence of a cure . . . it is traditional medical practice to attempt to ameliorate the symptoms or effects of the disease, and to rehabilitate the patient as far as possible to a plausible way of life. . . . Methadone maintenance therapy offers an effective means of managing the illness of heroin addiction—not to cure it, but to counter its effects.[43]

Possible Hazards and Side Effects

The main hazards of methadone are overdosing and use by nonde-pendent children and adults. Making the drug available only in tablet form (to be taken orally) can cut down on the danger of overdosing, since it is very difficult for a user to overdose on orally ingested methadone, even in high doses. Labeling and putting the methadone in hard-to-reach locations in the refrigera-tor when used by the patient at home should protect unknowing adults and children. Making the substance available only in powder form also cuts down on illicit intravenous injection, since the powder is potent only in oral form.

Various side effects have been reported with initial methadone intake, especially during the first one to six weeks, when the body adapts to the continu-ing presence of the drug. Uncomfortable side effects usually occur in the even-ing, at least eight hours after methadone ingestion, and can include constipation, delayed ejaculation, more frequent urination, numbness in the hands and feet, hallucinations, insomnia, nausea, vomiting, muscle pains, anorexia, and exces-sive perspiration. Weight gain and the need to drink more fluids can also occur, as can the feeling of oversedation and confusion. Side effects are usually mini-mal, however, and very seldom warrant the discontinuance of treament. If side effects do become too unpleasant, a dose reduction of ten milligrams followed by a buildup to the desired therapeutic dose level will usually solve the problem, since side effects occur in response to specific dose levels.[44]

Though some side effects may appear, premethadone symptoms (caused by street heroin use) show improvement once the user begins to stabilize on methadone. Headaches, joint pains, hiccups, diarrhea, loss of sexual desire, nervousness, runny nose, urination difficulty, and a general feeling of unhappi-ness either lessen or disappear. The patient's expectations once treatment has begun also play an important role in the reduction of symptoms and his or her general feeling of well-being.

How methadone use affects pregnancy is still uncertain. Carl Zelson, pro-fessor of pediatrics at New York Medical College, has reported that babies born to methadone users are likely to be more severely hurt than those born to heroin users. Dr. Zelson lists the findings of a study of ninety-one infants born to heroin- and methadone-dependent mothers at New York's Metropolitan Hospital Center:

1. More methadone babies (42) than heroin [babies] developed withdrawal signs, and symptoms of the former were more severe. . . .
2. Five methadone babies suffered convulsive seizures compared to two of the heroin babies.
3. Twelve of the methadone babies and five of the heroin babies had jaundice. In the methadone group, five of these were serious as opposed to only two in the heroin group.
4. Almost one-half of both groups had sub-average birth weights and abnormal sleep patterns.[45]

In another study, however, M. E. Strauss of Johns Hopkins University's department of psychology found that in a compared-subject controlled study of seventy-two nondependent pregnant women and seventy-two methadone-dependent pregnant women (all receiving prenatal care), the rates of pregnancy illness, pregnancy complications, and labor and delivery characteristics of the two groups did not differ.[46]

Withdrawal from congenital drug dependence usually occurs within forty-eight hours of birth. Since newborn infants are not as heavily dependent on the drug as their mothers, brief medication to relieve the withdrawal and detoxification stress usually returns such infants to a normal state. Increasing tolerance or psychological dependence is not evident.

The Process

Methadone maintenance is divided into three phases. During phase 1 low doses—30 to 40 milligrams of methadone are given with fruit juice. Physiological responses are monitored to determine the patient's tolerance level. For three to six weeks, dosage is increased until a level of stabilization is reached—a point where the patient is comfortable, has no craving for opiates and experiences no euphoria following an opium injection. When stabilization is reached, the dosage level is usually 60 to 100 milligrams a day.

In phase 2, the patient comes to the clinic daily to receive his or her methadone and to leave a urine sample that will be tested for methadone level and the presence of other drugs, such as alcohol, other opiates, amphetamines, or barbiturates. During this time, the patient may obtain continuous medical care and social rehabilitation along with job consultation, vocational training, educational guidance, and counseling.

Phase 3 begins after a year of stabilized behavior. At this point, the patient is considered partially rehabilitated and may begin taking several days' worth of methadone home for self-administration. The patient need only visit the clinic weekly for urine tests and to receive a new methadone supply, taking a full dose there under staff supervision. Any sign of opiate use, illegal trafficking, or undermedication returns the patient to phase 1 and daily clinic-administered doses. If instructions are followed, however, the patient may be able to find employment and rejoin the community at this point.[47]

Most clinicians in the field believe it is desirable to gradually reduce the dose of methadone needed for maintenance over a period of time. This process would determine the lowest dose possible that would still assuage the patient's cravings for opiates. Reductions of ten milligrams per week could be made until the lowest dose level is found. At this point, some patients might request total detoxification and abstinence.

In many cases, however, total discontinuance of methadone has led to postwithdrawal syndrome, a resurfacing of the desire for heroin. Clinical evidence indicates that such a desire can return even to patients who have been stable more than five years.

Rate of Success

Just how successful is methadone maintenance? There are several reasons why the program should meet with success: Because the drug can be obtained legally, it lessens the patient's guilt about desiring and taking narcotics, and reduces the need for self-punishment; it is relatively inexpensive compared with street heroin, and this often eliminates the need to steal to pay for it; since it is fully effective when taken orally, it eliminates the possibility of needle infections and blood vessel damage; it breaks up the ritual of injecting, which is often the high point of heroin use; and because it is long-acting, it will not subject the user to the psychological "bouncing" reported by many heroin users.

Early findings from an independent evaluation team from the Columbia University School of Public Health, charged with evaluating the success of methadone programs, *were* very favorable. A later five-year follow-up study on the Santa Clara County Methadone Program indicated that fully one third of those who participated in the program (drinking at least one methadone dose) were still abstaining from heroin five years later. Furthermore, the overwhelming majority of these people were no longer using methadone.[48]

But there are a number of criteria on which to base program evaluations. The first, of course, is the percentage of reduced opiate use. Others are the amount of substitution of alcohol, barbiturates, or amphetamines for heroin, patient return to employment or to a job-training program, improvement in physical and psychological health, and degree of continuing criminal activity. In other words, one should consider not only reduced drug use but also the participating patient's overall quality of life.

Many feel the relationship between methadone maintenance and reduction in criminal activities is an important indicator of progress for both patient and program. A *Consumers Union Report* states that in one treatment program

91% of the patients had been in jail [prior to treatment], and all of them had been more or less continually involved in criminal activities. . . . Since entering the treatment program, 88% of the patients show arrest-free records. The remainder have had difficulties with the law . . . the only possible conclusion is that the great majority of addicts placed on methadone, despite pre-existing handicaps such as poverty, poor health, little education, prison records, and years of addiction, became self-supporting as well as law-abiding while on mehadone. . . . [49]

Others, however, feel that crime reduction is not a true indicator of methadone-maintenance effectiveness. These critics feel that many dependents are criminals and that, drug use or not, it is reasonable to assume they will remain criminal. "Various studies of known addicts have shown that between one-half [and] three-fourths were known to be delinquent before turning to drugs. . . . [50]

Admissions criteria for early methadone-mainenance programs may have led to the idea's initial success statistics. Program participants were carefully selected, with psychotics and multiple-drug users specifically excluded. Patients needed to be particularly enthusiastic about joining the program. In some clinics, patients had a good employment record and a stable family record prior to dependency. By eliminating adolescent users and choosing only those users with the highest potential for success, the programs denied help to the people most in need of treatment. Success rates may have been high because harder-to-treat individuals did not participate.

Programs now have only limited success. To begin with, it is very difficult to encourage opiate users to come into the system and begin treatment. Another major problem is methadone's ability to induce dependency. Treatment programs have looked into this situation, using Darvon-N as a methadone detoxicant. This mode of therapy has been sharply curtailed, however, since a number of deaths have been related to its abuse.

A second problem is the illicit diversion of methadone to the street market, resulting in the same potential harm and types of problems that heroin diversion brings about. Reports indicate that the illicit methadone street market became well established because of an increase in illicit methadone diversion.[51]

A final problem may be the type of staff running the program. Rules may be established that favor staff convenience rather than patient needs. Staff members may adhere rigidly to unrealistic standards and punish or exclude patients whose behavior does not meet these standards. A successful program requires that those who run it be highly skilled and highly trained, and have continuous access to relevant updated data. Staff functioning and attitudes have a strong bearing on the success of treatment.[52]

It is easy to see that methadone maintenance is not a panacea for opiate dependency. It is, however, widely used, and *can* help rehabilitate a dependent. With a large and dedicated staff, adequate facilities, sufficient funding, various diversified therapy programs (group and individual), educational-improvement opportunities, vocational-training and job-placement services, and health care (medical and nutritional), methadone maintenance can be effective.

Social Implications of Methadone-Maintenance Programs

Critics charge that methadone-maintenance programs gloss over the social and economic conditions that drive people to opiate use and work only at controlling and pacifying addicts. Some feel that the programs are a potential form of group repression and covert social control, and reported accounts of methadone-linked sexual impotence arouse fears of population control and seemingly indefinite periods of chemotherapy. John Chappel writes:

Chemotherapy, including methadone, can be used in detrimental ways. It is reprehensible and destructive to treatment goals to use medication as a source of external control to muffle protest and stifle individual or collective attempts to alter oppressive aspects of the environment. Treatment [should] free the patient from internal blocks of problems that interfere with his ability to deal effectively with his environment. . . . when chemotherapy is used in the context of mutual participation in goal-directed treatment, it can contribute to the eventual achievement of an examined, responsible, self-determined, drug-free life.[53]

Methadone treatment is also thought of as a further step in a dangerous pattern of chemotherapy. When opium was determined to be dependency-producing, morphine was developed to treat it, but was soon found to be even more addictive. Heroin was then developed to treat morphine dependence, and finally methadone was developed to treat heroin dependence. In each instance, stronger chemical agents were substituted for weaker ones, and though the intent was improvement, the result was an intensified degree of addiction. Critics feel that chemotherapy may not be the answer to biochemical addiction, and that methadone maintenance is simply another step in the wrong direction.

Further criticism is voiced concerning the lack of readjustment techniques methadone-maintenance programs offer. Stephen Pittle, director of the Berkeley Center for Drug Studies, states that

the addict will still face a major hurdle in entering [or reentering] the work-day world, not unlike what Alice faced in Wonderland. The world of employers and employees, of coffee breaks and chitchat around the water cooler, is to the addict an unreal place, filled with eccentrics who make bizarre suggestions and unreasonable demands.
. . . Pittle advises giving addicts whatever help they need to meet the expectations of the straight world, without taking for granted their knowledge of even the most basic tricks and social skills that middle-class folks learn from childhood.[54]

This methadone-maintenance programs often do not do.

Pittle and his colleagues have devised a program—the Drug Abuse Treatment and Referral System (DATRS)—that assesses a user's strengths and needs and then matches them to a reentry program that is complementary and likely to be of service to him or her. The system is based on the assumption that those with fewer strengths and greater needs will require a more highly structured approach than those with greater strengths and fewer needs. According to Pittel, assessing the nature and severity of each user's drug involvement, as well as his or her personal and social resources, may enhance treatment.

NARCOTIC ANTAGONISTS

For some time, efforts have been made to develop a possible alternative to methadone maintenance—opiate-antagonist administration. Treatment programs involving antagonists have been widely heralded because these chemical agents are believed to have nondependency-producing properties but are still able to block opiate euphoria. Optimism concerning antagonists is especially high for treatment of: (1) heroin users who refuse or are not selected for methadone maintenance; (2) the casual user, whose level of dependency is minimal; and (3) individuals whose potential for developing dependencies is high—for example, teenagers in high schools in which drug use is already widespread, and members of the armed forces.[55]

Cyclazocine and Naloxone are two agents that have been tested, but their uncomfortable side effects and short period of effectiveness led researchers to the development of EN-1639. An acceptable length of action and little resulting discomfort make this blocking agent an attractive agent for clinical use.[56]

Research has also been focusing on the construction of time-release antagonists. Plastics have been suggested as the housing for such substances, but plastic-encased capsules would require surgical implantation and removal. Capsule casings that disintegrate, which have been tested, allow time-release action for one week.[57]

Despite wide interest in antagonists, some critics are questioning their effectiveness. But proponents believe that because antagonists block the rush and high of heroin, over a period of time users will lose their desire for opiates. Behaviors associated with drug use will also eventually be extinguished.

Psychological Considerations

Though antagonists can block the euphoria opiates produce, critics feel they do not assuage the biophysical desire and need for opiates following detoxification. There are those who suggest that while on narcotic antagonists the user will still feel the psychophysiological symptoms known as postwithdrawal or abstinence syndrome. Following drug-free periods, a user may begin to experience anxiety and general depression that may precipitate a subtle and prolonged desire for heroin. Such effects may continue for years, but would be especially pronounced the first year after detoxification. If relief from these effects cannot be provided, narcotic-antagonist treatment programs may be very short lived.

The Young User

A young, novice user, whose physiological adaptation to heroin may be minimal or nonexistent, may feel little or no postwithdrawal craving following detoxification. Early stages of novice use result predominantly from curiosity to experience the rush or high. As a result of his or her age and lack of experience, the young user hasn't seen and felt the severity of the street lifestyle of the opiate user. Therapy is less than desirable to such users because of the fascination of running and hustling in the streets. Attempts at treatment often present themselves as threatening coercion.

The task of therapy must transcend basic detoxification techniques because physiological dependence rarely constitutes the sole problem. The major problem is not dependence on the drug but infatuation with the heroin lifestyle.

DOES ANY TREATMENT WORK? _____

Despite the limited success of some opiate-dependency treatment programs, individuals in the field feel that no rehabilitation program can really help a user with a long-term habit, someone whose lifestyle is totally identified with a drug-using subculture. A review of clinical treatment at the U.S. Public Health Service hospitals in Lexinton, Kentucky, and Ft. Worth, Texas, backs up this theory, showing that users treated at these facilities were antisocial prior to dependence.[58] Various other studies attempting to assess psychopathology in opiate users point to numerous cases of inappropriate anger, distrust, disbelief in "real" relationships, immaturity, passivity, dependency, low pain threshold, inability to perceive delayed gratification, and a strong ability to manipulate others.[59] Such ingrained tendencies and characteristics make rehabilitation difficult.

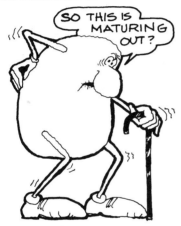

Maturing Out

On the other end of the spectrum, the absence of treatment can sometimes result in a cure. For reasons that remain vague and unsubstantiated, a large percentage of individuals who need clinical services but don't seek or receive them seem to recover on their own. For opiate users, time may be the answer. By the time users reach their mid thirties, they often become spontaneously abstinent. The onset of middle age may make their previous lifestyle unwarranted. "Addiction [that] begins in late adolescence when the person is faced with multiple inner drives and major decisions [may burn] out when his life becomes more stabilized through 'some process of emotional homeostasis.' "[60] This may be true for as many as one third of known users.[61]

If many users end up relinquishing opiates in their mid thirties, is much of drug-abuse treatment a waste of time? George Henry of the University of Kentucky's College of Medicine states that

for all the elegant studies which have brought us to the present state of knowledge concerning the mechanism of action of opioids and opioid antagonists and their effects on behavior, and for all the money and energy we have spent on treating the drug-dependent, we still do not know what happens to drug dependent persons who are not treated or incarcerated. Because we do not know the effect of "no treatment," there is no baseline for comparing the results of existing treatment programs.[62]

Even without an evaluation baseline,

results [from a multiplicity of treatment approaches] have been generally disappointing. [But it] should . . . be obvious that no single or simple approach could possibly satisfy all the complexities contributing to narcotic addiction, including the serious socio-economic problems of poverty, unemployment, lack of opportunities, and an adequate educational system; personality disturbance of major proportion involving conditioning to antisocial behaviors and difficulties in tolerating anxiety and frustration; the ingenuity of organized crime, reinforced by enormous profits; the rigidity of legislative and judicial structures; and the powerful pharmacologic effects and adaptive biological and psychological responses to the opioid drugs themselves.[63]

SUMMARY

Opium has existed for centuries. The class of opium drugs known as opiates have tremendous pain-relieving properties as well as the ability to produce one of the most powerful euphoric states known. Opiates often lead to psychophysiological dependence, and their legal use in the United States is therefore restricted to prescribed medical situations.

Morphine was the first pain-killer to be derived from opium. Heroin soon followed, but both drugs were found to produce dependence with regular use. However, because of heroin's effectiveness, there is increasing legislative support for legalizing heroin for terminally ill cancer patients. In recent years, methadone, a synthetic opiate, has been used to treat heroin dependency. Methadone blocks the euphoria of and desire for heroin, but unfortunately also leads to dependence. Under proper medical supervision and with proper counseling, however, methadone can be an effective treatment for heroin dependence.

Until recently, Darvon, a dependence-producing synthetic drug very similar to methadone, was easy to obtain and was routinely prescribed by most physicians for virtually every pain or physical discomfort. Recently, however, various government agencies and the medical community have become aware of its abuse and its propensity for contributing to overdose. Prescription of the drug is now greatly curtailed.

On the legal side of drug use, the National Addiction Rehabilitation Administration represented the first attempt to address drug abuse in medical rather than judicial terms. For the first time in recent history, drug dependents were thought of as needing medical treatment, not punishment. The passage of the NARA was the beginning of more positive attitudes toward the problem of drug dependency.

A number of treatment options are available to drug dependents. These include psychotherapy, peer pressure, chemotherapy, detoxification, job training, narcotic antagonists, and self-control, monitoring, and aversive stimuli. All of these treatment approaches can meet with varying degrees of success, depending on the sincerity of the individual in treatment, the training and attitudes of the staff, and the factors precipitating use and dependency states.

NOTES

[1]John B. Williams, *Narcotics and Hallucinogens* (Encino, Calif.: Glencoe Press, 1967), p. 129.

[2]Norman Taylor, *Narcotics* (New York: Dell Pub. Co., Inc. 1966), p. 38.

[3]Louis S. Goodman and Alfred Gilman, eds. *The Pharmacological Basis of Therapeutics*, 4th ed. (New York: Macmillan, 1970), p. 243.

[4]Williams, *Narcotics and Hallucinogens*, p. 134.

[5]Goodman and Gilman, *The Pharmacological Basis of Therapeutics*, p. 248.

[6]*Final Report of the Commission of Inquiry into the Nonmedical Use of Drugs* (Ottawa: Crown, 1973), p. 318.

[7]"U.S. Heroin Addicts Bear 10,000 Babies a Year," *Journal* 10, no. 1 (1981).

[8]Ibid.

[9]Jerome H. Jaffe, "Drug Addiction and Drug Abuse," in *The Pharmacological Basis of Therapeutics*, 5th ed., Louis S. Goodman and Alfred Gilman (New York: Macmillan, Co. 1975), p. 296.

[10]J. Stewart, H. de Witt, and R. Eikelboom, "Role of Unconditioned and Conditioned Drug Effects in the Self-Administration of Opiates and Stimulants," *Psychological Review* 91 (1984):251–68.

[11]Ibid.

[12]J. F. Maddox and D. P. Desmond, "Residence Relocation Inhibits Opiate Dependence," *Archives of General Psychiatry* 39 (1982):1313–17. Copyright © 1982 American Medical Association. Used with permission.

[13]Edward M. Brecher et al., *Licit and Illicit Drugs* (Boston: Little, Brown, 1972), pp. 104–5.

[14]Quoted in ibid., p. 104.

[15]Quoted in ibid., p. 108.

[16]Quoted in ibid., p. 113.

[17]Quoted in ibid., p. 113.

[18]John Strang and Les Kay, "How the Media Abuse Heroin," *New Scientist*, Oct. 18, 1984, p. 62.

[19]See Allen M. Mondzac, "In Defense of the Reintroduction of Heroin into American Medical Practice and H.R. 5290: The Compassionate Pain Relief Act," *New England Journal of Medicine* 311 (August 23, 1984):532–35. Copyright © 1984 Massachusetts Medical Society. Reprinted with permission of the *New England Journal of Medicine*.

[20]Ibid.

[21]*Codeine* (New York: Marc K and Company, 1969), p. 4.

[22]Williams, *Narcotics and Hallucinogens*, p. 25.

[23]Saul Blatman, "Neonatal and Follow-up," in *Proceedings of the Third National Conference on Methadone* (1970), p. 82.

[24]Leonard Class and Hugh E. Evans, "Narcotic Withdrawal in the Newborn," *American Family Physicians* 6, no. 1 (July 1972):76.

[25]Deborah Sternlicht, "The Prescribing of Darvon," *Street Pharmacologist* 2, no. 3 (June–July 1979):4–8.

[26]"Stir over Darvon," *Time,* 112, no. 23 (December 4, 1978):96.

[27]National Institute of Mental Health, *The Narcotic Addict Rehabilitation Act of 1966* (Washington, D.C.: Public Health Service, 1969), p. 2.

[28]National Institute of Mental Health, *Narcotics: Some Questions and Answers* (Washington, D.C.: Public Health Service, 1970), p. 3.

[29]Deena D. Watson, *National Directory of Drug Abuse Treatment Programs* (Washington, D.C.: National Institute of Mental Health, 1972), pp. 146–47.

[30]Brecher et al., *Licit and Illicit Drugs,* p. 69.

[31]Ibid., p. 13.

[32]Quoted in ibid., p. 57.

[33]Brecher et al., *Licit and Illicit Drugs,* p. 71.

[34]*The Challenge of Crime in a Free Society: A Report by the President's Commission on Law Enforcement and Administration of Justice* (New York: Avon Books, 1968), pp. 518–19.

[35]George M. Henry, "Treatment and Rehabilitation of Narcotic Addiction," in *Research Advances in Alcohol and Drug Problems,* volume I, ed. Robert J. Gibbins et al. (New York: John Wiley, 1980), pp. 267–68.

[36]Ibid., p. 268.

[37]Jerome D. Frank, *Persuasion and Healing,* 2nd rev. ed. (Baltimore: Johns Hopkins, 1973).

[38]M. D. Rosenthal, S. Mitchell, and Bias D. Vincent, "Phoenix House: Therapeutic Communities for Drug Addicts," *Hospital and Community Psychiatry* 20, no. 1 (January 1969):29.

[39]Brecher et al., *Licit and Illicit Drugs,* p. 82.

[40]James Q. Wilson, "Heroin Solution, The Fix," *New Republic,* October 25, 1982, p. 24.

[41]Ira Mothner and Alan Weitz, "Get Off Coke," *Rolling Stone,* June 7, 1984, p. 29.

[42]Marie E. Nyswander, "Methadone Therapy for Heroin Addiction: Where Are We? Where Are We Going?" *Drug Therapy* 1, no. 1 (January 1971):23.

[43]Quoted in Brecher et al., *Licit and Illicit Drugs,* p. 139.

[44]Ibid., p. 24; and Brecher et al., *Licit and Illicit Drugs,* pp. 153–54.

[45]Carl Zelson, "Methadone and Heroin," *Archives of Internal Medicine* 132 (July 1973):9.

[46]M. E. Strauss et al., "Methadone Maintenance during Pregnancy: Pregnancy, Birth and Neonate Characteristics," *American Journal of Obstetrics and Gynecology* 120, no. 7 (December 1, 1974):895–99.

[47]Nyswander, "Methadone Therapy for Heroin Addiction," 25–26.

[48]Avram Goldstein, "Heroin Maintenance: A Medical View," *Journal of Drug Issues* 9, no. 3 (Summer 1979):344.

[49]Quoted in Brecher et al., *Licit and Illicit Drugs,* pp. 142–43, 148.

[50]James Q. Wilson, Mark H. Moore, and I. David Wheat, Jr., "What Public Policy toward Heroin?" *Current Health* 147 (January 1973):16, 19.

[51]See, for example, Robert Y. Bazell, "Drug Abuse: Methadone Becomes the Solution and the Problem," *Science* 179, no. 4075 (February 23, 1973):772; Richard C. Stephens and Robert S. Weppner, "Legal and Illegal Use of Methadone: One Year Later," *American Journal of Psychiatry* 130, no. 12 (December 1973):1392–93.

[52]Barry S. Brown, Donald R. Jansen, and Urbane F. Bass III, "Staff Attitudes and Conflict regarding the Use of Methadone in the Treatment of Heroin Addiction," *American Journal of Psychiatry* 131, no. 2 (February 1974):216.

[53]John N. Chappel, "Methadone and Chemotherapy in Drug Addiction: Genocide or Lifesaving?" *Journal of the American Medical Association* 228, no. 6 (May 6, 1974):278. Copyright © 1974, American Medical Association.

[54]Quoted in Jack Horn, "Addicts in the Wonderland of Work," *Psychology Today* 8, no. 12 (May 1975):22. Reprinted with permission from *Psychology Today Magazine.* Copyright © 1975 American Psychological Association (APA).

[55]Henry, "Treatment and Rehabilitation of Narcotic Addiction," p. 281.

[56]Thomas H. Maugh II, "Narcotic Antagonists: The Search Accelerates," *Science* 177, no.4945 (July 21, 1972):250.

[57]Ibid.
[58]Henry, "Treatment and Rehabilitation of Narcotic Addiction," p. 283.
[59]Ibid., p. 284.
[60]Ibid., p. 291.
[61]Ibid.
[62]Ibid., pp. 293–94.
[63]Ibid., p. 289.

10

HALLUCINOGENS

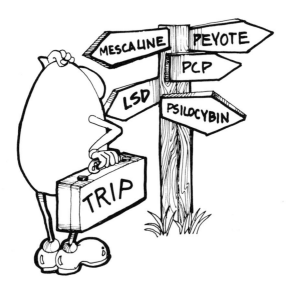

LSD

Introduction

LSD (Lysergic Acid Diethylamide-25) is the most potent psycho-active drug available. Originally synthesized by a Swiss chemist named Albert Hoffman in the mid 1940s, LSD was to be used as a headache remedy. From the time Dr. Hoffman discovered the drug, it quickly became a psychological research tool. Its hallucinogenic properties weren't discovered for several years, until Dr. Hoffman accidentally inhaled the substance and began to experience peculiar psychological changes.[1] Further tests revealed other potentially dangerous effects, such as chromosome damage, fetal abnormalities, and psychotic reactions. In 1965, after widespread experimental use by young people, purchase and use of LSD was made illegal.

The LSD subculture includes a colorful jargon: LSD is acid. The experience is a trip. A user is an acid head. The mind doesn't expand, it flips out. The acid head doesn't hallucinate, he freaks. Anybody who goes along on a trip is a co-pilot. If he has tripped before, he's a *guru*. A friend who keeps an acid head from jumping out a window is ground control. The acid supply man is a travel agent. A group of acid heads makes an Explorers' Club. And if an acid head dumps some acid in the punch at a party, the party becomes an Acid Test.[2]

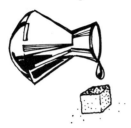

Psychophysiological Effects

Whereas most drugs are taken in milligrams (thousandths of grams), LSD is taken in micrograms (millionths of grams), usually 50 to 300 micrograms. Depending on the dose, effects may last from six to twelve hours. If LSD were taken on a continuous basis over a long period of time, increased dosages would be required to achieve desired effects. However, because LSD is so powerful a drug, most users do not take it frequently.

Researchers theorize that LSD works by stimulating the raphae nuclei. This section of the brain uses a neurotransmitter called serotonin that LSD chemically resembles, and is responsible for regulating incoming sensory information and outgoing muscular impulses. Researchers hypothesize that LSD increases the sensitivity of this brain region and allows more information to flow to higher brain regions, including those responsible for vision and emotion. Users may therefore experience heightened sensitivity to environmental stimuli, which can lead to distortions in perception (depth, touch/texture, color, sound, and balance). Synesthesia, or a blending of the senses, may also occur.

A secondary action of LSD is to increase activity in the sympathetic nervous system which results in pupil dilation and a rise in body temperature, blood pressure, and heart rate. In addition to a slight rise in blood-sugar levels, users have also reported on occasion nausea, headaches, loss of appetite, dizziness, and mild tremors.

The effects of LSD vary with the dose, purity, setting, expectations, and motivations of the user. Smaller doses (25 to 75 micrograms) may cause slight perceptual alterations; large doses (300 to 600 micrograms) may result in mystical experiences or severe paranoia. Pleasant expectations and planned use help to increase the chances of having a pleasant experience, but unexpected or unwanted use can have serious consequences. Many people never fully recover from bad trips. Many bad trips, which may be induced by sensory overload or unresolved emotional problems, can be resolved if a person acting in an nonthreatening manner "talks down" the individual in a supportive environment.

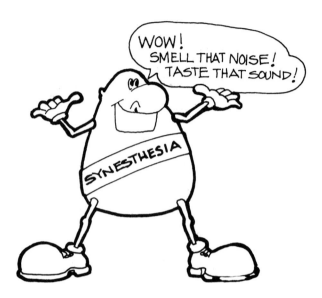

Occasionally, severe anxiety reactions may require mild tranquilization or psychiatric follow-up after the drug effects have ended.

Another possible adverse reaction to LSD is the flashback, a spontaneous reoccurrence of feelings that may have been experienced during an LSD trip weeks, months, or even years earlier. It has been estimated that flashbacks occur in approximately 5 percent of LSD users, although severe flashbacks or psychotic reactions are considerably rarer. Flashbacks, most of which are of short duration, are not always a negative: some users report them to be an unexpected bonus of the LSD experience. Many of the flashbacks that have been studied clinically center in unresolved problems, repressed fears, or frightening experiences while under the influence of the drug.

Finally, it was alleged for years that LSD can damage chromosomes. Although this is a widely touted claim, more recent analytical techniques indicate that the claim was exaggerated.

Society

It was Timothy Leary who raised LSD to national prominence with talk of mystical visions, egoless states, and trips within the mind. The drug was quite popular during the early 1960s, and articles depicting its evils—chromosome breakage, birth defects, insanity, and death and physical harm caused by users on bad trips—did little to discourage the acid's use. In 1965, however, concern over the drug's use grew, and the Drug Abuse Control Amendments were passed, putting federal controls on LSD manufacturing. LSD, along with depressants, stimulants, and other hallucinogenic drugs, were placed under the heading *dangerous drugs,* and their manufacture, processing, and distribution or sale became a federal offense.

The 1965 amendment sparked the beginning of a decrease in LSD use. From 1970 to 1980 dramatic reductions were noted, and current government surveys show that no more than 1 percent of the teenage/young-adult population uses LSD.

AN LSD CASE STUDY

About five years ago five friends drove from Seattle, Washington, to Eugene, Oregon, to attend a rock concert at Autzen Stadium. During the concert the group used blotter acid. One of the members decided to leave the concert. He got into a car and drove approximately twenty miles south on the freeway and turned off at a town named Cottage Grove. He got out of the car at the freeway exit and left the vehicle there. An older couple approached him and asked if he was okay. He asked them for a gun and they promptly left and contacted the state police. He entered the community and went from house to house requesting a gun. One of the houses where he stopped belonged to an off-duty state policeman, whose wife answered the door and told the man she did not have a gun. When the man left she told her husband, who was in another part of the house. He picked up his gun and went after the man, who had picked up a claw hammer from the policeman's garage. When the police officer caught up with the young man he noticed he had captured a small child and was swinging the hammer downward toward the child's head. The policeman reacted quickly and shot the young man through the heart, killing him. An autopsy indicated the young man had swallowed blotter acid and also had some back at his unattended vehicle. The policeman was cleared of any wrongdoing, and the child survived the ordeal.[3]

LSD seems to be making a name for itself again. The revival has been especially prevalent in California and in large urban centers in the East and Midwest. Involvement seems to center in some of the old organizations and old-timers getting back into the business.[4] Some drug-abuse experts believe the slight increase is due to the unusual amount of new publicity about LSD in the media, along with a fascinating variety of brands now available. More people are taking notice of a subject that has not been newsworthy in recent years.

LSD use in the 1980s is very different from the "vintage" LSD use of the 1960s and 1970s. In the early days, sugar cubes and animal crackers were among the favored ways of delivering doses of the drug, but these fell from favor because of their bulk. From the mid 1960s to the mid 1970s, LSD in the form of tablets dominated the street acid market. Eventually these gave way to increasingly smaller formats, particularly small gelatin chips known as *windowpanes,* tiny pellets knows as *microdots,* and the dominant format—*blotter.*[5] In the last-named format, diluted drops of the drug are placed on blotter paper. Usually the paper has been printed with some sort of artwork, such as dragons or popular comic-strip characters. It is then cut up into tiny pieces, usually one-quarter to one-half the size of a small postage stamp. Some blotters have slot-type perforations for easy separation.[6]

The idea behind smaller forms of the drug is to make it as undetectable as possible. The smaller-is-better ethic in LSD marketing is due to the minuteness of effective psychoactive doses of LSD. As little as 25 micrograms can produce noticeable perceptual and cognitive changes. One key difference between today's LSD and that of the past is potency. Most acid today is not as strong as it was in previous years. The average LSD dose now ranges from 40 to 60 micrograms, the average being 60. This compares with an average dose of 150 to 200 micrograms a decade ago. Some feel the lower dosage produces a more manageable reaction and may account for the increasing use of LSD.

Medical Research

Research into possible LSD uses has been carried out in several areas. In 1949, the CIA and various military agencies began exploring the use of drugs and other exotic methods for mind control. On April 3, 1953, Richard Helms proposed to CIA director Allen Dulles that a program for covert use of biological and chemical materials be set up.[7] It was approved and called MKULTRA.

In the early days, six Technical Services Staff professionals investigated possible uses of LSD. A small amount, these agencies felt, could turn strong-willed individuals away from their most basic perceptions and to a state of mind in which they could be manipulated. In November 1953, they "tested" a group of scientists from the Army Chemical Corps Special Operations Division at Fort Detrich in Maryland. One of the scientists, Frank Olson, became psychotic and jumped from a hotel window to his death. Because of this type of problem and the extensive cover-up it entailed, the CIA decided to experiment with underworld prostitutes and drug dependents, who would be less likely to draw attention to the experiment.[8] Safe houses were set up in New York and San Francisco where drugs were disguised in food, drink, and cigarettes. Despite the extensive testing, however, the agencies came up with no positive results. LSD-initiated mind control was impossible because of the many differences among the people tested. After all these years the Frank Olson case, among others, is now being uncovered and placed in front of the public by television, newspapers, and radio.

Investigators have also researched LSD use in a number of other situations. Some success has been noted in the use of LSD in attempts to help terminally ill patients cope with death, and one researcher has hopes for the drug's use in other areas of life stress, such as major decision making, psychosomatic illness, and dealing with reality.[9] LSD has been used in the treatment of neurosis and as an aid to therapy and self-concept in the treatment of sexual deviancy, mental illness, pain in cancer patients, and frigidity. Thus far, however, LSD does not appear to be a highly desirable therapeutic agent.

One of the most controversial issues surrounding LSD use is its alleged capacity to damage chromosomes. While *in vitro* (test tube) studies may be of questionable value, they do add to the data concerning possible harmful LSD effects. Maiman Cohen of the State University of New York at Buffalo reported in one such study that LSD-damaged white-blood-cell chromosomes are a conclusive index of genetic damage. Researcher Ralph Metzger states results of another study:

> A group of 22 LSD users is reported to have a mean of 13.2% chromosomal breakage, compared to a mean of 3.8% in a group of 12 non-users. However, we note that of the 22 "LSD users" not one had used only LSD, all except 3 had used amphetamines, most had used heroin and many phenothiazines (tranquilizers).[10]

LSD's relation to birth defects has also been under study. In cooperation with a pediatrician, three researchers studied 120 infants born to a sample of LSD users.[11] They concluded that "there is no evidence of a relation between parental LSD exposure and major congenital defects in their offspring." *However, no chemical known to science has been proved to be entirely harmless for all pregnant women and their babies during all stages of pregnancy.*[12]

Psychotherapists have used LSD in experiments on increasing the receptivity of patients to therapies or to dealing with personal problems. Most of their research, however, has failed to document significant therapeutic benefits other than an increase in patient morale. The drug has *not* proved to be the long-sought chemical key to schizophrenia. LSD has been shown to be of some value in treating autistic children, but the improvement rapidly reverses when the use of the drug is stopped. Similarly, attempts at treating chronic alcoholics with LSD have not met with long-term success, and in what limited successes there were, it was not thought that LSD was the decisive factor. Some successes have been obtained in treating cancer patients and amputees.

MESCALINE (PEYOTE)

Introduction

Mescaline is a hallucinogen derived from peyote "buttons," the dried tops of several species of cactus. Long in use as a part of American Indian religious ceremonies, peyote is said to have first become known through a revelation in a woman's dream. The substance is similar to strychnine and morphine, but is not physiologically active in humans.

Once dried, peyote buttons can be ingested in raw form, but they are usually extremely bitter and can cause nausea and vomiting. Synthetically produced mescaline has a better taste and less intense side effects, and can be liquefied, encapsulated, or made into tablets.

Peyote was first studied in the United States by Lewis Lewin, who extracted mescaline and adrenaline alkaloids from the plant. Lewin categorized mescaline as a "phantasticant" substance "capable of exercising [its] chemical power on all senses, but . . . particularly the visual and auditory spheres as well as the general sensibility."[13] Study of the plant, Lewin felt, would aid in the understanding of psychotic mental states.

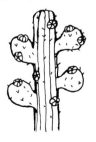

Though LSD was at the heart of the psychedelic drug movement, mescaline use became popular too, since its "trip" was not as intense and was therefore more manageable. Use has been curtailed, however, since mescaline is now classified as a dangerous drug under state and national drug laws. It may still be used in religious practices of the Native American church, and medically it is used as a tincture for angina pectoris, as a respiratory stimulant for pneumonia patients, and as a cardiac tonic.

Some of the Native American church rites were influenced to a degree by early Christianity, but slices of peyote have replaced the sacramental bread and wine. Native Americans regard the cactus as God's special gift to the Indians and equate its effects with the workings of the divine spirit. Their use of mescaline is limited to healing religious services only; the drug is not to be used for recreational purposes.

Psychophysiological Effects

Mescaline's primary effects are similar to those of LSD, focusing on sensory perception, particularly the audio-visual realm. With eyes closed, numerous colors and images may be visualized. With eyes open, mescaline users may be attracted to one particular object, and may focus on it for a long period of time. Synesthesia may occur, and the sense of time diminish or vanish. Thoughts that are ordinarily suppressed may come to the surface, and users are sometimes quite sensitive to new ideas. Mood swings usually occur soon after ingestion.

Mescaline users may experience visual distortion as well as acuity. Spatial relationships and objects may seem to increase or decrease in size, and depth perception can become distorted. One unknown user described the effect this way:

Confusion was suddenly becoming an issue. I pointed to the wall in an attempt to ask if it was as far away as it seemed and I noticed my hand and fingers appeared to have diminished in size. They too seemed farther away than normal. I knew my arms were not four feet long and, at the moment, it became apparent the mescaline had me firmly in its chemical grip. I gazed across what now seemed like a small-sized football field of a living room. The wallpaper seemed to writhe and undulate in a circular up and down manner much in the fashion that an amoeba moves under a microscope. The ceiling lowered and raised as if it were the membrane of a lung in the process of breathing. Of course, these were not grotesque perceptual distortions, but, nonetheless, they were readily apparent at that point. Sigrid said she did not share these perceptions and I said yes, that was to be expected. The couch seemed especially soft, like a goose-down filled bed as I spied the carpet. It too was moving amoeba-like.

Words had become equally impossible and unimportant. It seemed that now was the time to leave . . . to go for a long walk! Sigrid looked at me with an understanding expression and I assured her I would call as soon as the roller coaster stopped and I got off. The distance from the couch to the front door seemed to take forever to cover. However, we eventually made it to the front door and as Sigrid walked me out of her sorority house we gave each other a gentle kiss good night. I walked into the pitch black rain of the night . . . and continued walking for seven hours.

When mescaline is taken orally, it is quickly absorbed, permeating the blood-brain barrier within thirty minutes to two hours. Though neither psychological nor physical dependence is caused by the drug, mescaline use can result in pupil dilation, increased EEG activity, slight tremors, and occasional shaking, the effects lasting up to twelve hours. There is some cross-tolerance between mescaline and LSD, though tolerance of mescaline seems to develop more slowly. Mescaline is excreted relatively unchanged in the urine.

The kind of trip a mescaline user experiences depends a good deal on his or her expectations and the setting. Perceptions may be particularly enjoyable or insightful, but the mescaline user is usually aware that a drug is producing the experienced effects. If a trip becomes too intense, however, fear and panic may set in.

PSILOCYBIN

Introduction

Psilocybin is the chemical derivative obtained from the *Psilocybe Mexicana* mushroom. Fifteen species of this mushroom can be found growing wild in the United States or Canada, usually in moist areas such as wet meadows, pastures, and forests.

The psilocybin mushroom was worshiped in Guatemala as long ago as 1000 B. C. ,[14] and it appears that Aztec Indians consumed it in the belief that it would help to establish communication with the spirit world. Currently the drug has no medical use, but it is being researched as a possible aid in experimental psychiatry and therapy. Psilocybin is usually taken orally, as dried mushrooms or in tablet form, or it may be dried, ground, and added to food.

Psychophysiological Effects

Once ingested, psilocybin is converted by an enzyme in the stomach into psilocin.[15] The effects of the drug, which are similar to those of LSD, usually begin twenty-five to forty minutes later, and generally last from three to eight hours. The central nervous system is affected, and changes in time and space perception, wakefulness, attentiveness, suggestibility, and distractability occur.

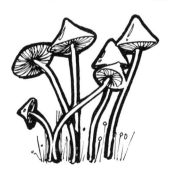

The physiological effects of psilocybin include dilation of the pupils, an increase in deep tendon reflex, and an increase in pulse rate, blood pressure, and body temperature.[16] The user may experience tingling sensations on the skin surface and weak to strong involuntary limb movements. Intoxication from psilocybin, much like intoxication from mescaline, may result in muscular relaxation and emotional dysfunctions such as extreme hilarity and loss of concentration. The user may smell pleasant but unfamiliar odors, and have illusions and hallucinations.

The use of psilocybin may also result in swings of emotion, from marked euphoria to marked depression or anxiety. Hazards of the drug include acute paranoia and accidental or deliberate death, though no deaths have been directly related to overdose.

Due to the increasing popularity of psilocybin, the number of people collecting the mushroom for use and sale has increased dramatically over the past few years. The increase in availability of the drug is a legitimate cause for concern. Property owners are becoming angry with trespassers. Increasing numbers of "shroomers" are being prosecuted for trespassing in the Pacific Northwest and the southeastern United States, where the mushrooms grow abundantly. Another danger is the high potential for mistaking a poisonous mushroom for psilocybin. It is estimated that toxic species outnumber psilocybin species by at least ten to one. Many mushroom pickers are not aware of this and so are especially vulnerable to mushroom poisoning.

PCP

Introduction

PCP (phencyclidine) is a difficult drug to classify. Many think of it as a hallucinogen, though it also produces depressant, stimulant, analgesic, and anesthetic effects.[17]

First synthesized in the late 1950s, PCP was intended for use as an animal tranquilizer and as an anesthetic in surgery on humans.[18] It produced such unwanted and unpleasant side effects, however, that experimental studies with humans were soon discontinued. In 1969, PCP became available "for veterinary use only," but as of April 1, 1979, all legal manufacturing of the drug in the United States was terminated.[19] Despite this restriction, PCP is relatively available because it is easy to produce. The drug can be injected, taken orally, or smoked.

Effects on Society

PCP, commonly known as angel dust, first came into popular street use in San Francisco in 1967. Many early PCP experimenters soon rejected it as undesirable. In spite of its reputation, however, PCP was increasingly seen on the street because of its cheapness, availability, and ability to masquerade as other popular street drugs, such as THC (tetrahydrocannabinol), mescaline, or cocaine. It is still cheap and available, and despite its dangers continues to be a drug of choice. Many take the drug simply to prove that they can handle it, and its use is spreading, some feel to epidemic proportions. A 1977 study revealed that PCP use had doubled among individuals aged twelve to seventeen and had increased 14 percent among those from eighteen to twenty-five.[20] PCP was on the decrease. However, today it has become an epidemic in many major cities. For example, in Washington, D.C., PCP has caused so many people to be admitted to Saint Elizabeth's Hospital "that it is called with grim irony the key to Saint E's."[21]

Psychophysiological Effects

PCP is a powerful drug even in small quantities. It has a particularly strong effect on the cerebral cortex, although it affects the entire body, and tolerance can develop quickly. In large doses the drug acts as a tranquilizing depressant, often inducing coma or comatose-like behavior. All too often, PCP results in psychotic episodes, seizures, violent behavior, and death.

PCP is most often smoked, but taking the drug in tablet or capsule form or snorting pure powder affords a larger dose. Injecting or snorting the drug produces almost immediate effects; effects from smoking may take fifteen minutes to appear.[22] The experience can vary: users report that PCP makes them feel as if they're in another world—a fantasy world that is sometimes pleasant, sometimes not. When the high wears off, users often feel mildly depressed, irritable, and alienated from their surroundings.

A PCP Case Study

One afternoon two high school boys, who were best friends, decided to use PCP. After ingesting the substance one boy felt tired and fell asleep on the davenport. In the meantime the other boy started hallucinating and thought his friend was a wild animal attacking him. He went into the kitchen and found a knife and proceeded to stab his friend in the chest twenty-one times. He killed his best friend, yet when the effects of the drug wore off he had no recollection of what had happened.[23]

This case study is just one example of the bizarre effects of PCP. People often hear about these emergency cases and think that a person who takes PCP will become a killer. PCP does cause adverse effects about 30 percent of the time and violent reactions somewhat less often. Two doctors who treat PCP patients have explained some of the reasons teenagers turn to drugs like PCP. They have found that in order to solve the drug problems of most kids it is necessary to try to solve the environmental and behavioral problems that lead them to use drugs. Most of the PCP users had been physically or emotionally battered. Of the female patients, 60 percent had had incestuous relationships. They also found that although the people who used PCP less frequently tended to become violent, they often didn't remember their behavior and so had little motivation to quit. Chronic users of PCP were more likely to act out sexually. PCP for many users is an escape, as one user explains:

PCP blocks out the whole world, and you are in your own world. That's always there anyway, but there's so much to interfere with yourself when you're straight that you can't deal with yourself.[24]

Most descriptions of PCP experiences are similar to this one. However, some users are looking for an intensification of emotion, stimulation, and sometimes a new experience. Also, users have reported they enjoyed the aphrodisiac effects of the drug.[25]

Though it is not really known how PCP affects the body, "the medical guess is that PCP acts on nerve cells, preventing stimuli from different parts of the body from being correctly processed by the brain."[26] Generalized numbness, blurred vision, muscular dysfunction, and dizziness may occur, and profuse sweating, flushing, increased blood pressure, and rapid heartbeat are typical. A mild dose of three to eight milligrams produces "spaciness," problems with perception and coordination, numbness, increased blood pressure, bloodshot eyes, and impaired speech. A dose of ten to twenty milligrams produces indifference to pain, sweating and flushing, drooling, distorted vision, bulging eyeballs, muscle rigidity, verbal inhibition, mental and physical retardation (a general slowing down), and a total inability to comprehend time and space.[27] Larger amounts of the drug may cause users to appear drunk, confuse their speech, and distort their vision. Thinking, remembering, and making decisions can be very difficult.

Long-Term Effects   Many users who take PCP regularly experience disturbances in memory, judgment, concentration, and perception long after they stop taking the drug.[28] Long-term users are also subject to recurring bouts of anxiety and depression and sporadic outbreaks of violent behavior.

Hazards   Though a PCP overdose may be lethal, more PCP users die from accidents caused by drug-induced behavior than from the drug itself.[29] People on PCP have drowned in shallow water because they weren't able to tell which way was up. Others have had auto accidents, fallen off roofs, and fallen out of windows because of the drug's intoxicating effects.[30] PCP use has also been linked to suicides, drowning from sedation, and self-inflicted wounds.

SUMMARY

LSD, mescaline, and psilocybin are hallucinogenic drugs that were particularly popular in the 1960s and early 1970s. They affect sensory perception and can lead to a variety of adverse psychological conditions. LSD causes the most severe effects and its action lasts the longest. All the drugs are illegal to purchase, except mescaline when it is used by the Native American church in religious services.

Another hallucinogenic drug, phencyclidine (PCP), was originally used by veterinarians as an animal tranquilizer. It is still popular today with young people, though it was deemed illegal in 1979. Use of PCP can lead to confusion, convulsions, psychosis, and even death. The hallucinogenic drugs seem to gain periodic popularity, then their usage decreases. When they are used it is with a somewhat clearer expectation of what to expect than in the past.

NOTES

[1]Bernard Aaronson and Humphrey Osmond, *Psychedelics* (New York: Doubleday, 1970).

[2]John Cashman, *The LSD Story*. Copyright © 1966 by Fawcett Publications Inc. With permission of the Fawcett Books Group, Consumer Publishing Division of CBS Inc.

[3]Presented to a drug class at the University of Oregon by Terry Beckkedahl, an Oregon State Police criminologist.

[4]*Drug Survival News*, November/December 1981, pp. 12–13. Reprinted with permission of Do It Now Foundation, Phoenix, AZ.

[5]Ibid. p. 13.

[6]Ibid.

[7]John Marks, "Sex, Drugs, and the CIA: The Shocking Search for an Ultimate Weapon," *Saturday Review* 6, no. 3 (February 3, 1979). Copyright © 1979 by *Saturday Review*. All rights reserved. Reprinted with permission.

[8]Ibid.

[9]Ralph Metzger, "Reflection on LSD Ten Years Later," *Journal of Psychedelic Drugs* 10, no. 2 (April–June 1978):137–40.

[10]Ralph Metzger, *Psychedelic Review* 10 (1969):48.

[11]William H. McGlothlin, Robert S. Sparkes, and David O. Arnold, "Effect of LSD on Human Pregnancy," *Journal of the American Medical Association* 212 (June 1, 1970):1483–87.

[12]Edward M. Brecher et al., *Licit and Illicit Drugs* (Boston: Little, Brown, 1972), p. 390.

[13]Quoted from A. Hoffer and H. Osmond, *The Hallucinogens* (New York: Academic Press, 1967), p. 2.

[14]Jeremy Sandford, *In Search of the Magic Mushroom*.

[15]R. Schultes and Albert Hofmann, *The Botany and Chemistry of Hallucinogens* (Springfield, Ill.: Chas. C Thomas, 1973), pp. 22–23.

[16]L. E. Hollister, *Chemical Psychoses: LSD and Related Drugs* (Springfield, Ill.: Chas. C Thomas, 1968), p. 52.

[17]Sidney Cohen, "PCP (Angel Dust): New Trends in Treatment," *Drug Abuse and Alcoholism Newsletter* 7, no. 6 (July 1978):1–3.

[18]National Institute on Drug Abuse, *PCP* (Washington, D.C.: Department of Health, Education and Welfare, 1977).

[19]Richard Geary, "PCP (Phencyclidine): An Update," *Journal of Psychedelic Drugs* 2, no. 4 (October–December 1979):265.

[20]"PCP: Alcohol and Drug Fact Sheet," *Drug Information Center (DIC)* (Eugene: University of Oregon, 1980), pp. 1463–66.

[21]William L. Chaze, "The Deadly Path of Today's PCP Epidemic," *U.S. News & World Report*, November 19, 1984, pp. 65–66. Reprinted with permission.

[22]"Phencyclidine: PCP," *National Clearinghouse for Drug Abuse Information* 14, no. 2 (March 1978):1–11.

[23]Presented to a drug class at the University of Oregon by Terry Beckkedahl, an Oregon State Police criminologist.

[24]Katherine Carlson, "PCP from the Other Side: Users Look at Phencyclidine," *Journal of*

Psychedelic Drugs 11, no. 3 (July–September 1979): p. 232. Reprinted with permission of Haight-Asbury Publications, San Francisco.

[25]Ibid.

[26]Peter Koper, "Angel Death," *New Times* 10, no. 6 (March 20, 1978).

[27]Mark L. Richards et al., "Phencyclidine Psychosis," *Drug Intelligence and Clinical Pharmacy* 13, no. 6 (June 1979):336–39.

[29]National Institute on Drug Abuse, *PCP.* p. 2.

[29]Ibid. p. 3.

[30]Ibid. p. 4.

11

MARIJUANA
still a controversy

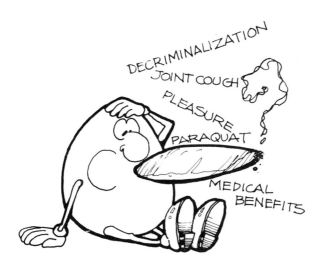

INTRODUCTION

Marijuana is a drug made from the chopped leaves, stems, and seeds of the cannabis plant. It has been used as an intoxicant and an herbal medication in various parts of the world for centuries, and is still used by many people today. Its variable effects and uncertain hazards, however, make it a most controversial drug.

Marijuana Use in the World

The first detailed description of cannabis appeared in a medical book prepared by the legendary Chinese Emperor Shen-Nung in 2700 B. C. ,[1] but archaeological data suggest that knowledge of cannabis's use goes back at least 6000 years.[2] Early uses of cannabis included smoking it as part of purification rituals and relieving pain during surgery. Hashish, the resin of the marijuana plant, was eaten and drunk in Arabian countries during the Middle Ages.

Cannabis use did not spread to western Europe until the late 1700s; its therapeutic uses were studied intently by a British physician named O'Shaughnessy in 1843.[3] Quasi-medical and medical use of a variety of cannabis preparations, including elixers and medicines, occurred in North America later in that century, but nonmedical consumption of cannabis in North America did not appear until the twentieth century. Presently, marijuana appears to be the fourth most popular psychoactive substance in the world,[4] preceded only by caffeine, nicotine, and alcohol. Some speculate that upcoming generations will feel the same way about marijuana as people today feel about cigarettes and alcohol—they'll accept using it as a way of life.

Marijuana Use in the United States

Though marijuana was used earlier in this century, it gained great popularity in the 1960s. It is still the fourth most widely used drug in the United States, with an estimated 30 million regular users.

Many young people are introduced to marijuana by their peers, usually acquaintances, friends, sisters, or brothers. People often try drugs such as marijuana because they feel pressured by peers to be part of the group. Students have reported some of the following reasons for using marijuana: to have a good time with friends, to get high, to relieve boredom, to enhance the effects of other drugs, and to cope with stress. It is interesting to examine some of the reasons former daily users have discontinued their habit: loss of interest in getting high, concern about harmful psychological effects, and concern about their loss of energy and ambition. At its peak, daily or nearly daily use of marijuana involved more than one in ten high school seniors, with nearly daily use of marijuana nonsubstantially more common than daily use.[5]

An increasing number of adults are using marijuana. It is estimated that about 44 percent of those from twenty-six to thirty-four smoke pot, but 7 percent of those over thirty-five.[6] Many young people continue to use their preferred drug as they grow older. Also, for a variety of reasons, some adults are being attracted to marijuana. However, the overwhelming preponderance of use is by those under thirty.

Though statistics are contradictory, it appears that American-grown marijuana is increasing and may now be enough to supply at least half of the nation's demand. The Department of Agriculture estimates the value of the nation's corn crop in 1984 at $19.5 billion, followed by hay at $11.5 billion and soybeans at $11.3 billion. The same year, the House Select Committee on Narcotics Abuse said the annual U.S. pot crop could be worth from $10 to $50 billion.[7] The West (California, Hawaii, Idaho, and Oregon) continues to be the leading marijuana-growing area. In addition to an increased supply, quality of the plant has improved through the application of selective cultivation. It appears that the U.S.-grown marijuana, some of the best in the world, is approximately five to twelve times more potent than it was three to five years ago. New research must be conducted to study the effects of the newer, high-potency plant. It is imperative that we learn more about marijuana since it is the most widely used of all the illicit drugs.

During the early 1900s, marijuana was *incorrectly* classified as a narcotic in popular and legal literature. No comprehensive scientific study of the drug had been done in this country, but it was *assumed* to be a narcotic and its use was linked to violent crimes and insanity by the media and federal narcotics officers. In 1932 the National Conference on Uniform State Laws included marijuana provisions in the Uniform Narcotic Drug Act. In late 1937 Congress adopted the Marijuana Tax Act, which prohibited the use of marijuana.[8]

With the escalation of opiate-use violations in the 1950s, corresponding marijuana penalties were increased at the request of federal drug officials. Eventually, first-offense possession of marijuana was made a felony punishable by lengthy imprisonment. Public opinion began to turn away from such heavy sentencing, however, and in 1973 the state of Oregon reduced the penalty for possession of less than one ounce of marijuana to a fine of no more than $100.[9] Marijuana was also reclassified as a Schedule I drug under the Comprehensive Drug Abuse Prevention and Control Act of 1970, and as such it cannot be marketed but it can be used for research. Currently the Department of Health and Human Services is considering a proposal to reclassify marijuana as a Schedule II drug so that it might become a prescribed medicine for glaucoma and chemotherapy.[10] Several states have already passed laws allowing marijuana to be used in the treatment of certain patients.

Paraquat

Mexico provided much of the best marijuana until a couple of years ago, when the Mexican government began to crack down on drug exporters and sprayed the marijuana crops with the herbicide Paraquat. Colombia moved rapidly to fill the gap. And as we have noted, the plant is increasingly being cultivated in the United States.

Paraquat is a toxic herbicide that has been used since 1975 in marijuana-

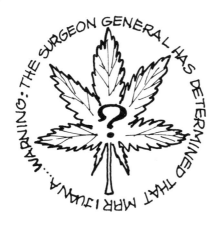

eradication programs conducted by the Mexican government. The chemical was patented in England and is manufactured in Mexico.[11] Spraying with Paraquat has significantly reduced marijuana production in Mexico, but the chemical is used in the United States only for weed control and as a desiccant of soybeans and cotton.

In 1978, there were reports that marijuana contaminated with Paraquat was being brought into the United States. Since Paraquat can cause irreversible lung damage and fibrosis (a scarring of the lung that inhibits oxygen absorption),[12] to those who inhale concentrated amounts of it, Congress requested that the Office of Drug Abuse Policy (ODAP) at the White House investigate the validity of such reports. The ODAP did find that Paraquat-sprayed marijuana was crossing the border, and it is said to be still doing so today.

PHARMACOLOGICAL CLASSIFICATION

The pharmacological classification of cannabis has been the subject of much public misunderstanding. Such controversy is most likely caused by the fact that under various conditions and doses, the drug may have stimulant, sedative, analgesic, and hallucinogenic effects. Scientists contributing to the First Report of the National Commission on Marijuana and Drug Abuse felt that marijuana should be listed in a category by itself.[13] The authors of the report stated that "pharmacologically speaking, cannabis is unique and distinct from psychomimetics [drugs that mimic a psychotic disorder], opiates, barbiturates and amphetamines."[14]

Marijuana (grass, pot, weed, dope, etc.) is the common name for a drug made from the plant *Cannabis sativa*. The psychoactive ingredient is delta-9-tetrahydrocannabinol (THC) although "there are more than 420 chemicals [in the] sixty-one cannabis plants."[15] The amount of THC in marijuana determines its potency. The type of plant, weather, soil, time of harvest, selective cultivation, and other factors determine this amount.

Hashish, or hash, is made by taking resin from the leaves and flowers of the marijuana plant and pressing them into cakes or slabs. Hash oil may contain 50 percent THC. Pure THC is almost never available, except for research.

PHYSIOLOGICAL EFFECTS

When marijuana is smoked, its effects usually last from two to four hours; if the drug is ingested, effects may last five to twelve hours. Physiological responses include mild dilation of the blood vessels in the extremities, a slight increase in blood flow to the arms and legs, and a slight reduction of body temperature through heat loss. Blood pressure is slightly elevated, and reddened eyes and a dry mouth can also be expected. Although appetite is usually stimulated, blood sugar levels remain largely unaffected.

The hazards of marijuana use are related both to the drug itself and to the method of administration. Acute effects, such as psychological dependence, can occur with high dose or chronic use. On occasion anxiety reactions have been reported, and more rarely, hallucination-caused physical harm with very large doses, especially if the drug is eaten.

The supportive evidence in this section is derived largely from the 1982 report *Marijuana and Health,* research by the Institute of Medicine of the National Academy of Sciences, studies by the Canadian Addiction Research Foundation for the World Health Organization, and current research reports. It is interesting to note that some of these findings are in conflict.

Effects on Body Functions

Marijuana is absorbed into the bloodstream through the lungs or intestines, depending on the route administered, and then distributed to different parts of the body. THC is highly fat-soluble and some of it is stored in the fatty tissue. *This means that it may stay in the body for as long as a month.* The metabolites are then slowly excreted from the body in urine and feces. THC and other cannabinols accumulate in the fatty linings of the cells and are released back into the bloodstream over many days. Studies of experienced users show that the half-life of THC is nineteen hours, and fifty hours for its metabolites.[16]

Though it is known that marijuana is an active intoxicant that affects body functions, the extent of its effects, both positive and negative, is difficult to determine. J. Thomas Underleider, presidential appointee to the Shaffer Commission, has stated that, "no intoxicant or, for that matter, no drug is totally safe or harmless. However, it is my opinion that marijuana involves only minimal harm to the user."[17] Backing up that theory are the findings of a careful review of the literature and testimony of health officials, which revealed that not a single human fatality in the United States has ever resulted solely from marijuana use.[18]

A 1970 National Institute of Mental Health Study on Jamaica (the Jamaican Study) also concluded that marijuana was a relatively harmless intoxicant.[19] The study revealed that marijuana did not cause amotivational syndrome, mental illness, or physical abnormalities in thirty individuals who were heavy marijuana smokers.[20] Similar studies in Jamaica, Greece, and Costa Rica indicated that marijuana causes amotivational syndrome. However, the small numbers used in these studies make it difficult to make generalizations that apply to a whole population.[21]

Pulmonary Effects

Marijuana smoking can have harmful pulmonary effects. Chronic marijuana use has been seen to impair lung function in otherwise healthy subjects.[22] Heavy marijuana and/or hashish use can also cause chronic bronchitis, emphysema, and fibrosis.[23] Residuals of smoked marijuana have been shown to be carcinogenic to animal skin.

Lung tissue continually exposed to marijuana smoke exhibits changes as serious as, or possibly more serious than, those found in tissues of heavy cigarette smokers. Though it has been argued that less frequent use of smaller quantities of marijuana might reduce this hazard, the custom of deep inhalation and the practice of consuming virtually all of each joint may more than offset any hazard reduction. Additionally, there is evidence that if marijuana is readily available, the number of marijuana cigarettes consumed (up to ten joints daily) may approach that of tobacco cigarettes.[24]

It is known that cigarette smoking can lead to various forms of cancer. Currently there is also concern that marijuana and cancer may be linked. "Marijuana smoke contains 50 percent more cancer causing materials than tobacco smoke," says Donald P. Tashkin, "so the potential for causing lung cancer is real." He also says that though the research evidence is still sketchy and even contradictory in some cases, much of it suggests that marijuana smoke induces inflammatory changes in the lining of the respiratory tract that may be precancerous. "The smoke also has toxic effects on cells which have an important role in protecting the lungs against infection and other noxious insults," Tashkin says.[25] That marijuana smoke can irritate the lungs and throat and result in "joint cough," strongly suggests that prolonged heavy smoking of marijuana, like that of tobacco, will lead to cancer of the respiratory tract and to serious impairment of lung function.[26]

It seems logical that the high amount of tobacco smoke that enters the average cigarette smoker's air passageways should put him or her at a higher risk than a marijuana smoker. However, according to Sidney Cohen, two factors equalize the risk:

1. Typical cigarette smokers do not inhale smoke deep into the bronchial passages, or if they do, it's for a short time. Marijuana is inhaled as deeply as possible.
2. In recent years, there has been an increase in the amount of marijuana smoked per individual.[27]

A large number of people view marijuana smoking as harmless, relaxing, and possibly beneficial. Decades ago, a strikingly similar belief prevailed about cigarette smoking. After the 1964 surgeon general's report came out that view changed dramatically. "In terms of knowledge about the effects of marijuana, I suspect we are now where we were 20 years ago in cigarette smoking," says Donald T. Frederickson, assistant dean at New York University's Post Graduate School of Medicine.[28] Of growing concern is the potentially harmful effects of today's marijuana, which is ten times stronger than that of the 1960s.

Cardiovascular Complications

Cardiovascular problems resulting from marijuana use may be relevant only to the elderly or to persons with preexisting cardiac disorders.[29] Recent American Medical Association reports emphasize that the use of marijuana by patients with impaired heart function may precipitate chest pain more rapidly, following less effort, than smoking of tobacco cigarettes.[30] "Marijuana accelerates the rate at which the heart contracts and may temporarily weaken the strength of contractions, making it potentially dangerous for people with certain cardiac conditions."[31] Though this and similar evidence is limited, warnings against marijuana use for heart patients and others who may have impaired cardiac function seem justified.[32]

There is good evidence that the smoking of marijuana typically causes acute changes in the heart and circulation. However, there is controversy surrounding the issue of how it affects the "normal," healthy individual. According to a study by the Committee of the Institute on Medicine, there is no evidence of a permanently deleterious effect on the cardiovascular system.[33] However, evidence shows that marijuana increases the work of the heart, usually by raising the heart rate—as much as 50 percent, depending on the amount of THC in the cigarette—and in some persons by raising the blood pressure. This work load poses a threat to persons with hypertension, cerebrovascular disease, and coronary artherosclerosis.

A similar warning may be in line for cardiac patients who combine marijuana with alcohol. A recent research paper indicates that this combination may be very dangerous for these individuals.[34] Intense nausea, vomiting, and a drop in heart rate from 150 to 36 beats per minute have occurred in subjects using both of these drugs.

Effects on the Immunology System

Marijuana may act as an immunosuppressant, substance that inhibits the body's response to disease. The data from hospital studies thus far are contradictory, however.

One recent study revealed that marijuana in doses equivalent to human use did suppress circulating antibodies in rats.[35] Other recent studies of chronic users of marijuana suggest a possible correlation between heavy and prolonged marijuana use and the user's immune response. The researchers noted, however, that the witnessed effects were transitory, varying significantly among subjects and closely related to the time the blood samples were obtained and tested.[36]

The data from animal studies suggest that marijuana has an immunosuppressant effect that is mild compared with those of known immunosuppressant drugs. The studies in humans are contradictory: some demonstrated mild immunosuppressant effects, but others, using the same or similar methods, found no differences in the immune system between normals and chronic marijuana smokers. No animal or human studies have yet determined if marijuana smokers are more prone to infections or other diseases.[37] Researchers are concerned that further research may not yield definitive findings, and because of the widespread use of marijuana, even weak immunosuppressive effects are alarming.

Effects on Endocrine Functioning

The issue of marijuana's possible effect on endocrine functioning was first raised in 1972. In 1974, experimental evidence suggesting that marijuana causes a reduction in serum testosterone, the principal male sex hormone, was first published. Low sperm counts in heavy marijuana users have also been indicated,[38] though the significance of this finding is yet to be evaluated. Further studies of chronic hashish users in Greece also indicate a diminution of sperm count and alterations in the cellular characteristics of the spermatozoa in otherwise normal young males.[39]

Several animal studies have found that relatively high doses of THC have caused reduced testicular weights and lowered levels of plasma testosterone. Nevertheless, since a range of factors influence testosterone levels in men (e.g., the time of day the assay is done and any drugs in the system) and since reduced levels have still been within normal limits, the clinical significance of endocrine studies may be limited to persons who are already impaired or of marginal fertility.

Although animal studies have shown that THC lowers the concentration of brain hormones that control reproductive functions, it is not known if there is a direct effect on reproductive tissues. THC appears to have a modest, reversible suppressive effect on sperm production in men, but there is no proof that it has a deleterious effect on male fertility. Although there is convincing evidence that marijuana interferes with ovulation in female monkeys, researchers are not convinced that this occurs in human females.[40]

To date, there is no conclusive evidence that the use of marijuana during pregnancy can harm the fetus in humans. However, it is highly recommended that women abstain from drugs during pregnancy to avoid any potential risk. THC is known to cross the placental barrier in animals and to cause birth defects when administered to animals in large doses.[41]

Psychomotor Impairment

The Department of Health, Education and Welfare's 1979 report *Marijuana and Health* states that there is clear-cut evidence that marijuana impairs reaction time, motor coordination, and visual perception, making it dangerous for people to drive, fly, or operate machinery while intoxicated by marijuana.[42] At the Fifth World Congress of Psychiatry in 1978, Danish investigators offered proof that cannabis reduces driving skills.[43] Braking time was shown to slow down after cannabis use, as was time of response to sound. Illusions were reported to occur and sudden flights of ideas caused confusion and anxiety in new situations. Responses involving eye–hand coordination were impaired, and the more complex the situation became, the slower the responses.

Research also indicates that with a severity directly related to dose, marijuana impairs motor coordination and affects tracking and the sensory and perceptual functions important for safe driving and the operation of other machines; impairs short-term memory; and slows learning. The drug appears to alter the sense of time, reduce one's ability to do things that require concentration, and affect the swift reactions and coordination that are so essential in driving a car or operating machinery. Driving experiments show that marijuana use affects a wide range of skills needed for safe driving. Thinking and reflexes are slowed, making it hard for the driver to respond to sudden, unexpected events.[44]

Also, the driver's ability to track (stay in lane) through curves, to brake quickly, and to maintain speed and the proper distance between cars is affected. Research shows that these skills are impaired for at least four to six hours after smoking a single marijuana cigarette, long after the high is gone. If a person drinks alcohol while using marijuana, the risk of an accident is greatly increased.

Despite such evidence that marijuana impairs driving ability, it is likely that more marijuana users than ever before now drive while high.[45] As use becomes increasingly common and socially acceptable, and as the risk of arrest for simple possession decreases, more and more users will probably risk driving while high. In limited surveys, 60 to 80 percent of those questioned indicated that they sometimes drive while high.[46]

Genetic and Brain Damage

Chromosome and Cell-Metabolism Alterations   Early reports of increased chromosomal breakage and human cell-culture abnormalities resulting from marijuana use have *not* been corroborated by recent research. Reports do indicate, however, that marijuana may increase the number of lung cells containing abnormal levels of chromosomes and may also increase the number of white blood cells showing abnormally low levels of chromosomes.

Early research has also indicated the possibility that cannabis, or one or more of its chemical components, inhibits DNA metabolism in abnormal (carcinogenic) animal cells while leaving normal cells unaffected. If such preferential inhibition also occurs in humans, marijuana may turn out to be of chemotherapeutic value as an anticancer agent.[47] Further study may also substantiate current indications that cannabis, its synthesized components, or chemically related drugs might prove useful in preventing organ rejection in human organ-transplant surgery.[48]

Effects on the Brain   According to some reports, it can be said with confidence that marijuana has acute effects on the brain, including chemical and electrophysiological changes.[49] Its most clearly established acute effects are on mental functions and behavior. However, other studies have concluded that there is no persuasive evidence that marijuana causes overt changes in the brain.[50] Computerized studies of users of marijuana reveal no gross changes in brain structure. Studies indicating marijuana-related structural changes in monkey brains utilized flawed methodologies and cannot be cited as evidence that marijuana affects electrical activity in the human brain. In any event, such changes have not been demonstrated to persist in humans after use of the drug has been discontinued. It appears that more research on the use of stronger marijuana needs to be conducted before a final decision can be made about the efects marijuana has on the brain.

Research on Brain Damage   When two samples of young men with histories of heavy cannabis smoking were studied in Missouri and Massachusetts, brain scans showed no evidence of cerebral atrophy. However, researchers Harold Kolansky and William Moore suggest that biochemical and even structural cerebral changes occur with chronic long-term cannabis use.[51] Symptoms of these changes include apathy, disturbed self-awareness, confusion, and unrealistic understanding, but such symptoms disappear three to twenty-four months after marijuana use has ended. Marijuana-caused intoxication also produces minimal and transient changes in brain waves, but results of brain-wave studies are still unclear and inconsistent.

Tolerance

Tolerance to marijuana has been demonstrated in both humans and animals. Although tolerance can develop rapidly after only a few small doses, it disappears at an equally rapid rate for many who are affected. Large doses administered to animals result in tolerance lasting for longer periods. Tolerance to marijuana does not necessarily have health implications unless it should lead to stronger and more frequent doses with adverse consequences, such as stronger respiratory effects.

PSYCHOLOGICAL EFFECTS

Small doses of cannabis generally elicit euphoria, enhanced congeniality, and a mood of relaxed passivity. At moderate doses these effects are intensified, and may be accompanied by some impairment of short-term memory, disturbances in thought patterns, lapses in attention, subjective feelings of unfamiliarity, depersonalization, and sensory distraction. Large doses bring on a further loosening of emotional and social restraints, a deeper feeling of relaxation or euphoria, stronger distortions of time and space, and illusions. Reports of individuals who have taken large doses also mention mental confusion, as well as rather terrifying paranoid thoughts and anxiety. When extremely large doses are taken, hallucinations may occur. Fortunately, anxiety and panic reactions begin to diminish shortly after the drug's effect wears off.

How marijuana affects the user depends not only on the dose taken but also on how experienced the smoker is. Quite often the new user experiences little if any chemical effect. Appreciation of the altered state may have to be acquired before the user can actually perceive it. Novice smokers may experience only protracted laughter or tears during their first marijuana experiences.

Psychopathology

The most common adverse psychological reaction to marijuana among American users is acute anxiety.[52] This reaction is an intense response to the perspective and distortion of reality marijuana generally produces. The reaction appears to be more common in relatively inexperienced users although unexpectedly high doses of cannabis can cause panic in the more experienced user as well. Symptoms of acute anxiety generally respond to sensitive assurance and diminish soon after the effects of marijuana recede.[53]

Transient mild paranoia is another adverse reaction common to marijuana users. Those who are characterized by more paranoid defense mechanisms are less likely to experience other acute adverse reactions. If users are concerned about their drug experience and/or the circumstances of use, anxiety and mild paranoid reactions to the drug are likely to occur. In a study of college student users, Naditch and colleagues found that those who were hypochondriacs, who felt less in control of their lives, and who were more at the mercy of external events were more likely to have adverse reactions to marijuana and other psychoactive drugs.[54]

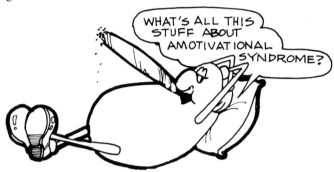

Amotivational Syndrome

There is still uncertainty over whether chronic marijuana use causes or results from apathy, listlessness, and associated personality difficulties. A much-disputed alleged effect of cannabis, however, the "amotivational syndrome," purports that individuals who smoke the drug become apathetic, lose interest in work, and suffer from a general lack of motivation.

Individuals and Society

Results of a two-year longitudinal study of university students who used marijuana indicated that marijuana use is common among students, and in fact it increased over the study period.[55] Results also showed that use was higher among students whose fathers had high-status occupations and among those undergoing psychological distress; that there was no significant relationship between marijuana use and sex, age, college year, or community size; and that involvement in conventional activities was not related to drug use. Researchers felt that smoking marijuana was not an antisocial act for students but one that enabled them to emulate others and to facilitate entrance into a group.

Melges and colleagues tested the effects of THC, including temporal disintegration and depersonalization (reduced ability to retain, coordinate, and serially index immediate memories and perceptions). Subjectively these effects are experienced as mild confusion; behaviorally they are related in the type of apparent responses disintegration produces. Subjects were tested on temporal distinction, goal directedness, and changes in emotion, including aggression and egotism. The findings were that (1) THC induces temporal disintegration and depersonalization and (2) changes in temporal disintegration correlated positively with changes in depersonalization (as each subject became more temporally disorganized, he or she simultaneously became more depersonalized).

Experiences with and reactions to marijuana differ from individual to individual. Two researchers report that experiences also differ from one culture to another.[56] For example, Jamaican field workers and fishermen have long used ganja, a more potent form of cannabis, to *prevent* hunger and cold. But for most American users, smoking marijuana *produces* hunger. The effects of marijuana, it seems, may more accurately reflect a subculture's expectations of the drug than the pharmacological course it takes.

Burnout is a term sometimes used by marijuana smokers themselves to describe the effect of prolonged use. Young people who smoke marijuana heavily over long periods can become dull, slow-moving, and inattentive. These "burned-out" users are sometimes so unaware of their surroundings that they do not respond when friends speak to them, and they often do not realize they have a problem.

Flashbacks

Marijuana flashbacks—spontaneous recurrences of feelings and perceptions similar to those produced by use of the drug—have been reported by some users.[57] Such experiences may range from the quite vivid re-creation of a drug-related experience to a much milder form of remembrance. A survey of U.S. Army personnel who used marijuana found that flashbacks occurred in both frequent and infrequent users and were not necessarily related to previous LSD use. It has since been reliably reported, however, that although flashbacks under the influence of marijuana are rare, individuals who have used LSD previously may be slightly more likely to have LSD-like flashbacks when they use marijuana afterwards.[58] The cause of flashbacks is still uncertain, but those who have experienced them usually require little or no treatment.[59]

THERAPEUTIC OR MEDICAL USES OF MARIJUANA

Though cannabis presently has limited medical application, studies indicate that the drug may have a bright future as a chemotherapeutic agent. Glaucoma and cancer are two diseases now undergoing experimental treatment with cannabis.

Glaucoma

Glaucoma is a disease in which the retina, the part of the eyeball that receives the image from the lens, degenerates. It is caused by intraocular pressure, which eventually reduces available intraocular fluids and secretions.

Because marijuana enables blood vessel membranes to relax and expand in an elastic fashion, it creates more space for the blood to flow and thus reduces pressure. When marijuana is used to reduce intraocular pressure, it allows intraocular fluids to remain at sufficient levels.

Though there has been a good deal of controversy over marijuana's use in glaucoma treatment, the recent *Randall* vs. *FDA* lawsuit in the District of Columbia has upheld the legality of that use. The suit determined that physicians could be licensed to prescribe cannabis for glaucoma treatment,[60] and at least four states (New Mexico, Florida, Illinois, and Louisiana) have passed laws legalizing marijuana for research and treatment purposes.[61]

Cancer

Studies at UCLA and other research centers have evaluated THC's capacity to alleviate various symptoms of cancer as well as side effects resulting from chemotherapy.[62] The drug compares very favorably with Compazine, the standard but pharmacologically inconsistent drug of choice for these side effects. Researchers at the Sydney Farber Cancer Institute have also substantiated THC's effectiveness as a therapeutic adjunct in the treatment of cancer.[63] Because it often induces relaxation, the drug may additionally find application as an antianxiety agent in cancer treatment. This use may be of great value because of the recognized link between emotional distress and cancer propagation. A large-scale study in California has found marijuana to be a safe and effective way of reducing the side effects of radial chemotherapy treatment given to cancer patients in the state.[64] Nine hundred patients who had failed to respond to normal antinausea treatments were given marijuana, to eat in capsules or to smoke in cigarettes. Almost 60 percent reported that the drug relieved the vomiting and nausea associated with chemotherapy.

Anorexia Nervosa

People suffering from this condition refuse to eat, or eat and then induce vomiting. Because marijuana genuinely enhances the appetite, it is hoped that the drug may prove effective in anorexia treatment. Marijuana's capacity to reduce tension may also help enhance the appetite during treatment.[65]

Other Applications

Cannabinoids, active agents in cannabis, have been used in the past and are presently being investigated or employed in some countries to reduce anxiety, stimulate appetite, reduce blood pressure, prevent convulsions, and act as diuretics, analgesics, sedatives, and anaesthetics. In South Africa and the United States, marijuana has been used to ease the discomforts of childbirth. Cannabis has also been used to reduce insomnia; to treat coughs, tetanus, burns, earaches, and migraine headaches; to ease opiate and alcohol withdrawal; and as an aid in obstetrics and psychotherapy.[66] Other past uses include the treatment of corns, warts, and hemorrhoids.

Recently, a synthetic analogue of THC—Nabilone—was discovered.[67] Nabilone produces less euphoria, less tachycardia, and less of an increase in blood pressure than THC. The drug has now been used by more than 100 patients in the United States in the treatment of nausea and vomiting. Though the development of Nabilone and the research done on potential medical uses of cannabis are encouraging, the extent to which marijuana may be used in medical context is still unclear. Research will continue, and more definite uses should be known in the near future.

SUMMARY

Marijuana use is on the upswing in the United States. The drug helps many users to feel euphoric and relaxed, though large doses may cause anxiety or paranoia. In some cases, marijuana has been shown to have therapeutic properties. Glaucoma patients have experienced relief from intraocular pressure after taking marijuana, and the drug shows promise for treatment of cancer-caused anxiety and chemotherapy side effects.

Despite its seeming therapeutic value, the effects of marijuana are not predictable. The following conclusions therefore seem reasonable:

1. Pregnant women should *not* use the drug.
2. Adolescents should be discouraged from use, especially heavy use.
3. The heart-accelerating property of cannabis may further impair people with heart problems.
4. People with lung disease should not use the drug because of its irritating effects.
5. The infrequent use of marijuana (less than once a week) probably will not result in ill effects.
6. Study of the therapeutic potential of cannabis should continue.[68]

Marijuana use continues to be quite high in the United States. Since it is easily harvested in many areas of the country it is more plentiful. Also, enforcement seems a difficult task.

NOTES

[1]Norman Taylor, *Narcotics: Nature's Dangerous Gifts* (New York: Dodd, Mead, 1966), p. 20.

[2]*Cannabis: A Report of the Commission of Inquiry into Non Medical Use of Drugs* (Ottawa: Crown, 1972).

[3]"Marijuana: Alcohol and Drug Fact Sheet," *Drug Information Center (DIC)* (Eugene: University of Oregon, 1979).

[4]John Kaplan, *Marijuana, the New Prohibition* (New York: World Publishing, 1972), p. 23.

[5]*Marijuana and Health,* Ninth Report to the U.S. Congress from the Secretary of Health and Human Services. (Rockville, Md.: National Institute on Drug Abuse, 1982), pp. 1–20.

[6]Nancy C. Doyle, "Marijuana and the Lung," *American Lung Association Bulletin,* November 1979.

[7]"Increasing U.S. Pot Crop," *Register Guard* (Eugene, Oregon), January 8, 1985.

[8]National Commission on Marijuana and Drug Abuse, *Marijuana: A Signal of Misunderstanding* (New York: New American Library, Signet, 1972), p. 21.

[9]"News Release: State of Oregon Marijuana Survey," *Grassroots*, April 1978, pp. 19–21.

[10]Stuart Nightengale and Seymour Perry, "Marijuana and Heroin by Prescription: Recent Developments at the State and Federal Level," *Journal of the American Medical Association* 24, no. 4 (January 26, 1979):373–75.

[11]National Commission on Marijuana and Drug Abuse, *Marijuana*.

[12]R. J. Smith, "Poisoned Pot Becomes Burning Issue in High Places," *Science* 200, no. 4340 (April 28, 1978):417–18.

[13]*Marijuana and Health*, First report to the U.S. Congress by the Secretary of the Department of Health, Education and Welfare (Washington, D.C.: U.S. Government Printing Office, 1972), p. 55.

[14]Ibid., p. 56.

[15]Milan Korocock, "News Report Underline Health Hazards," *Focus on Alcohol and Drug Issues, Marijuana Update*, September/October 1982, p. 4. See also National Commission on Marijuana and Drug Abuse, *Marijuana: A Signal of Misunderstanding.*

[16]Ibid.

[17]Quoted in Norman E. Zinberg, "The War over Marijuana," *Psychology Today* 10, no. 7 (December 1976):102. Reprinted from *Psychology Today Magazine*. Copyright © 1976 American Psychological Association (APA).

[18]Zinberg, "The War over Marijuana," p. 102.

[19]Edward M. Brecher et al., "Marijuana: The Health Question," *Consumer Reports* 40, no. 3 (March 1975).

[20]G. G. Nahas et al., "Inhibition of Cellular Mediated Immunity in Marijuana Smokers," *Science* 183, no. 4123 (February 1, 1974).

[21]*Marijuana and Health*, First Report to the U.S. Congress by the Secretary of Health, Education and Welfare (Washington, D.C.: U.S. Government Printing Office, 1979), p. 3.

[22]Ibid., p. 20.

[23]R. L. Henderson, F. S. Tennant, and R. Guerny, "Respiratory Manifestations of Hashish Smoking," *Archives of Otolaryngology* 95 (March 1972):248; and Sidney Cohen, "Marijuana: A New Ball Game?" *Drug Abuse and Alcoholism Newsletter* 8, no. 4 (May 1979).

[24]S. Cohen et al., "A 94-Day Cannabis Study," in *Pharmacology of Marijuana*, ed. M. C. Braude and S. Szara (New York: Raven Press, 1976), p. 621.

[25]Quoted in Nancy C. Doyle, "Marijuana and the Lungs," *American Lung Association Bulletin* 65, no. 9 (November 1979):4.

[26]*Marijuana and Health*, Ninth Report, pp. 1–20.

[27]Sidney Cohen, "Marijuana: Pulmonary Issues," *Drug Abuse Newsletter* 9, no. (January 1980).

[28]Quoted in Doyle, "Marijuana and the Lungs," p. 4.

[29]Zinberg, "The War over Marijuana"; Cohen et al., "A 94-Day Cannabis Study."

[30]R. Prakash et al., "Effects of Marijuana and Placebo Marijuana on Hemodynamics in Coronary Disease," *Clinical Pharmacology of Therapeutics* 18, no. 1 (July 1975):94.

[31]"The Medical View," *Time* 113, no. 5 (January 29, 1979):27. Reprinted by permission from *Time*, The Weekly Newsmagazine; Copyright Time Inc. 1979.

[32]Ibid.

[33]Institute on Medicine, *Marijuana and Health* (Washington, D.C.: National Academic Press, 1982), pp. 50–52.

[34]A. Sulkowski and L. Vachon, "Side Effects of Simultaneous Alcohol and Marijuana Use," *American Journal of Psychiatry* 134, no. 6 (June 1977):691.

[35]*Marijuana and Health*, p. 18.

[36]Ibid., p. 20.

[37]Institute on Medicine, *Marijuana and Health*, pp. 50–52.

[38]*Marijuana and Health*, p. 18.

[39]W. C. Hembree et al., "Marijuana Effect upon the Human Testis," *Clinical Research* 24, no. 3 (1976); C. N. Stefanis and M. R. Issidorides, "Cellular Effects of Chronic Cannabis Use in Man," in *Marijuana: Chemistry, Biochemistry and Cellular Effects*, ed. G. G. Nahas (New York: Springer-Verlag, 1976).

[40]Institute on Medicine, *Marijuana and Health*, p. 3.

[41]*Marijuana and Health*, Ninth Report, p. 30.

[42]*Marijuana and Health*, p. 18.

[43]"Cannabis and Driving Skills," *Canadian Medical Association Journal* 107 (August 19, 1978):269–70.

[44]National Institute of Mental Health, *Marijuana* (Washington, D.C.: Department of Health and Human Services, U.S. Government Printing Office, 1983).

[45]P. Thompson, "Stoned Driving Is Unpleasant, Say Marijuana Smokers," *Journal* 4, no. 1 (1975):13.

[46]H. Klonoff, "Effects of Marijuana on Driving in a Restricted Area and on City Streets: Driving Performance and Psychological Changes," in *Marijuana: Effects on Human Behavior*, ed. Loren L. Miller (New York: Academic Press, 1974).

[47]*Marijuana and Health*, p. 23.

[48]Ibid.

[49]*Marijuana and Health*, Ninth Report, p. 2.

[50]Institute on Medicine, *Marijuana and Health*, p. 3.

[51]Harold Kolansky and William T. Moore, "Toxic Effects of Chronic Marijuana Use," *Journal of the American Medical Association* 222, no. 1 (October 2, 1972):35–41.

[52]J. A. Hilikas, "Marijuana Use and Psychiatric Illness," in *Marijuana*, ed. Miller; R. E. Meyer, "Psychiatric Consequences of Marijuana Use: The State of the Evidence," *Marijuana and Health Hazards: Methodologic Issues in Current Research*, ed. J. R. Tinklenberg (New York: Academic Press, 1975).

[53]*Marijuana and Health*, p. 27.

[54]M. P. Naditch, P. C. Alker, and P. Joffe, "Individual Differences and Setting as Determinants of Acute Adverse Reactions to Psychoactive Drugs," *Journal of Nervous and Mental Disease* 284 (1971):792.

[55]Irving Ginsberg and James R. Greenly, "Competing Theories of Marijuana Use: A Longitudinal Study," *Journal of Health and Social Behavior* 19, no. 1 (March 1978):22–34.

[56]Glenn R. Eichel and Richard Troiden, "The Domestication of Drug Effects: The Case of Marijuana," *Journal of Psychedelic Drugs*, 10, no. 2 (July–September 1978):133–36.

[57]*Marijuana and Health*, p. 29.

[58]Institute on Medicine, *Marijuana and Health*, p. 126.

[59]M. D. Stanton, J. Mintz, and R. M. Franklin, "Drug Flashbacks, II: Some Additional Findings," *International Journal of the Addictions* 11, no. 1 (1976).

[60]Norman E. Zinberg, "On Cannabis and Health," *Journal of Psychedelic Drugs* 112, no. 1–2 (January–June 1979):135.

[61]Perry Bethesday, "Marijuana and Heroin by Prescription?" *Journal of the American Medical Association* 241, no. 4 (January 26, 1979): 373–75.

[62]Sidney Cohen, "Marijuana as Medicine," *Psychology Today* 11, no. 11 (April 1978):60.

[63]Donald Sweet, "Marijuana for Drug-Induced Nausea and Vomiting," *Journal of the American Medical Association* 243, no. 12 (March 28, 1980):1265.

[64]"Cancer Patients Turned On," *New Scientist* 96 (December 16, 1982): 709.

[65]Zinberg, "On Cannabis and Health," p. 139.

[66]Cohen, "Marijuana: A New Ball Game?" p. 32.

[67]Beverly J. Montgomery, "High Interest in Medical Uses of Marijuana and Synthetic Analogues," *Journal of the American Medical Association* 240, no. 14 (September 29, 1978):1469–70.

[68]Adapted from Cohen, "Marijuana: A New Ball Game?"

12

OVER-THE-COUNTER DRUGS
what you can get without a prescription

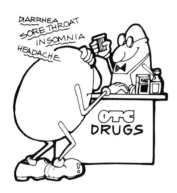

INTRODUCTION

One of the traditions we have inherited from our ancestors is self-medication. The advertising industry has taken advantage of this tradition by promoting thousands of drugs that can be purchased without prescription "over the counter." Cold and cough medications, vitamins, laxatives, analgesics, and an assortment of potions, ointments, and balms are big over-the-counter sellers, as well as antihistamines, which are the most commonly used sedative-hypnotics.[1] Over-the-counter (OTC) drugs are readily obtained and are believed by consumers to be safe as well as helpful in the treatment of a disease or in the alleviation of some of its symptoms. Each year, Americans spend billions on close to 300,000 OTC drugs.

Despite their popularity, OTC drugs can be hazardous if directions for their use are not followed and if improper self-diagnoses are made. The FDA

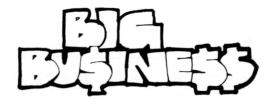

enforces laws to protect consumers from danger, but consumers can best protect themselves by taking only the drugs they need, not overbuying or keeping drugs for long periods of time, not combining drugs carelessly, not continuing to use a drug if symptoms of illness persist, reading and following directions for use, and seeking professional advice before combining drugs.[2] To help consumers use products properly, manufacturers should list the common or generic names and quantities of active ingredients, instructions for using the drug, and simple, direct warnings of possible side effects as well as limitations of the drug's effectivness (many drugs are not effective except as placebos).

Because OTC drugs are sold in a competitive market, much depends on how they are advertised, as well as how effectively they relieve symptoms. Advertisers appeal to consumers in every possible way—through emotions, faddism, bias, fear, envy, greed, even lust. Researcher Lois Debakey lists the following classical techniques that are used to promote over-the-counter drugs:

1. Bandwagon—Every mother I know buys brand X children's aspirin, so why don't you?
2. Testimonial—I drank antacid and I feel great; next time you need an antacid try the one I use.
3. The Down Home Approach—Standing by his barn Grandpa tells you about the analgesic he uses for his arthritis; if it's good enough for him, it's good enough for you.
4. The Authority Figure—A man in a white coat who looks like a doctor says he knows what is best and if you're smart you'll use what he suggests.[3]

Self-indulgence is another emotional appeal that is coupled with the implication of instant relief and the idea that people should feel perfect every day. Announcement of a new scientific breakthrough is still another way advertisers try to win consumers.

The strongest technique of all may be the "I understand" attitude many advertisements take when promoting cures. Smoking, drinking, eating, and staying out late are all Okay, they tell us, just as long as we take their product afterward. Another appeal to consumer psyches is made through references to tests, documents, and evidence, with the intent of lending "scientific credibility" to products. But not only do most advertisements fail to mention exactly what test was done, they also fail to mention if the company itself sponsored or financed the research.[4]

Development of OTCs in the United States

Patent medicines popular in England were imported to the American colonies soon after British migration to this country. The first American-patented medicine was Samuel Lee's "Bilious Pills," registered in 1796. Other medicines soon followed, many of which contained opiates. Alcohol too was a major constituent of patent drugs, often constituting 25 to 50 percent of the products.[5] Other ingredients found in these patent medicines included morphine, cocaine, caffeine, and belladonna.[6] Claims of the drugs' effectiveness were grossly overstated, and many advertisements stated that the medicines were cure-alls available from doctors, pharmacies, general grocery stores, and traveling shows and by mail.[7]

As pioneers moved westward and doctors and pharmacists were in short supply, self-medication became a widespread method of health care. Early settlers had to rely on European folklore, Indian remedies using domestic plants, and the word of traveling entertainers. Patent medicines were an $80-million-a-year business by 1900.[8]

By the 1980s, the number of nonprescription preparations and the popularity of self-medication had increased greatly, but so had the incidence of adverse reactions. Though these drugs are more sophisticated than early patent medicines, they are still potentially dangerous, for several reasons:

1. Most OTC medications have unclear label instructions.
2. Most OTC medications contain several ingredients.
3. Many of the medications can be used for multiple symptoms.
4. The public considers OTC medications to be safe.
5. The public believes the government would never allow the sale of a dangerous product.[9]

Reform

Other possible dangers associated with over-the-counter drug use include adverse reactions that can occur even when one is using the medication precisely according to the instructions on the label. Drug toxicity can be caused by excessive use or overdosage. Finally, people can use a drug inappropriately because of their own misdiagnosis of their medical problem, or by mixing an over-the-counter drug with another medication, resulting in an adverse drug interaction.[10]

At the turn of the century, health hazards from patent medicines were a political issue. Outcry at effects of adulterated foods eventually resulted in the passage of the 1906 Food and Drug Act, which affected OTC drugs by lowering their alcohol content to 17 percent and limiting opiates to prescription medicines. The act also divided drugs into proprietary (over-the-counter) drugs and ethical (prescription) drugs. It was intended to stop misleading advertising and consumer ignorance, but these problems remain a major concern today.

Since 1972 the FDA has had panels of nongovermental experts reviewing more than seventeen major classes of over-the-counter preparations. In 1984, after reviewing the 300,000 or so drug products marketed under various names, the advisory panels report that only about one third of the ingredients are effective as well as safe for their intended use.[11] The remaining ingredients required additional proof if manufacturers were to be allowed to continue to market them. The report did not imply that only one third of all over-the-counter drug products contain ingredients that are safe and effective. Instead it meant that although many products contain ingredients that are safe, they may also have other ingredients whose safety has not yet been determined.

The panel recommendations are currently being incorporated into regulatory action, but already this review has allowed some new products to be sold over the counter to consumers (cortisone, fluoride rinses, new antihistamine and cold ingredients, and new nighttime sleeping aids). It has also quickly removed other ingredients that were deemed obvious hazards (Methapyrilene in sleep aids, hexachlorophene in soaps).

Earlier panel recommendations included placement of an ingredient into one of three categories. Category I contains ingredients considered safe and effective. Category II includes ingredients definitely shown to be unsafe or ineffective (panels have the power to recommend removal of any ingredient from the market that is viewed dangerous). Category III is for ingredients that seem to need further testing. The pharmaceutical industry has supported such categorization and review, and on its own initiative has removed several proposed Category II ingredients from the market.

SALICYLATES (ASPIRIN)

History

The modern history of salicylates began in 1852, when salicylic acid was first synthesized and found to have many useful properties. In 1874, Kalbe and Lauteman developed a procedure to produce the acid.[12] Its antiseptic properties enabled it to be used as a preservative to prevent milk and meat spoilage. During surgery it was used as an antiseptic and to treat infectious diseases.

Acetylsalicylic acid, commonly known as aspirin, was produced by the reaction of acetylchloride and sodium salicylate. For years it was an obscure chemical with no known therapeutic applications. Such therapeutic use was finally discovered in Germany when a man suffering from chronic rheumatoid arthritis approached his son, who was working with Bayer, to help find relief. Several different salicylate compounds were concocted, and finally acetylsalicylic acid proved successful. Salicylates were then used to treat a wide variety of diseases during the late nineteenth century.

It was not long, however, before the strong analgesic action of aspirin was recognized. Its greatest use soon became that of pain relief, particularly muscular pain and headache. Today it is the most popular of all drugs, both prescription and over-the-counter. "Americans alone ingest more than 50 million tablets of aspirin a day,"[13] and acetylsalicylic acid is an integral component of approximately 400 different drug preparations sold in this country. Aspirin is considered a miracle drug by many, since it is an effective fever reducer as well as an analgesic for a myriad of common ailments. Aspirin is big business. Sales of aspirin-based products in the United States amount to approximately $700 million per year.

Physical Effects

Salicylates are absorbed from the stomach and intestinal tract, then selectively distributed to the nervous system.[14] When they affect the hypothalamus, they reduce fever. When they affect certain sites in the upper spinal cord, they bring pain relief. Salicylates also block production of pain-producing plasma particles, causing further pain relief. As the chemicals move through the system, they dilate blood vessels, causing mild heat loss and sweating as well as a reduction in blood pressure.

Respiration is not normally affected by therapeutic doses (300 milligrams to 1 gram). Larger doses, however, are capable of stimulating brain respiratory-control centers, resulting in hyperventilating and excessive levels of oxygen and carbon dioxide in the body. If high dosages are continued over prolonged periods, severe potassium depletion may result, leading to general fatigue and dizziness.[15]

Long-term salicylate use can also produce serious gastric disturbances. Irritation of the protective mucosal stomach lining and mild to severe abdominal bleeding are often associated with prolonged salicylate therapy.[16] Since aspirin can also decrease blood coagulability, its use can also aggravate existing abdominal bleeding.

Intoxication from salicylates may be mild or severe, depending on the dosage. Mild intoxication, termed salicylism, is characterized by tinnitus (ringing in the ears), dizziness, headache, and disorientation. Severe intoxication produces marked mental confusion and gastric irritation, and internal tissue bleeding may be noted. Toxic doses—approximately 20 grams—produce changes in the body's acid-base balance, shifting the pH of body fluids. Death from overdose is possible, especially for children five and younger. Approximately 15 percent of all childhood poisoning deaths are aspirin-related.

Some individuals experience adverse responses to salicylates even after small doses. Users can occasionally fall victim to severe allergic shock reactions to the drugs, as well as severe asthma attacks if they are particularly hypersensitive. For these individuals, aspirin substitutes such as acetaminophen are advised.

Salicylates apparently do not produce discernible tolerance or physical dependence, nor do they result in withdrawal symptomatology following discontinuation. Many individuals do appear to be psychologically disposed to compulsive salicylate use, however, for either real or imagined pains, and such use can have mild toxic effects.

Side Effects

Extensive use of aspirin can cause numerous side effects. These may include gastrointestinal bleeding, nausea, vomiting, activation of peptic ulcer, bone-marrow depression, hepatitis with jaundice, and after a prolonged time, kidney damage. When aspirin interacts with other drugs, such as alcohol, Vitamin C, some diuretics, antidiabetic drugs, insulin, and penicillin, it can increase or decrease these drugs' effectiveness, and in combination with some of them it can cause toxicity and increased stomach sensitivity.

Therapeutic Effectiveness

Aspirin is recommended for four therapeutic uses: (1) as an analgesic, to relieve mild to moderate nonspecific pain; (2) as an antipyretic, to reduce fevers of over 101° F (though this may mask the need for more elaborate treatment); (3) as an antiinflammatory agent, to reduce inflammation in arthritis and other inflammatory conditions; and (4) to decrease platelet aggregation—to keep platelets from adhering and clotting. Aspirin's effectiveness in these four areas has been applied to many diseases, but the drug is particularly useful in relieving the effects of rheumatoid arthritis. It may also prove to be critical in preventing heart attacks.

Rheumatoid Arthritis   Most doctors agree that the salicylates, particularly aspirin, are effective in relieving arthritis. A member of the committee of the American Rheumatic Association states that "either in the form of aspirin or sodium salicylate, the salicylates are the most useful drugs in the treatment of rheumatoid arthritis, and in a considerable proportion of patients, aspirin is the only drug needed. . . ."[17] The most effective dose is approximately seven to ten grams per day, unless side effects necessitate a dose reduction. Aspirin's antiinflammatory action is the main reason aspirin is used to treat arthritis, a disease in which joints become inflamed. Aspirin also successfully treats other effects of arthritis, however, relieving pain, reducing morning stiffness, and lessening swelling and immobility.[18] Aspirin's success in relieving arthritis symptoms is thought to be achieved by direct blocking of the "pain" receptors, as well as reduction of the production of inflammatory agents at the disease site.

Heart Attacks   Though the value of using aspirin to prevent heart attacks has not been completely determined, aspirin is known to hinder blood clotting, which is a cause of heart attacks.[19] In 1974, a British study found that out of 600 heart-attack patients who ingested one aspirin daily, 25 percent had fewer subsequent heart attacks than those who took placebos.[20] Another study by the Boston Collaborative Drug Surveillance program found that heart attack was half as common to regular aspirin takers as it was to individuals who seldom took aspirin. It also concluded that first as well as recurrent nonfatal heart attacks were less likely among regular aspirin takers. The study warned, however, that evidence "fell short of establishing that ASA [aspirin] prevents heart attacks."[21]

By 1978, aspirin was known to be effective in preventing strokes. This knowledge prompted its use in the treatment of atherosclerosis, a narrowing of the blood vessels that can lead to myocardial infarctions. The exact dose needed to prevent heart attacks is still uncertain, but an extensive myocardial-infarction study nonetheless recommended routine aspirin use for the prevention of myocardial infarctions. Other recent studies have also indicated that aspirin is of value in the treatment of coronary disease.

Toxicology

Though aspirin appears to rank as one of the safest drugs used today, it can cause gastric hemorrhage, bronchial asthma, and mild bleeding. These adverse reactions can be serious and even fatal, and some consumers feel that all medications that contain aspirin should be available only by prescription. Efforts have been made to have warning labels placed on containers of aspirin medications, and the recently introduced childproof top is another attempt at preventing adverse reactions.

Reye's Syndrome   A recently formulated warning by the Food and Drug Administration indicates that children who have chicken pox, flu, or late-winter fluline symptoms should not be given aspirin. A high percentage of children who suffer or die from a rare liver disorder known as Reye's syndrome turn out to have been treated with aspirin for chicken pox or flu symptoms.[22] Whether or how aspirin enhances this risk is not currently known, but acetaminophen does not have this risk.

Gastrointestinal Bleeding   Aspirin seems to have an affinity for the stomach. It accumulates there after oral dosages and increases gastric salicylate levels following intravenous infusion.[23] As we have noted, aspirin is believed to have an effect on the protective mucus lining of the stomach,[24] and "ingestion of aspirin, in doses of 1 to 3 g. day [three to twelve tablets], will induce acute gastrointestinal bleeding in about 70 percent of normal individuals."[25] Such bleeding can result in iron-deficiency anemia and, more seriously, massive gastric hemorrhage. Hemorrhage is especially possible in aspirin takers suffering from peptic ulcers.

Bleeding Tendency   In relatively high doses—3 grams (about twelve tablets) or more per day for a week—aspirin prevents clotting.[26] Even the

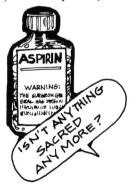

ingestion of a single dose of 0.3 to 1.2 grams prolongs clotting time by several minutes in normal persons and to a much greater degree in people with bleeding disorders. The tendency to bleed may last for four to seven days, and though this would normally be of little significance, during surgery it could produce serious complications. Aspirin should therefore be avoided prior to surgical procedures, especially by people with bleeding disorders.

Hypersensitivity Reactions Hypersensitivity (allergic) reactions to salicylates are commonly manifested as skin eruptions, edema, and asthma. The symptoms are generally characterized either by sudden weakness, sweating, fainting, and collapse, as in an asthmatic attack, or by an acute rash.

Allergy to salicylates seems somewhat mysterious. Aspirin-sensitive patients are rarely sensitive to salicylic acid or sodium salicylate,[27] yet aspirin is the chief culprit in 83 percent of allergic "poisonings" caused by salicylates.[28] One study estimated that approximately 1 to 500 are sensitive to aspirin, and that of these only a small percentage experience severe reactions.[29] Fatalities have occurred, however, after the ingestion of only a small dose of aspirin.

Asthma is the allergic reaction to aspirin that has received the most attention. "In a review of drug sensitivity [it was] found that 19 drugs or groups of drugs may precipitate asthma. Of these, aspirin is the only one to do so commonly."[30] Despite these findings, it appears that aspirin is rarely the sole cause of asthmatic attack.

Acetaminophen

For people who cannot take aspirin, acetaminophen is an acceptable substitute. The drug is marketed in the United States under approximately fifty brand names—Tylenol, Datril, Liquiprin, and others. Acetaminophen is effective in reducing fever and decreasing pain, and does not produce gastric irritation or intestinal bleeding or appear to have any affect on platelet formation.[31] Despite this benign appearance, the drug can still cause serious liver damage and even death if an overdose is taken.[32] Symptoms of an overdose may include nausea, vomiting, diarrhea, abdominal pain, and drowsiness.

Is acetaminophen better than acetylsalicylic acid? Despite the claims made by advertising agencies, both drugs are very good pain relievers. Aspirin is less expensive,[33] but for patients with gout, patients taking anticoagulants, pregnant women, and persons with allergies to aspirin or asthma, acetaminophen is the better choice. For those who need an antiinflammatory medicine, however, aspirin is the better choice, since it is much more effective in reducing inflammation.

LAXATIVES*

Introduction

There is a durable attitude, spanning many centuries and many cultures, that associates excrement with evil and its elimination with the expiation of guilt. The practical result is that most people of our society still regard even transitory constipation as something to be directly and promptly treated with a cathartic.[34]

Today, advertisements constantly state that for good health and well-being we should be "regular" in our bowel movements. Irregularity (constipation), aftermeal discomfort, and headaches will disappear if we just take a laxative. To help us on our way, over 700 proprietary drugs that promote defecation are manufactured and made available each year. Over $200 million are spent on these nonprescription laxatives and other elimination aids, and between 15 and 30 percent of people over sixty take more than one laxative dose per week.[36]

Despite laxative popularity, taking a laxative is rarely appropriate for children and only occasionally appropriate for adults. It is not true that daily defecation is necessary for good health. Many people in perfect health have bowel movements every two to three days or longer without ill effect.[37] Supposed constipation may simply be slow movement of feces through the large intestine—slow but perfectly adequate for the particular system. A panel of scientists who reviewed OTC laxative products for the FDA stated that "there is widespread overuse of self-prescribed laxatives. . . . The Panel is concerned because many people are using laxatives that don't need them."[38]

This overuse can be dangerous. Continued unnecessary doses can lead to dependence on laxatives for normal bowel movements, a need for stronger medication, or a malfunctioning of the gastrointestinal tract. If a laxative is taken to relieve abdominal pain, cramps, nausea, or vomiting, the intestinal activity the laxative produces can cause further irritation. Laxatives can also rupture an inflamed appendix, greatly increasing the risk of serious illness.[39]

Understanding Constipation

True constipation—a condition in which the feces become hard and dry because fluid is not absorbed quickly enough to produce softer stools—is a rare condition found primarily in aged or infirm patients. Occasional irregularity may occur, however, though such instances are believed to result from behavioral, rather than physiological, causes.

*Though drugs that cause evacuations of the intestine (bowel movements) are generally referred to as laxatives, cathartics and purgatives are often incorrectly included in this category. A laxative causes increased peristalsis (wavelike contractions of the intestine) by (increasing or decreasing) water content, producing a soft, well-formed stool. A cathartic, on the other hand, causes a more drastic fluid evacuation and is almost always associated with increased motor activity in the intestines. A purgative is a more energetic agent that a cathartic or a laxative.[35] Despite these differences, and for purposes of simplicity and consistency, only the term *laxative* will be used in this text.

One source of constipation is an improper diet that leaves too little residue in the intestinal tract for a bowel movement. Not eating breakfast can occasionally cause constipation, since eating or drinking in the morning (coffee and tea are potent laxatives) sometimes triggers the "gastrocolic reflex," the urge to defecate. Not responding to this urge can also produce constipation. So can insufficient fluid intake, since dry feces have difficulty descending through the colon.

Certain drugs, particularly sedatives, codeine, and aluminum hydroxide or calcium used as antacids, are also causes of constipation.[40] So are irritating laxatives which, ironically, are the most common cause of nonorganic chronic constipation.

Certain stress-producing situations or emotions may also produce bowel discomfort, as can pregnancy, when the enlarged uterus puts pressure on the intestine.[41] Lack of adequate exercise can be a final source of constipation.

Types of Laxatives

Just as there are different sources and reasons for constipation, there are different types of laxatives to use in treatment. Each group exerts its effect through a different mechanism and can conceivably serve different laxative needs.

Stimulant Laxatives   The strongest and most abused laxatives are the stimulant (irritant) laxatives. These drugs promote bowel movements by directly stimulating the small intestine, colon, or both. Results often appear in less than eight hours, their intensity and rapidity dependent on the dose.[42] Stimulant laxatives are usually divided into three subcategories: anthraquinones (powders responsible for the cathartic action), purgative oils, and a miscellaneous group.

Bulk-Forming Laxatives   These are among the safest of all laxatives. They contain synthetic or natural polysaccharides and cellulose derivatives, including bran and psyllium. They also contain hydrophillic compounds that bind and hold water and form a jellylike mass in the intestines, inducing bowel contractions.[43] Their effect is much less dramatic than other types of laxatives and may not be apparent until twelve to seventy-two hours after use. Bulk-forming laxatives are not digestible and therefore are not absorbed in the digestive tract. They remain in the gut until mixed with the intestine contents, after which they are expelled together with the fecal matter. This type of laxative is considered the ideal drug for patients with bulk-forming problems, such as the elderly or the infirm.[44]

Saline Laxatives   Saline laxatives are salts (magnesium, phosphate, and glycerin) that are freely soluble in water. They seem to have a number of effects on the gastrointestinal tract and promote evacuation by increasing the amount of water in the intestines.[45] Some saline laxatives are effervescent and should be taken with large quantities of water. Depending on the dose, these drugs usually take effect three to six hours after use.

Stool-Softener and Lubricant Laxatives   The active ingredients of stool-softener laxatives and lubricant laxatives are particularly useful when stools are hard and dry, or when disease of the anus makes passage of stools painful. These products should be used only occasionally, however, or no longer than a week when taken daily, since they may interfere with the absorption of a number of nutrients, including some vitamins.

Though most of the laxatives that make up these categories are likely to aid in constipation relief, a laxative with just a single active ingredient is more likely to produce fewer unwanted side effects and undesirable interactions between drugs.[46] When purchasing a laxative, look for labels that state the product is for the "short-term relief of constipation." Labels should not say the product will result in good health, the relief of indigestion, headaches, or excessive belching. They also should not warn against the hazards of constipation, because such warnings are "unproven and thus unacceptable."[47]

Laxative Use

Constipation will generally alleviate itself if it isn't perpetuated with continual laxative use. Before resorting to chemical relief for constipation, people should be aware of the range of normal bowel function; respond to the need to defecate when it is first felt; add fiber to their diet; resist hurrying breakfast; exercise, and have patience. If a laxative is truly needed, a doctor or pharmacist should be consulted, because evidence suggests that individuals purchasing proprietary laxatives do not receive proper counsel concerning the merits and toxicity of these products. "There is no class of nonprescription drugs in which professional guidance is needed more than with the use of laxatives."[48]

COUGH RELIEVERS (ANTITUSSIVES) ——————————————

The Cough

A cough can be defined as a sudden expulsion of air from the lungs. In the clinical sense it is a form of protection, because it is an automatic attempt to release foreign matter from the esophagus. Coughs can result from a number of causes, from an irritation to pulmonary fibrosis. Cough suppressants have been developed because coughing can be an acute respiratory ailment.

Reducing the Severity

Effective antitussives reduce the severity of a cough several ways. First, the cough reliever depresses the medullary center. Second, it tends to block impulse transmission in the nervous system. Third, it interferes with the impulses of the cough reflex. Fourth, it removes irritants by facilitating bronchial drainage.

Codeine is the most effective opiate for reducing the severity of a cough. It can lead to tolerance and physical dependency, but in small doses it is rated high as an antitussive because it is rapidly absorbed following administration. Effects are generally felt fifteen to thirty minutes after use, and relief is maintained for between four and six hours. Codeine combined with aspirin appears to be the most effective antitussant, but choosing the best product from the 50,000 non-prescription items now marketed for coughs, colds, allergies, and bronchial conditions can be complicated.

For those who don't wish to use codeine, a number of nonopiate substitutes are available. The most commonly used is most likely dextromethorphan, because it is as potent as codeine but does not produce dependency. Such nonnarcotic antitussives also do not lead to significant abuse problems, which codeine preparations can.

ANTIHISTAMINES

In 1910, a naturally occurring hormone named histamine was discovered. The hormone was found to release valuable antibodies that attack various bacteria, viruses, chemicals, and antigens (foreign bodies). Though this pharmacological action was both remarkable and necessary for protecting the body from disease, it was often found to result in vasodilation and blood vessel permeability; increased secretions that cause sneezing, runny nose/eyes, congestion, and itching; nausea; and changes in various smooth muscles, glands, and connective tissue.[49] To combat these side effects, antihistamines were developed; they offered relief by temporarily reducing histamine release.*

Antihistamines are most commonly found in "cold," "allergy," or "hay fever" preparations, since pollen, dust, bee stings, and enzymes are notable promoters of histamine release. They are also employed in tranquilizers, decongestants, antitussives, anticonvulsants, local anesthetic, and antinausea and motion-sickness medicines,[50] because their action can relieve sinus congestion, itching, nausea, insomnia, and restlessness and can reduce skin eruptions.

Not all antihistamine effects are beneficial, however. Side effects include drowsiness, a sense of weakness, dryness of the nose, mouth, and throat, and constipation. Rare, adverse reactions, which indicate the drug is not working properly and for which a physician should be quickly consulted, include allergic reactions (hives, itching), headaches, dizziness, inability to concentrate, ner-

*In 1947, a pregnant woman attending the Johns Hopkins allergy clinic was given a new drug to control her hives. It so happened that she suffered from car sickness as well. When reporting to the clinic the following week, she mentioned that not only had the new medicine taken care of her hives, she had also noticed that it prevented her usual sickness when she traveled in the streetcar. Stimulated by this observation, Leslie N. Gay, chief of the allergy department, and Paul E. Carliner sought other victims of motion sickness to test the new drug. Later, when the drug proved itself, it was given the name Dramamine.

vousness, blurred or double vision, and difficulty urinating. A physician should also be consulted if a person develops signs of nausea or vomiting; severe behavioral disturbances such as confusion, excitement, or delirium; or any signs of unusual bleeding or bruising.

Although antihistamines alone can be obtained only with a prescription, when combined in low dosages with other drugs they are available over the counter. Because they often cause drowsiness, all products containing them must have a warning label to that effect.[51] Antihistamines should not be taken by individuals who need to be alert, are hypertensive, have severely dry mucous membranes, are taking certain other drugs, particularly depressants, or are pregnant.[52]

VITAMINS AND MINERALS

Introduction

Vitamins are organic compounds necessary in small amounts for normal growth and maintenance of life. They transform foods into energy, but do not provide energy or build or maintain body parts. There are thirteen or more of them, occurring naturally in foods and synthetically in vitamin preparations.

The vitamins and minerals sold over the counter in the United States are a billion-dollar business.[53] Though a well-balanced diet will usually meet all the body's vitamin needs (see Table 12–1), anyone who feels the need for vitamins or minerals can get them in drugstores, supermarkets, and health-food stores, from door-to-door salespeople, or through the mail. Despite their popularity, some vitamins and minerals may be dangerous if taken by the wrong people or in excessive dosages.

Vitamin and mineral products are sold in the United States with one of two labels: dietary supplement (intended to increase total dietary intake of one or more essential vitamins or minerals) and nonprescription drug (sold to prevent or treat a specific vitamin or mineral deficiency, such as one resulting from pregnancy, nursing, alcoholism, or intestinal disease).

Recently, a nongovernmental panel created by the FDA evaluated the safety and effectiveness of all over-the-counter vitamin and mineral products sold as drugs. According to the panel, only nine vitamins and three minerals are safe and effective as over-the-counter drugs. The nine vitamins are C, B_{12}, folic acid, niacin, B_6, riboflavin, thiamine, A, and D. The panel determined that biotin, choline, vitamin E, and pantothenic acid should not be sold as single-ingredient, nonprescription drugs because deficiencies of these vitamins are virtually nonexistent. The panel also felt that vitamin K should be available by prescription only, since it is particularly dangerous for people taking anticoagulants.

More than a hundred miscellaneous ingredients, including apricots, brewer's yeast, buckwheat, comfrey root, hesperidin, kelp, lecithin, malt extract, molasses, rose-hips powder, and wheat germ, some of which are natural sources of vitamins and minerals, were considered inappropriate by the panel for inclusion in vitamin-mineral preparations. Such ingredients were excluded be-

TABLE 12–1 United States Recommended Daily Allowances

	Unit	Infants (0–12 months)	Children under 4 Years	Adults and Children 4 or More Years	Pregnant or Lactating Women
**Vitamin A	IU	1500	2500	5000	8000
**Vitamin D	IU	400	400	400	400
**Vitamin E	IU	5	10	30	30
Vitamin C	mg	35	40	60	60
Folacin (folic acid)	mg	0.1	0.2	0.4	0.8
Thiamine (B₁)	mg	0.5	0.7	1.5	1.7
Riboflavin (B₂)	mg	0.6	0.8	1.7	2.0
Niacin	mg	8	9	20	20
Vitamin B₆	mg	0.4	0.7	2	2.5
Vitamin B₁₂	mcg	2	3	6	8
Biotin	mg	0.05	0.15	0.3	0.3
Pantothenic acid	mg	3	5	10	10
*Vitamin K					

IU = international unit
mg = milligram
mcg = microgram

*Source: FDA Consumer, U.S. Government Publication, Washington, D.C. (April 1979).
**fat soluble vitamins.

cause they do *not* contribute to the product's effectiveness to treat or cure deficiencies. Combination products were deemed appropriate, however, because conditions that cause deficiencies usually involve more than one nutrient. Combinations that include any of the approved vitamins or any of the approved vitamins plus approved minerals were classified safe and effective as over-the-counter drugs. Pantothenic acid and vitamin E, which should not be sold as single ingredients, can be included in vitamin-mineral combinations that do not contain any other fat-soluble vitamins.

As for minerals, the panel said that calcium, iron, and zinc are safe and effective for single-ingredient use. Copper, fluoride, iodine, magnesium, manganese, phosphorous, and potassium were deemed inappropriate for over-the-counter sales because deficiencies are rare and because some of the minerals can be dangerous in high doses. The panel also pointed out that there is no need for multimineral preparations. This recommendation was made because multiple mineral deficiencies rarely occur as a result of one condition.

Specific Use

The nongovernmental panel found that many manufacturers listed unverifiable claims and did not post adequate warnings on their products. They felt labels should be reworded to state that preparations should be used only "when the need for such therapy has been determined by a physician." They

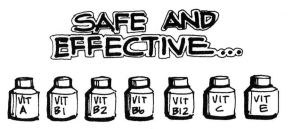

also recommended that labels include specific doses to be taken, and that listings be required of all ingredients in these preparations.

There are a number of claims that the panel felt labels should not be allowed to make:

1. claims of special effectiveness, such as "high" or "super" potency
2. claims that a product is "natural," because there is no evidence that natural forms of vitamins and minerals are better than synthetic ones
3. claims that vitamin C is useful for treating such conditions as the common cold, atherosclerosis, allergy, mental illness, corneal ulcers, thrombosis, anemia, or pressure sores
4. claims that vitamin A is of value against warts on the bottom of the feet, acne or other skin diseases, dry and wrinkled skin, stress ulcers, respiratory infections, or eye disorders
5. claims that vitamin D is effective in lowering blood cholesterol levels or in preventing or curing osteoporosis in the elderly
6. claims that any preparation is specially effective in geriatric use
7. claims that folic-acid preparations can prevent folic-acid deficiency in women taking oral contraceptives
8. claims that vitamin B_6 is useful for preventing kidney stones or controlling vomiting in pregnant women
9. claims that vitamin B_1 (thiamine) helps stimulate mental response or is useful in treating skin disease, multiple sclerosis, infections, cancer, or impotence

Recommendations by the vitamin-mineral panel were received by the FDA as part of the agency's effort to review all nonprescription drugs. The recommendations and a proposed monograph or "recipe book" for vitamin-mineral preparations were published in the March 16, 1979 *Federal Register*. A final monograph is expected in 1986, and six months after its publication manufacturers who sell vitamin and mineral preparations as drugs must reformulate and relabel their products to comply with the monograph. If compliance is not achieved, products must be removed from the market.[54]

Specific Vitamins

Vitamin A (Retinol)   Vitamin A is an oil-soluble vitamin that is stored in the liver. It is necessary for new cell growth and healthy tissues and is essential for seeing in dim light. Besides night blindness and other eye maladies, a vitamin A deficiency can cause dry, rough skin that may become more susceptible to infection.

Vitamin A is found in foods in two forms: as carotene, a yellow pigment in green and yellow vegetables and yellow fruits that the human body converts to vitamin A, and as vitamin A itself, found in animals who have formed it from carotene and store it in body tissues. Good sources of vitamin A are liver, eggs, and milk.

Large doses of vitamin A can cause increased pressure inside the skull. This pressure so mimics symptoms of a brain tumor that tumors have been suspected in several patients whom hospital personnel later discovered consumed high quantities of vitamin A. Carotene, on the other hand, is practically nontoxic.

Vitamin B$_1$ (Thiamine)   This vitamin is water-soluble, as are all vitamins in the B complex. It is required for normal digestion, growth, fertility, lactation, the normal functioning of nerve tissue, and carbohydrate metabolism. B$_1$ can be found in abundant quantities in pork, soybeans, beans, peas, nuts, and enriched and whole-grain breads and cereals.

A deficiency of vitamin B$_1$ can cause beriberi, a dysfunctioning of the nervous system. Other deficiency effects include loss of appetite, body swelling (edema), heart problems, nausea, vomiting, and spastic muscle contractions throughout the body.

Vitamin B$_6$ (Pyridoxine, Pyridoxal, Pyridoxamine)   Vitamin B$_6$ is necessary for the utilization of protein. It is found abundantly in liver, whole-grain cereals, potatoes, red meats, green vegetables, and yellow corn. Deficiency symptoms include mouth soreness, dizziness, nausea, weight loss, and severe nervous disturbances.

Vitamin B$_{12}$ (Cyanocobalamin)   Vitamin B$_{12}$ is necessary for the normal development of red blood cells, as well as the functioning of all cells, particularly in the bone marrow, nervous system, and intestines. Good sources of this vitamin are organ meats, lean meats, fish, milk, eggs, and shellfish. Since most vegetables do not contain any measurable amounts of B$_{12}$, strict vegetarians should supplement their diets with this vitamin. A deficiency can cause pernicious anemia and, if the deficiency is prolonged, degeneration of the spinal cord.

Vitamin C (Ascorbic Acid)   This least stable of the vitamins promotes growth and tissue repair, including the healing of wounds. It also aids in tooth and bone formation and when used as a food additive acts as a preservative. Vitamin C can be found in turnip greens, green pepper, kale, broccoli, mustard greens, citrus fruits, strawberries, currants, tomatoes, and other vegetables. Just one three-to-four-ounce serving of any of these foods will supply all your daily vitamin C needs.

Lack of vitamin C can cause one of the oldest diseases known to humans—scurvy. Signs of scurvy include lassitude, weakness, bleeding of the gums, loss of weight, irritability, and ease of bruising.

Vitamin D (Calciferol)   Vitamin D is necessary for bone formation: it aids in the absorption of calcium and phosphorus. To accomplish this work, the body—through the liver and kidneys—converts the vitamin to a hormonelike material.

Abundant sources of vitamin D include canned and fresh fish (particularly the saltwater varieties), egg yolk, and vitamin D–fortified foods such as milk and margarine. People who regularly expose their skin to the sun can get vitamin D that way, since it is formed in the skin by the ultraviolet rays. The daily requirement is very small, and excess amounts are stored in the body.

Too much vitamin D can cause nausea, weight loss, weakness, excessive urination, and the more serious conditions of hypertension and calcification of soft tissue, including the blood vessels and kidneys. Bone deformities and multiple fractures are also common. Too little vitamin D can cause rickets, a bone-deforming disease that can result in bowed legs, a deformed spine, "pot-belly" appearance, flat feet, or stunted growth.

Vitamin E (the Tocopherols)   Vitamin E is one of the most talked about vitamins, and to some extent the exaggerated and unsubstantiated claims made for it result from a combination of hope and misinterpretation. In actuality, vitamin E helps to prevent oxygen from destroying other substances. In other words, it is a preservative, protecting the activity of other compounds such as vitamin A and polyunsaturated fat. Abundant sources of vitamin E are vegetable oils, beans, eggs, whole grains (the germ), liver, fruits, and vegetables.

No clinical effects in humans have been associated with very low intake of vitamin E. A rather rare form of anemia in premature infants, however, responds to vitamin E medication.

Vitamin K   There are several natural forms of vitamin K, which is needed for blood clotting. There is also a synthetic form of vitamin K, menadione, which may be obtained only by prescription. Vitamin K is found in several foods, including spinach, lettuce, kale, cabbage, cauliflower, liver, and egg yolks. A deficiency can cause hemorrhage and liver damage.

Niacin   Niacin is necessary for the healthy condition of all tissue cells. It is one of the most stable vitamins, and can be found in liver, lean meats, peas, beans, enriched and whole-grain cereal products, and fish. A deficiency of niacin causes pellagra, a once-common disease characterized by rough skin, mouth sores, diarrhea, and mental disorders.

Pantothenic Acid   Pantothenic acid is needed to support a variety of body functions, including proper growth and maintenance. It is found abundantly in liver, eggs, white potatoes, sweet potatoes, peas, whole grains (particularly wheat), and peanuts. A deficiency can cause headache, fatigue, poor muscle coordination, nausea, and cramps.

Folic Acid   Folic acid helps the body manufacture red blood cells and is essential in normal metabolism. The most abundant sources of this vitamin are liver, navy beans, and dark green leafy vegetables. Other good sources are nuts, fresh oranges, and whole-wheat products. A deficiency of folic acid causes a type of anemia.

Biotin   Once called vitamin H, biotin is now the sole term for this vitamin, which is actually a member of the B complex. It is important in the metabolism of carbohydrates, proteins, and fats, and can be found in eggs, milk, and meats. Raw egg white contains a substance that is known to destroy biotin.

Most deficiency symptoms involve mild skin disorders, some anemia, depression, sleeplessness, and muscle pain. A deficiency is extremely rare, however, probably because bacteria in the intestinal tract produce biotin.

Misconceptions

Even though the fairly common vitamin-deficiency diseases of forty years ago have all but disappeared, the typical American consumer is still concerned about the true "need" for vitamin supplements. Is there really any need? Each person should answer this question only after examining his or her regular diet and learning what vitamins can and cannot do.[55] The following list of myths and facts may help this learning process:

MYTH: Organic or natural vitamins are nutritionally superior to synthetic vitamins.
FACT: Synthetic vitamins, manufactured in the laboratory, are identical to the natural vitamins found in foods. The body cannot tell the difference and gets the same benefits from both sources. Statements to the effect that "Nature cannot be imitated" and "Natural vitamins have the essence of life" are without meaning.
MYTH: Vitamins give you "pep" and "energy."
FACT: Vitamins yield no calories. By themselves they provide no extra pep or vitality, nor an unusual level of well-being.
MYTH: The more vitamins the better.
FACT: Taking more vitamins than are necessary is a waste of money and time. In fact, in some cases excess amounts can be harmful.
MYTH: You cannot get enough vitamins from the conventional foods you eat.
FACT: Anyone who eats a reasonably varied diet should not need supplemental vitamins under normal circumstances.[56]

Megavitamin Madness

Because individuals vary in nutritional needs, it is difficult to know the exact amount of vitamins that is "too much." Some individuals, however, take extremely large doses of vitamins, and evidence is accumulating that such megavitamins can be harmful. When large doses are taken, vitamins stop acting like vitamins and begin acting like drugs.

[Mega]vitamins are being used . . . to treat everything from schizophrenia and cancer to the common cold. . . . Most scientists agree that massive doses of vitamins do have pharmacological effects on the body. They act like drugs and have drug-like effects. . . . [They also have] hazardous long-term effects. Vitamin C at 500 mg. actually destroys vitamin B_{12}, which is necessary to prevent red blood cell abnormalities and pernicious anemia. Excessive vitamin C falsifies blood sugar levels in testing diabetes. Prolonged use of large doses can be implicated in gout, hemorrhaging of ulcers, formation of kidney stones, severe diarrhea, and liver and genetic abnormalities.[57]

DIET PILLS

Phenylpropanolamine (PPA) is the appetite suppressant found in most diet pills, which manufacturers claim to be a safe and effective way to lose weight. PPA is one of the main drugs found in nasal decongestants such as Sineoff and Vick's Day Care. Although manufacturers claim PPA to be safe and effective, many organizations, physicians, and public agencies have expressed concern about the safety of OTC drugs containing it. The results of studies of biological effects of PPA have been conflicting, but reports have surfaced of adverse reactions in some people. The FDA has not made an official ruling on the relative safety and effectiveness of PPA, but a 1978 FDA advisory panel approved it as safe and effective when used for up to twelve weeks as an adjunct in weight reduction.[58] The controversy over PPA's safety as an OTC drug stems from its close chemical resemblance to amphetamines and its sympathomimetic effects in the body. As consumers, we should be aware of studies done on the biological effects of PPA, the FDA's delay in deciding PPA's safety and effectiveness, and the labeling and use of PPA in children's OTC medications.

Theoretically, PPA depresses the appetite and mimics the effect of amphetamines by stimulating the central nervous system.[59] Cardiac stimulation, high blood pressure, nervousness, headache, and insomnia are some of the common side effects. PPA also appears to pass into the breast milk of nursing mothers.[60] Acute temporary mental derangement is another side effect. A number of studies have indicated that PPA may cause anxiety, dizziness, hallucinations, and acute psychotic episodes.[61] Some individuals are taking OTC drugs containing PPA as amphetamines to get high.

Another consideration regarding the safety of PPA is the possible synergistic effects of PPA taken with other drugs. Over 50 percent of the diet pills in the United States OTC market contain both PPA and caffeine, which have synergistic effects on cardiac stimulation.[62] Imagine taking the recommended dosage of your favorite diet pill, which contains 50 milligrams of PPA and 200 milligrams of caffeine. You take the pill after getting up so you won't want breakfast. In addition, you consume your usual two to three cups of coffee before going to work. After about two hours you have 50 milligrams of PPA and 380 to 500 milligrams of caffeine in your system! This continues throughout the day, during coffee breaks and lunch hour. Stimulation of the CNS to this degree can bring tachycardia (fast heart rate) and aggravate hypertension (high blood pressure), not to mention having lesser effects such as headaches and insomnia. Most people who are taking diet pills are overweight, which has been associated with cardiac problems and high blood pressure, so taking PPA and caffeine together is a threat to a person's health.

SUMMARY

OTC drugs account for over $2 billion in sales every year. In general, they may provide relief, but many feel these drugs are used too often and may have serious side effects or complications.

One of the most popular of these drugs is aspirin, which helps to eliminate headache, reduce pain, and lessen inflammation in arthritis sufferers and may eventually prove effective in reducing heart attacks. Unfortunately, aspirin often has undesirable intestinal side effects and may also hinder platelet production. Acetaminophens may be used as an alternative, but they are more expensive, lack aspirin's antiinflammatory capability, and may damage the liver.

Laxatives are another popular OTC product. Though their use is largely unnecessary if proper foods, adequate fluids, and regular exercise are taken, many people employ them almost habitually. Laxatives are available as stimulant, bulk-forming, saline, and stool-softener products.

Cough relievers are still another high-selling OTC drug. The most effective of these suppressants are codeine-based, but they also cause dependence if used on a regular basis. Antihistamines are also potent medicines and should be taken with caution. Some antihistamines are effective in cold and allergy treatment and in the prevention of motion sickness.

The use of phenylpropanolamine (PPA) has increased in the form of diet pills. Our weight conscious society views this drug as a way to help lose weight. Its help in reducing the appetite makes it a very popular drug. However, caution must be practiced because there is some concern about the safety of PPA.

NOTES

[1] Richard Hall et al., "Psychiatric and Physiological Reactions Produced by Over-the-Counter Drugs," *Journal of Psychedelic Drugs* 10, no. 3 (July–September 1978):423–26.

[2] Food and Drug Administration, *Current and Useful Information from the Food and Drug Administration: Self Medication* (Washington, D.C.: Department of Health, Education and Welfare, 1973).

[3] Lois DeBakey, "Happiness Is Only a Pill Away: Madison Avenue Rhetoric without Reason," *Addictive Diseases: An International Journal* 3, no. 2 (1977):274.

[4] Ibid.

[5] W. H. Post and J. H. McGrath, "Patients and Potions," *Journal of Drug Issues* (Winter 1972), p. 54.

[6] White Rabbit, *Drug Information Center (DIC),* (Eugene: University of Oregon, 1975).

[7] Edward M. Brecher et al., *Licit and Illicit Drugs* (Boston: Little, Brown, 1972), p. 3.

[8] Post and McGrath, "Patients and Potions," p. 52.

[9] Hall et al., "Psychiatric and Physiological Reactions," p. 423.

[10]"Judging OTC's: Science Narrows it Choices," *American Pharmacy* NS19, no. 5 (May 1979):242. Reprinted with permission American Pharmaceutical Association, Washington, D.C.

[11]"OTC Review Milestone," *FDA Consumer*, February 1984, p. 32.

[12]Martin Gross and Leon Greenberg, *The Salicylates: A Critical Bibliographic Review* (New Haven: Hillhouse Press, 1948), p. 5.

[13]"Relieving the Analgesic Headache," *Time* 110 (August 1, 1977). Reprinted by permission from *Time*, The Weekly Newsmagazine; Copyright Time Inc. 1977.

[14]White Rabbit, *DIC*, p. 10.

[15]"Acetylsalicylic Acid (Aspirin): Alcohol and Drug Fact Sheet," *Drug Information Center (DIC)* (Eugene: University of Oregon, 1980).

[16]Howard A. Pearson, "Comparative Effects of Aspirin and Acetaminophen on Homeostasis," *Pediatrics,* November, 1977.

[17]Quoted in Gross and Greenberg, *The Salicylates,* p. 5.

[18]"Drug Induced Diseases," *Excerpta Medica* 4 (1972):70.

[19]Dan Shapiro, "Aspirin Flunks a Coronary Test," *Newsweek,* February 18, 1980.

[20]John C. Krantz, "The Jury Is Still Out: Aspirin Medication for Heart Attack Prevention," *American Pharmacy* NS19, no. 1 (January 1979):14–15.

[21]Paul E. Shindler, "Aspirin: Marvel Drug," *Science Digest* 84 (December 1978):14–18. From *Aspirin Therapy: Cutting the Risk of Heart Disease* by Paul E. Schindler, Jr. Copyright © 1978 by Paul E. Schindler, Jr. Used with permission from the publisher, Walker and Company, NY.

[22]David R. Zimmerman, *The Essential Guide to Non-Prescription Drugs* (New York: Harper & Row, Pub., 1983).

[23]M. J. H. Smith and Paul K. Smith, *The Salicylates: A Critical Bibliographic Review* (New York: Interscience Publishers, 1966), p. 215.

[24]Hugh H. Hussey, "Aspirin Can Be Dangerous," *Journal of the American Medical Association* 228 (April 29, 1974):609.

[25]Harvey J. Weiss, "Aspirin: A Dangerous Drug?" *Journal of the American Medical Association* 229 (August 26, 1974):1221.

[26]Hussey, "Aspirin Can Be Dangerous," p. 609.

[27]"Allergy to Aspirin," *British Medical Journal* 3 (July 27, 1974):217.

[28]Gross and Greenberg, *The Salicylates,* p. 5.

[29]Ibid.

[30]"Drug Induced Diseases," p. 70.

[31]Pearson, "Comparative Effects of Aspirin and Acetaminophen."

[32]Jan Koch-Weser, "Acetaminophen," *New England Journal of Medicine* 17 (December 2, 1978).

[33]"Is Tylenol (et al.) Any Better than Aspirin?" *Consumer Reports* 142 (October 1977).

[34]Walter Modell, *Drugs of Choice* (St. Louis: C. V. Mosby, 1960), p. 370.

[35]Erwin Di Cyan and Lawrence Hessman, *Without Prescription* (New York: Simon & Schuster, 1972), p. 72.

[36]J. H. Cummings, "Progress Report: Laxative Abuse," *GUT* 15 (September 1974):58.

[37]Charles Beck, "Laxatives: What Does Regular Mean?" *FDA Consumer* (May 1975):1.

[38]Quoted in ibid., p. 2.

[39]J. H. Cummings, G. E. Sladen, and O. F. W. James, "Laxative Induced Diarrhea: A Continuing Clinical Problem," *British Journal of Medicine,* March 23, 1974, p. 539.

[40]Marvin L. Corman, C. Malcom, and John A. Collier, "Cathartics," *American Journal of Nursing* 75, no. 2 (February 1975):71.

[41]Cummings, Sladen, and James, "Laxative Induced Diarrhea," p. 73.

[42]Ibid.; Barbara Smith and Bruce White, "U. T. Student Forum: Review of Laxatives and Cathartics," *Tennessee Pharmacist* 9, no. 12 (December 1973):1.

[43]M. D. Derezin, "Laxatives and Fecal Modifiers," *American Family Physician* 10, no. 1 (July

[44]Melva Weber, "Laxatives: Overused and Undersafe," *Vogue,* June 1975, p. 60.

[45]"Over-the-Counter Drugs," *Federal Register* 40, no. 56 (March 21, 1975):12, 910; Pearson, "Comparative Effects of Aspirin and Acetaminophen," p. 509.

[46]Corman, Malcom, and Collier, "Cathartics," p. 510.

[47]Beck, "Laxatives," p. 4; Corman, Malcom, and Collier, "Cathartics," p. 510; Weber, "Laxatives," p. 16.

[48]Griffenhagen and Hawkins, *Handbook of Non-prescription Drugs* (Washington, D.C.: American Pharmacological Association, 1973), p. 62.

[49]Betty Bergersen and Elsie E. Krug, *Pharmacology in Nursing,* 14th ed. (St. Louis: C. V. Mosby, 1979); Corman, Malcom, and Collier, "Cathartics," p. 426.

[50]Walter Modell, *Drugs of Choice: 1968–1969* (St. Louis: C. V. Mosby, 1967), p. 440.

[51]Annabel Hecht, "Drugs and Driving" *FDA Consumer* 12 (September 1978):17–19.

[52]*Physician's Desk Reference to Pharmacological Specialties and Biologicals,* 28th ed. (Oradell, N.J. Medical Economics, 1974).

[53]Annabel Hecht, "Vitamins Over-the-Counter: Take Only When Needed," *FDA Consumer* (April 1, 1979):17.

[54]Ibid.

[55]"Some Facts and Myths of Vitamins," *FDA Consumer* (1979):17.

[56]Hecht, "Vitamins Over-the-Counter," p. 17.

[57]Jean Mayer, "Megavitamin Madness: How Much Is Too Much?" *Family Health* 12, no. 2 (February 1980):48–49.

[58]American Pharmaceutical Association, *Handbook of Non-Prescription Drugs,* 6th ed. (Washington, D.C., 1979), pp. 221–24.

[59]Albert Dietz, "Amphetamine-Like Reactions to Phenylpropanolamine," *Journal of the American Medical Association* no. 205, 6 (February 13, 1981):601–2.

[60]James Long, *Essential Guide to Prescription Drugs,* 3rd ed. (New York: Harper & Row, Pub., 1982).

[61]Dietz, "Amphetamine-Like Reactions to Phenylpropanolamine," pp. 601–2; Gunnar Norvenius, "PPA and Mental Disturbances," *Lancet* 2 (1979):1367–68.

[62]APA, *Handbook of Non-Prescription Drugs,* p. 221.

13

PRESCRIPTION AND OTHER DRUGS OF INTEREST

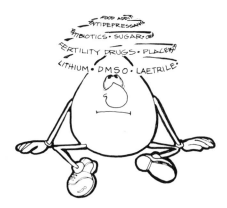

PLACEBOS

Introduction

A potent analgesic such as morphine can ease the suffering of severe injuries, but it sometimes fails to relieve mild pain. Give a man a sugar pill, and his agonizing ache will vanish because he believes the doctor's medicine will help him. Bite on a bullet, receive a shot of morphine, or swallow a sugar pill. Which will relieve pain best? Each can reduce pain better than the others under appropriate conditions.[1]

Placebos, substances that are used in medical treatment but have no pharmacological effect on the problem they are supposed to treat have existed for ages. But as placebos appear in more and more medical procedures, many are questioning the validity of their use. Is the practice harmful or beneficial? Because a sugar pill can relieve a pain through the user's belief in it, should it be given? If patients do gain relief from placebo effects, perhaps placebos are a viable treatment option. But in order to formulate an answer, it is necessary to know the mechanisms of the placebo process and the possible factors in negative and positive responses to treatment.

When a patient receives medical treatment, he or she assumes the treatment will be of physiological benefit, though it may not directly cure his or her symptoms or illness. The intent of giving a placebo is to change the patient's physiological condition by changing his or her attitude. Improvement occurs because of what the individual expects or desires, based on what he or she was told would occur.

The reliability of placebos is the subject of much scientific research, which indicates that a sizable percentage of most groups receiving placebos will show positive effects on any given trial. However, there is conflicting evidence on whether the same individual will react to the placebo in a consistent manner with repeated trials.

Individual Differences

Placebos are not necessarily inert. They may be fully effective drugs but they may not directly affect the problem they are given to treat. Placebos are capable of producing positive or negative effects, depending on the individual, the social milieu, and situational variables.[2] People likely to be most affected by placebos are usually those who are more open to the influence of others, are less critical of self and others, are more trusting of physicians and medicines, inhibit direct expression of hostility, and communicate socially desirable things about themselves. Individuals who are acutely distressed or anxious are also likely to experience placebo effects because of their need to obtain relief.

Social Environment and Situational Variables

When a patient takes a placebo, the degree of social support he or she receives from family members for reacting positively to the placebo will influence its potency. Situational variables, such as the physician's behavior, stimulus characteristics of the placebo, and treatment milieu exert a certain influence as well.

Administration, Frequency, and Cost

The method by which a placebo is administered, plus the placebo's visual and sensory characteristics, affects the patient's perception of how well the "medicine" will work.[3] Many people believe that injection of a drug has a more pronounced effect than oral administration because they consider injection to be the faster method, and they therefore expect almost immediate relief from it. Also, the mechanism of injection is impressive: invariably the patient feels that the needle coming nearer contains the much-awaited cure-all. The more

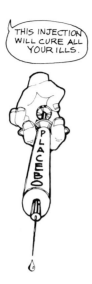

impressive the visual and sensory characteristics of the placebo, the more impressive the placebo is deemed by the patient.

It is no accident that specific artificial colors and flavorings are used in brand-name drugs. Studies have indicated that if a person takes a placebo in pill form, a large brown or purple pill or a small bright red or yellow pill may produce better results than those of other colors.[4] Other studies indicate that two pills are more effective than one, and, if chewed or dissolved in the mouth, a pill with an unpleasant taste produces better effects. In one of these studies, subjects were separated into two groups and instructed to swallow a pill. Some of the pills contained lactose and some ascorbic acid. The first group of students reacted negatively or had no reaction to the lactose pills, saying they felt they had been given placebos because the pills tasted so sweet. The second group swallowed the pills containing ascorbic acid and said they felt they had received actual medicine—a positive effect.[5]

Several other factors that influence placebo effectiveness are how often the dose is administered and how much the placebos cost. If a physician prescribes several doses during the day, the patient may feel a responsibility to follow the instructions and may experience greater effects. If the cost of the medicine is high, greater results are often experienced, because many believe that costlier drugs work more effectively.

Placebos are perceived as having a limited role in modern medicine, and only in situations where the physician has a good feel for the medical history, current condition, and potential responses of the patient.[6] It is preferable to have a good doctor-patient relationship based on honest disclosure of medical conditions. If patients are being given placebos, the success of a placebo to reduce symptoms should not be a reliable basis for determining that those symptoms were all in the patient's head.

ANTIBIOTICS

Classification

Antibiotics are metabolic compounds produced by microorganisms such as molds and soil bacteria that inhibit the growth of other microorganisms; their synthetic derivatives have the same effect. The three most important groups of antibiotics are penicillins, tetracyclines, and streptomycins, but there are over a dozen lesser-used antibiotics as well.[7] When at work in the body, antibiotics act either as a bacteriostatic (bacterial-growth-inhibiting) or bactericidal (bacterial-destruction) agent, or both.[8]

History

Penicillin, the first antibiotic, was discovered in 1928 by Alexander Fleming. When a culture of staphylococci was accidentally contaminated with a green mold, *Penicillin notatum,* Fleming noticed that the culture ceased to grow and was destroyed. It wasn't until 1940, however, when clinical researchers at Oxford developed a procedure for isolating and purifying the antibiotic, that its widespread use began.[9] Penicillin became known as the Wonder Drug because of its great ability to control disease-producing bacteria in the body.

Effects

Antibiotics destroy or inhibit the growth of infectious bacteria in many ways. Penicillins can destroy bacteria by interfering with their production of new protective cell walls as they multiply and grow.

The three groups of antibiotics also have different ranges of effectiveness. Penicillin is effective in low concentrations, though this effectiveness depends on the type of administration: generally an oral dose is only about one-fifth as effective as the same dose administered by injection. The amount of food in the stomach as well as the rate at which that organ empties are also factors that influence effectiveness, since food can slow absorption of the drug and decrease effectiveness.

Streptomycins are not absorbed into the bloodstream from the gastrointestinal tract. They are most effective when taken orally, but lose their effectiveness if taken with milk or other dairy products.

Tetracyclines are generally considered bacteriostatic agents and have bactericidal properties only in large doses. They are successful orally against a wide range of organisms. This family of antibiotics usually results in a modification of the infectious bacteria by slowing down or reducing the effectiveness of infectious bacteria.

Antibiotics are generally unable to affect certain regions of the body, such as the brain, the eye, and abscesses. Abscesses must be drained before antibiotic therapy will be of value.[10] Nor are antibiotics effective against viral infections, such as the common cold, influenza, measles, and mumps.

True toxic reactions to penicillin occur rarely. A number of individuals, however, do exhibit marked hypersensitivity to this drug. Symptoms of hypersensitivity include rashes, fever, skin eruptions, and more severe reactions capable of causing death. Severe symptoms may include joint pain, asthma, anaphylactic shock, and bone-marrow depression.

Though there are few toxic reactions to penicillin, toxic reactions to other antibiotics can occur with large doses. Occasional side effects may also be experienced, including hearing loss, vertigo, gastrointestinal upset, nausea, vomiting, and diarrhea. Permanent staining of developing teeth in young children, fetuses, and developed teeth of the elderly may be caused by tetracycline.

Resistance to Antibiotics

The number of antibiotic-resistant species of disease bacteria is increasing throughout the world. Penicillin, for example, used to be 100 percent effective against staphylococcus; its effectiveness has now diminished to less than 30 percent because of resistance.[11] Such growth of resistant species can be attributed to the passing on of resistance capabilities to ensuing generations of bacteria. Drug-resistant bacteria apparently manufacture a resistance-transfer chemical that enables bacteria never exposed to an antibiotic to become immune to it.[12] This resistance-transferring system is a limitation in all antibiotic therapy, and the problem will perhaps be solved only through the development of new antibiotic forms.

Resistance transferring may also be taking place outside the human body. Animals are often given antibiotics because for unknown reasons, they stimulate growth in chickens, pigs, and cattle, resulting in tastier meat with more fat. Antibiotics also inhibit animal diseases that threaten when large numbers of stock are kept in close confinement. This practice may be contributing to a potentially serious health problem. Though the evidence remains inconclusive, critics of the antibiotic-feeding programs are concerned that drug-resistant bacteria within animals will transfer their resistance to human disease bacteria. In response to this possibility, British scientists have convinced the British government to place controls on the kinds of antibiotics used in their animal feeds.[13] Similar controls are also in effect in the United States.

Changes in the human body caused by antibiotics may also lead to an increase in the number of infections unresponsive to antibiotic actions. Termed *alterations in the host,* these reactions to antibiotics range from changes in the body's normal microorganism population to interference with nutrition and the development of *superinfections.* When microorganism level is changed, normal bacteria decrease and abnormal bacteria or fungi increase. When this condition becomes extreme, a superinfection develops, and organisms not affected by antibiotics are able to grow rapidly.

Misuse

Misuse of antibiotics may involve improper dosage, improper administration, inadequate duration of treatment, or use by inappropriate patients. The patient must be sure to take the prescribed amount as well as the prescribed number of doses even though the symptoms of the infection may disappear before that number has been reached. Generally, antibiotic therapy is continued over a period of ten days; after that time any remaining doses should be disposed of.

Proper administration is very important in antibiotic use. Penicillin can be attacked by destructive secretions in the stomach, so it should be taken before meals, when there are less such secretions. Five times as much penicillin must be taken orally as intravenously in order to have therapeutic effectiveness, but care must be taken during intravenous injection if other drugs are present; for the combination could cause a chemical reaction that would alter the effectiveness of both drugs.[14]

Age and physical condition are other important factors in antibiotics use. Since newborns do not have mature livers, they are unable to metabolize antibiotics as well as adults and should not receive them. Adults with liver or kidney damage also should not take antibiotics. Pregnant women should not be given these drugs, since antibiotics cross the placental barrier and also have been found in the mother's spinal fluid and milk. One antibiotic, streptomycin, has been linked to fetal abnormalities when taken during pregnancy.[15]

ANTIDEPRESSANTS

Introduction

Depression—a condition of low spirits, gloominess, dejection, and decreased activity—is a very common complaint today. It is estimated that 15 percent of the American population suffer from symptoms of depression each year.[16] Fortunately, in most cases, this condition is situation-specific and of short duration. For some individuals, however, depression continues, and if help is not received they may sink into a deep pathological depression. This state is characterized by (1) great sadness associated with hopelessness and helplessness, and possible suicidal tendencies, (2) anxiety, and (3)inhibition.[17] Because the danger of suicide exists, chemical treatment of depression is often necessary.[18]

Amphetamines and electroconvulsive therapy (ECT) were early means of treating depression. But with the discovery of antidepressants in the 1950s, a new epoch in the treatment of mental illness began. Researchers discovered that antidepressants were able to elevate a patient's mood without also accelerating his or her heartbeat and causing insomnia or other unpleasant amphetamine side effects. Antidepressants also did not cause the relapses, confusion, and loss of memory ECT treatment often did. Antidepressant drugs soon became a "more pleasant, less traumatic form of treatment and one more suited to outpatient use."[19]

Despite the popularity of antidepressants, a great deal of controversy surrounds their use. A study of fifty-one consecutively admitted depressed patients at the National Institute of Mental Health found that many depressed patients are admitted to a hospital before they have received adequate chemotherapy as outpatients.[20] Researchers speculate that this lack of adequate drug treatment may result from the "physician's unfamiliarity with or bias against use of [antidepressants]."[21] But studies also show that these drugs are often prescribed too frequently as well.

Antidepressants should be used only when a biochemical cause for depression has been established. They are not meant for use in treating the mild and transient symptoms of depression associated with many life situations.

Classifications

Antidepressants fall into two categories: Monoamineoxidase inhibitors (MAOI), and tricyclics. Other drugs, such as amphetamines, caffeine, barbiturates, tranquilizers, and sedatives, have also been used to treat depression, but they are not classified as antidepressants.

Psychophysiological Effects

Antidepressants act on the central nervous system by increasing the availability of the chemicals (neurotransmitters) responsible for transmitting nerve signals at critical sites (nerve synapses) in the brain and throughout the central nervous system. The primary neurotransmitter that antidepressants are thought to act on is the chemical norepinephrine (or noradrenaline). Research has established that when norepinephrine levels in certain portions of the brain are low, chronic depression can occur. It is thought that when a natural deficiency of norepinephrine exists in certain portions of the brain, antidepressants, by increasing the rate of norepinephrine use in the nerves, can gradually increase mood and alleviate depression.[22]

As with all drugs, however, the action of antidepressants is not entirely specific, and they may produce adverse effects, such as dry mouth, blurred vision, faintness, nasal stuffiness, chills, drowsiness, and tremors. In addition, weakened libido, confusion, gastrointestinal distress, skin eruptions, weight increase, sweating, and urinary retention may occur.

With continued use, tricyclics and MAOI drugs can impair kidney and liver functions in some individuals.[23] Tricyclics can also lower a person's seizure threshold, and should therefore be used with caution in seizure-producing illnesses or disabilities. Both types of antidepressants are known to cross the placental barrier,[24] but they are not thought to produce physical or psychological dependence.

Monoamineoxidase-inhibiting drugs increase one's chemical sensitivity to a large number of foods and other drugs, a condition that may persist for many days following MAOI discontinuation. These drugs react unfavorably with such foods as cheese, beer, wine, pickled herring, chicken livers, and foods containing yeast extracts (tyramine-rich foods). Administration of MAOIs is especially hazardous during any drug-induced central-nervous-system depression, since it may cause an unexpected CNS-depressant overdose.[25] Though the acute overdose level of MAOIs in humans has not been firmly established, symptoms of acute toxicity are known. They include agitation, delirium, tremors, sweating, neuromuscular irritability, and hyperthermia, which can progress to a coma and even death.

MAOIs are no longer employed routinely. Instead, almost all the antidepressants used are tricyclics. MAOIs have stronger side effects and can interact with tyramine-rich foods to dangerously increase blood pressure.

NITROUS OXIDE (N₂O)

Nitrous oxide (laughing gas) is an artificial compound of nitrogen and oxygen. It is colorless, has a sweet odor and taste, and works as an anesthetic when inhaled. Nitrous oxide affects the central nervous system, impairing memory, the ability to concentrate, and the ability of the senses to function. It is considered to be one of the safest and least expensive of all general anesthetics,[26] since it is nonaddictive and nonallergenic and may be used concurrently with sedative agents, local-anesthetic injections, or other inhalants.

The anesthetic properties of this drug were first noted in 1779, but the gas was not employed for pain relief until 1884, when it was used during tooth extractions. Today, it is administered along with a supply of pure oxygen. This mixture prevents the lungs from becoming oversaturated with the drug.

The effects of nitrous oxide vary with the dose. Increasing amounts of the gas will cause the user to pass through stages of anesthesia and intoxication to unconsciousness. Though moderate doses generally produce a euphoric, dreamlike state, with sensations of driving, flying, and floating, some individuals may experience more extreme reactions, including violent physical activity, heart convulsions, and/or delirium. Side effects include nausea, vomiting, and amnesia, and current research speculates that prolonged use may cause a reduction in white blood cells.[27] Other findings have linked nitrous oxide to spontaneous abortion[28] and various malignant conditions.[29]

LITHIUM

Classification

Lithium is a metallic salt that can be administered as a strong antimanic tranquilizer in individuals who are suffering from a biochemical imbalance in portions of the brain that causes violent or manic behavior.

Pharmacology

Lithium helps to normalize mood and behavior in those with chronic manic-depressive illness by correcting chemical imbalances in certain nerve-impulse transmitters that can influence emotion and behavior.[30] Current thinking is that excessive levels of norepinephrine in certain sections of the brain can lead to excessive behavior characterized by emotional instability and potential violence.[31] Lithium helps reduce excessive norepinephrine firings so as to bring a person back to more normal behavior.

Lithium possesses one quality that makes it completely unlike any other drug used in psychiatry. It does not metabolize—it retains its physical integrity in the body and does not bind to any blood or tissue protein. This unique characteristic enables a physician to precisely monitor the amount of the drug in the brain or kidney. This can be done by simply determining lithium's concentration in the blood.

Medical Use

Lithium's unique psychoactive qualities are of great significance in the treatment of manic depression, a disease consisting of sudden and intense mood swings. Not only does the drug inhibit depression, it curbs hyperexcitability (mania) without producing the "blanket suppressions of behavior characteristic of the standard sedatives."[32] Continuous daily treatment with lithium brings patients to more "normal" moods and even makes it possible for some hospitalized patients to return home on only a maintenance dosage.[33]

Lithium has a very narrow margin of safe use. The level of drug required to be effective is quite close to the level that can have adverse effects. Careful dosage adjustments based on periodic measurements of blood levels are mandatory.[34]

Though lithium has many beneficial qualities, it can have adverse effects in some patients. These may include nausea, tremors, tiredness, dry mouth, and difficulty in organizing thoughts. Such effects, though, are generally mild and short-lived.[35] An overdose will affect the central nervous system, resulting in hypertonic or rigid muscles, gross contraction of skeletal muscles,[36] and possibly coma.

LAETRILE

Laetrile, an extract of apricot kernels, was widely boosted as an anticancer drug during the past two decades. Promoters of the drug claimed that laetrile spontaneously decomposes in the body into hydrogen cyanide, which immediately stops cancer cells' chemical respiration. To date, objective testing has never found laetrile to produce such a chemical reaction, and the vast majority of reputable scientists consider the use of laetrile dangerous for several reasons.[37]

First, cancer patients who decline standard anticancer therapies in favor of laetrile will likely see their cancers continue to grow, to the point where conventional anticancer therapies can no longer be effective. In addition, laetrile taken orally, can break down into forms of cyanide that can be toxic. Symptoms of cyanide poisoning that patients should be alert for include giddiness, nausea and vomiting, heart palpitations, and the skin turning blue from lack of oxygen.

Finally, the FDA has found many deficiencies in laetrile marketed to the public.[38] Some laetrile products were found to contain microbial contamination, other dangerous chemical adulterants, and subpotent tablets. To date, most scientists are in agreement that laetrile has no ability to inhibit cancerous growths, and is not a harmless therapy, as some of its promoters allege.

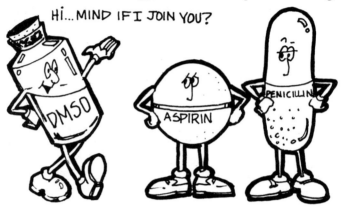

DIMETHYL SULFOXIDE (DMSO)

History

Dimethyl sulfoxide was first synthesized in Russia in 1866. A byproduct of paper-pulp processing, it initially aroused excitement because of its capacity as a solvent, an antifreeze, a hydraulic fluid, and a reagent that could speed up many chemical reactions.[39] Little testing of the substance was carried out until well into the twentieth century, however, when Stanley Jacob of the University of Oregon's Health Sciences Center conducted research in 1964 on the freezing and thawing of membrane tissue. During that research, Jacob and Robert Herschler, Crown Zellerbach's chemical-applications supervisor, found DMSO to have cryoprotective properties (the capacity to protect something from cold) for living tissues. They also reported its unique capacity to penetrate tissue in plants and animals and to dissolve other drugs and aid their absorption through the skin.

Jacob's first report, made in 1964, caused increasing interest in DMSO.[40] Reports of the drug's ability to relieve inflammation, sprains, strains, bruises, and a variety of skin conditions soon became common. Clinical investigation of DMSO continued until a report associated the drug with disturbances in the lens of the eye and with myopia (nearsightedness) in experimental animals. The FDA immediately halted further clinical study, even though tests of patients being treated with DMSO revealed no changes in their lenses. Further findings concluded that "the lens toxicity findings originally reported in dogs and later confirmed in certain other species have no equivalent or counterpart in human therapy. . . ."[41]

Even though data presented at two world conferences made it apparent that allegations of toxicity from clinical use of DMSO were infrequent and lacked severity, federal roadblocks still hamper the use of DMSO nationwide. The drug may be used only by veterinarians in the treatment of musculoskeletal injuries and inflammation in animals; for interstitial cystitis (a bladder condition) in humans; and as a commercial solvent. Researchers must submit an Investigational New Drug request to the FDA to carry out controlled studies that the FDA may monitor. However, several states have passed or are in the process of passing laws allowing its use, and clinical application of the drug in Europe has met with very apparent success.

Clinical evidence gathered from the United States and Europe from the 1960s to date indicates that DMSO may be an effective drug for some conditions. DMSO is inexpensive to produce; it can be manufactured in its pure form for as little as three to four dollars per gallon (but it retails for as much as eighteen dollars a pint).

Physical Effects

DMSO may be administered topically, subcutaneously, intramuscularly, intravenously, orally, and by inhalation. It has wide-ranging properties, not all of which are clearly understood.[42] The chemical penetrates tissue membranes easily, and effectively transports other molecules with it. Skin absorption of certain hormones, allergens, and antitumor agents is increased when those substances are diluted with DMSO. Substances such as hydrocortisone, when diluted with DMSO, remain as reservoirs beneath the skin, staying effective and resisting depletion for two weeks or more. Washing the skin surface with soap and water or alcohol does not destroy the reservoir. People who take DMSO often develop an oysterlike breath.

Under specific conditions, DMSO has protected test animals from cellular damage from extreme cold or irradiation. The drug is known to possess certain antibacterial and antiviral properties and appears to reduce bacterial resistance. When certain specific antibacterial drugs are diluted with DMSO, the amount of antibiotic required for treatment is reduced.

Dimethyl sulfoxide also displays analgesic properties. When injected, it blocks the conduction of nerve impulses. No apparent ill effects from this condition have been demonstrated in animal tests, and the effect is reversible.

Clinical Side Effects   Very few side effects, besides breath odor, have been observed in humans using DMSO. Among 4180 patients receiving topical DMSO treatment, some of whom longer than one year, the incidence of localized dermatitis was 3.5 percent; generlized dermatitis, less than 0.1 percent; and headache and nausea, 1.6 percent.[43] In another study, mild scaling dermatitis was observed in some subjects after their skin was swabbed twice daily for twenty-one days with 90 percent DMSO. This mild epidermal damage regressed as treatment continued, and the skin eventually returned to normal.[44]

Fate and Metabolism   How DMSO is metabolized, and what becomes of the drug after administration into the body, have been evaluated in humans by means of radioactive-labeling techniques. Hucker et al. found that DMSO reached peak blood serum levels in four to eight hours.[45] This indicates to many that a simple oxidation-reduction system exists. The drug is eliminated through the kidneys, with half of most doses eliminated within fourteen days of cutaneous application. "The most perplexing problem to those who have studied the fate and metabolism of DMSO is the fact that 100 percent recovery of the initial drug has not been achieved."[46] Poorest recovery yields have resulted in studies in which the drug was applied cutaneously; the best recovery results followed intravenous injection.

ORAL CONTRACEPTIVES

History

The capacity of hormones to prevent ovulation was first noted in animal experiments in 1921. Further experiments in the 1930s and 1940s clearly demonstrated that daily doses of female sex hormones, especially estrogen and progesterone, would prevent ovulation in laboratory animals.

In 1960 the first oral contraceptive, consisting of a combination of synthetic female hormones, was marketed in the United States. The Pill was heralded as a major breakthrough in the field of birth control, and was first viewed by most as the ideal contraceptive. Not only did the Pill appear to be nearly infallible as a contraceptive, but it also helped women feel secure about their birth-control method. The Pill was also easy to use, and increased independent behavior. By 1970, about 19 million women around the world were using oral contraceptives, which soon became the most popular means of birth control.[47]

Extensive controversy concerning the Pill's safety did not arise until the late 1960s, when various side effects of the drug gained world-wide prominence. Many women began to feel uneasy about taking the Pill, yet in the minds of many others the Pill's advantages still far outweighed its possible adverse effects. Today, use of oral contraceptives continues, but physicians are required to describe the drug's side effects and risks prior to use.

Composition and Use

The oral contraceptive is composed of synthetic estrogens designed to prevent ovulation, thus making pregnancy impossible, and progestins, which allow the menstrual cycle to continue. The quantities of progestin and estrogen used in the various brands differ markedly, although current trends indicate a reduction in dose size to reduce the risk of blood clotting. In addition to birth-control applications, oral contraceptives are used to treat certain disorders of the Fallopian tubes, menopausal stress, and menstrual irregularities.

Mechanism of Action

The estrogen in oral contraceptives inhibits factors involved in ovulation; progestin prevents ovulation itself and regulates the growth of the uterine lining, which is discharged as "menstrual bleeding."[48] According to Philip Corfman, director of the U.S. Center for Population Research at the Department of Health and Human Services, oral contraceptives appear to inhibit conception in six different ways:

> First, by acting on the pituitary gland, oral contraceptives inhibit the production of certain reproductive hormones. Second, [they] alter the state of the endometrium, which is the mucus coat of the uterus. Third, the progestins may alter the cervical mucus and thus create a plug to prevent the ascent of the sperm. Fourth, the oral contraceptives may alter the motility of the Fallopian tubes, again making it difficult for sperm to meet egg. Fifth, the progestogen factor may prevent capacitation, which is the ability of the sperm to enter the egg. Sixth, the pill may have a direct inhibiting effect on the ovaries' release of eggs—apart from the effect it exercises through the pituitary hormones.[49]

Theoretically, any method having only one of these effects would prevent pregnancy. If all six actions are taken, as they are by some contraceptive preparations, the chance of pregnancy is extremely remote. Statistics show that if the Pill is taken regularly for a year, less than one pregnancy per 1000 women results, making oral contraception the most effective method of birth control.[50] The failure rate of the intrauterine device (IUD) is 19 pregnancies per 1000 women, that of the condom 26 per 1000, and for the diaphragm 179 per 1000.[51]

Possible Side Effects

All drugs routinely have side effects that patients should be aware of. On rare occasion they may have adverse reactions, which indicate they are not working properly, and a physician should be promptly consulted. Routine side effects in users of oral contraceptives include some retention of fluid with possible weight gain, spotting in the middle of the menstrual cycle, a change in the menstrual flow, breast tenderness, and an increased susceptibility to yeast infections.

Adverse reactions include pain or tenderness in the leg, which could indicate thrombophlebitis (an inflammation of a vein in the leg, with a resulting blood clot.[52] Shortness of breath, chest pain, or coughing could indicate a pulmonary embolism (the movement of a blood clot into the lungs). In some women the risk of stroke (a blood clot in the brain) is increased, so strong headaches, blackouts, sudden weakness, or paralysis of any part of the body should be immediately reported to a physician. Other rare circulatory problems with oral contraceptives can include retinal thrombosis (a blood clot in the eye), which manifests itself as a sudden impairment of vision, and heart attacks, which show up as a sudden pain in the chest, neck, or arm accompanied by weakness, sweating, and nausea. Other rare adverse reactions include a rise in blood pressure in some sensitive individuals, impairment of the liver, and depression.

Effects from Smoking while Taking the Pill   A recent study of the effects of smoking while taking birth-control pills found that women over forty who take these pills but do not smoke have a mortality rate of 11 per 100,000; women in the same age group who use oral contraceptives as well as smoke have a mortality rate of 62 for every 100,000. Users who smoked but were in their twenties and thirties also had a higher death rate than users who didn't smoke.

Cancer and Tumors   Medical experts are still arguing over whether the hormones found in oral contraceptives (which create changes in the tissue lining of the uterus and cervix) cause cancer, stimulate an already existing cancer, or encourage the development of a future cancer. Since some cancers take as long as fifteen to twenty years to develop, and since oral contraceptives were not put on the market until 1960, conclusive evidence is still unavailable. However, increased hormonal secretions may stimulate malignant growths. Regular Pap smears and breast examinations will greatly reduce the chance of such growths going undetected.

A study of the relationship between liver tumors and oral-contraceptive use in young women found that clinical symptoms of tumors were more severe among users. The study also confirmed the association between oral-contraceptive use and focal nodular hyperplasias (excessive formations of tissue due to an increase in the number of cells). These results may be somewhat subjective because of researcher interpretation, but they do appear to indicate probable relationships between tumors and oral-contraceptive use.[53]

Birth Defects and the Pill

The majority of babies born to mothers who became pregnant while taking the pill appear to be entirely normal at birth.[54] In a New York State Health Department study, only 14 percent of 108 women who gave birth to infants with limb defects had taken hormones during pregnancy; in a control group of 118 women who gave birth to normal-appearing infants, only 4 percent had taken the Pill. A British Royal College of General Practitioners report agrees with the Health Department's general findings. The report states that "there is no evidence that oral contraceptives have any adverse effects on the outcome of pregnancies following their use."[55]

A Pill for Males

Chinese scientists have developed and are now testing a male birth-control pill that has been 99 percent effective for the 10,000 men tested so far.[56] The pill, called gossypol, is a compound extracted from cotton seed. It apparently works directly on the testes, impairing sperm production, but must be taken for at least two months before infertility occurs. The effects of the pill are reversible, with sperm counts generally returning to normal three months after the pill's discontinuation.

During a fifteen-month study period, male sex hormone levels remained normal and little difference was observed between androgen (male hormone) levels before and after the experiment. Though some men complained of reduced sex drive, none complained of impotency. With so many apparent advantages, this contraceptive may prove to be of great value.

FERTILITY PILLS

Introduction

Until the late 1950s, methods used to induce ovulation in women who were not ovulating remained largely unsuccessful. With the discovery of the two major fertility pills, clomiphene citrate (Clomid) and the human menopausal gonadotropin (Pergonal), the success rate improved. Clomiphene citrate is a synthetic estrogen that was originally expected to act as a contraceptive, and the human menopausal gonadotropin (HMG) is a substance originally isolated from the urine of postmenopausal nuns.[57] HMG is usually more effective in producing ovulation than clomiphene: one study found that two thirds of all anovulatory women treated with HMG become pregnant, compared with 20 to 30 percent who become pregnant following clomiphene-citrate treatment.[58] Even so, clomiphene is often preferable: it has fewer side effects, is fairly inexpensive, and is taken for fewer days.

Method of Effect

Normal ovulation depends on a functioning relationship among the hypothalmus, the pituitary gland, and the ovaries. Any disturbance in this relationship may result in anovulation, the failure of an ovum to be released. When used to treat anovulation, clomiphene citrate enlarges the ovaries and triggers the increased release of ovary-stimulating hormones. The amount of clomiphene citrate used in infertility procedures must be carefully monitored, however, because too small a dose will only supplement natural estrogens and have no evident influence on the ovaries.

When infertility treatment begins, one 50-milligram dose per day, taken orally or intravenously, is given to the patient for five days, generally from the fifth to the tenth day of the menstrual cycle. (Approximately half the drug is excreted within five days after it is taken.) After five days of treatment, instructions are given for the timing of intercourse, which for optimal results should take place every other day between the fifth and fifteenth day following the last dose of clomiphene. During this time, the basal body temperature must be carefully checked because a rise in temperature is one indication that pregnancy has taken place.[59]

If the first treatment with clomiphene is ineffective, the dose may be cautiously raised to 100 milligrams after a thirty-day interval and five days of doses are again administered. If this second treatment is also ineffective, one more treatment may be tried, although this decision and subsequent ones should rest solely in the hands of the patient and the physician.

Women who do not respond to three series of 100-milligram-per-day treatments may then be put on the human menopausal gonadotropin, a more power-ful fertility drug. HMG doses are generally administered for nine to twelve days, and are thought to stimulate follicles that encourage the development of imma-ture ova, though this is still uncertain.

Possible Side Effects

Ovarian enlargement, with or without cyst formation, occurs in 14 percent of all clomiphene citrate–treated women and is considered the major side effect of the drug.[60] Pelvic tenderness or discomfort from cysts can be diminished with estrogen treatment and reduced doses of clomiphene. Women with ovarian cysts prior to treatment should not use clomiphene, and those with enlarged ovaries should take only small doses. Cysts usually subside following discontinuation of clomiphene, but if left untreated, they may burst, leading to internal hemorrhaging and death. Ovarian cysts are an even greater risk for women using Pergonal.[61]

Hot flashes are another side effect, prevalent in 10 to 11 percent of clomi-phene users; they are similar to hot flashes experienced during menopause.[62] This intermittent flushing is thought to be caused by the antiestrogen effect of clomiphene and is usualy painless, dissipating once clomiphene intake ceases.

Side effects involving vision occasionally occur in clomiphene patients. Though these reactions are generally minimal, some persons have blurred vision or see spots or flashes of light. Such occurrences should be given special consid-eration since they may be dangerous if experienced during activities requiring motor skills. Side effects involving sight are generally reversed once clomiphene treatment ceases.

Though most side effects of fertility-pill treatment are generally minimal, some more adverse reactions have been experienced. These include nausea, vomiting, increased nervous tension, headaches, allergic dermatitis, loss of hair, depression, fatigue, breast soreness, weight gain, increased appetite, increased urination, and heavy menstruation. When clomiphene is used to treat infertility in men (something which is rarely done), baldness, vision difficulties, and skin rashes may develop with long-term use.

Multiple Births

Though fertility-pill treatment often results in pregnancy, more than one child sometimes results from that pregnancy. Between 8 and 10 percent of clomiphene-treated patients give birth to two or more children in one delivery.[63]

One theory holds that excessive dosage levels cause many ova to ripen simultane-ously, but most experts agree that imprecise timing is the real problem. In natural ovulation, they say, the ovary has a way of signaling the presence of a single ripe ovum to the pituitary gland, which responds instantly by producing hormones that trigger the ovary to ovulate and cause further maturation of ova to cease. But apparently, chemicals that stimulate ovulation disrupt this delicate mechanism.[64]

The infants are not identical in drug-induced multiple births since each child develops from a separate egg. Identical offspring are more likely to result from natural ovulation when one fertilized egg separates.

FOOD ADDITIVES

Introduction

Food additives are chemicals, primarily nonnutritive ones that are added to foods during growing or processing. These chemicals are added to maintain or improve nutritional value, to maintain freshness, to help in processing or preparation, or to make food more appealing.

> Food additives are so much a part of the American way of eating today that most of us would find it difficult to put together a meal that did not include them.
> Take a typical lunch, for example: sandwich, instant soup, gelatin dessert, and a cola drink. The bread has been fortified with vitamins and also contains an additive to keep it fresh. The margarine has been colored pale yellow—or, if you use salad dressing, it has been made with emulsifiers to keep it from "separating." The luncheon meat contains nitrite; the soup, an additive to keep it from becoming rancid; the gelatin, red coloring to make it pretty. Finally, the cola to wash it all down: without coloring, flavoring, sweeteners, or artificial carbonation, the pause that refreshes is nothing more than plain water![65]

Agents that modify the appearance of foods are called thickeners, firmers, stabilizers, or emulsifiers. They are found in such products as peanut butter, in which they keep the oils from separating from the water-soluble components. Chemicals such as monoglycerides and diglycerides are used to increase volume or add uniformity and fineness to products. Antispoilants, such as calcium and sodium propionate, butylated hydroxyanisole (BHA), and butylated hydroxytoluene (BHT) which was determined to be unsafe, are used to preserve foods and lengthen their shelf life by preventing deterioration. Substances such as glycerine are added to foods to control moisture content, and other substances are added to alter natural processes. Examples of such additives are ethylene, used to quick-ripen bananas, and malic hydroazide, used to prevent potatoes from sprouting.

Although chemicals with hard-to-pronounce names are common food additives, the most widely used additives are sugar, salt, and corn syrup. These three, plus such other substances as citric acid (found in oranges and lemons), baking soda, vegetable colors, mustard, and pepper, account for more than 98 percent, by weight, of all food additives used in this country.[66] A summary of these and other food additives are shown in Table 13–1.

History

The use of food additives to preserve and enhance the flavor and appearance of food is not new. Salt was used to preserve meats and spices to

TABLE 13-1 Additives: What, Where, Why They Are . . .

PURPOSE: To Aid in Processing or Preparation
CLASS: Emulsifiers

Some Additives	Where You Might Find Them
Carrageenan	Chocolate milk, canned milk drinks, whipped toppings
Lecithin	Margarine, dressings, chocolate, frozen desserts, baked goods
Mono/diglycerides	Baked goods, peanut butter, cereals
Polysorbate 60, 65, 80	Gelatin/pudding desserts, dressings, baked goods, nondairy creams, ice cream
Sorbitan monostearate	Cakes, toppings, chocolate
Dioctyl sodium sulfosuccinate	Cocoa

Their Functions
Help to evenly distribute tiny particles of one liquid into another, e.g., oil and water; modify surface tension of liquid to establish a uniform dispersion or emulsion; improve homogeneity, consistency, stability, texture.

PURPOSE: To Aid in Processing or Preparation
CLASS: Stabilizers, Thickeners, Texturizers

Some Additives	Where You Might Find Them
Ammonium alginate	Dessert-type dairy products, confections
Calcium alginate	
Potassium alginate	
Sodium alginate	
Carregeenan	Frozen desserts, puddings, syrups, jellies
Cellulose derivatives	Breads, ice cream, confections, diet foods
Flour	Sauces, gravies, canned foods
Furcelleran	Frozen desserts, puddings, syrups
Modified food starch	Sauces, soups, pie fillings, canned meals, snack foods
Pectin	Jams/jellies, fruit products, frozen desserts
Propylene glycol	Baked goods, frozen desserts, dairy spreads
Vegetable gums; guar gum, gum arabic, gum ghatti, karaya gum, locust (carob) bean gum, tragacanth gum, larch gum (arabinogalactan)	Chewing gum, sauces, desserts, dressings, syrups, beverages, fabricated foods, cheeses, baked goods

Their Functions
Impart body, improve consistency, texture; stabilize emulsions; affect appearance/mouth feel of the food; many are natural carbohydrates which absorb water in the food.

PURPOSE: To Aid in Processing or Preparation
CLASS: Leavening Agents

Some Additives	Where You Might Find Them
Yeast	Breads, baked goods

Baking powder, double-acting (sodium bicarbonate, sodium aluminum sulfate, calcium phosphate)	Quick breads, cake-type baked goods
Baking soda (sodium bicarbonate)	Quick breads, cake-type baked goods

Their Functions
Affect cooking results; texture and increased volume; also some flavor effects.

PURPOSE: To Aid in Processing or Preparation
CLASS: pH Control Agents

Some Additives	Where You Might Find Them
Acetic acid/sodium acetate	Candies, sauces, dressings, relishes
Adipic acid	Beverage/gelatin bases, bottled drinks
Citric acid/sodium citrate	Fruit products, candies, beverages, frozen desserts
Fumaric acid	Dry dessert bases, confections, powdered soft drinks
Lactic acid	Cheeses, beverages, frozen desserts
Calcium lactate	Fruits/vegetables, dry/condensed milk
Phosphoric acid/phosphates	Fruit products, beverages, ices/sherbets, soft drinks, oils, baked goods
Tartaric acid/tartrates	Confections, some dairy desserts, baked goods beverages

Their Functions
Control (change/maintain) acidity or alkalinity; can affect texture, taste, wholesomeness.

PURPOSE: To Aid in Processing or Preparation
CLASS: Humectants

Some Additives	Where You Might Find Them
Glycerine	Flaked coconut
Glycerol monostearate	Marshmallow
Propylene glycol	Confections, pet foods
Sorbitol	Soft candies, gum

Their Functions
Retain moisture.

PURPOSE: To Aid in Processing or Preparation
CLASS: Maturing and Bleaching Agents, Dough Conditioners

Some Additives	Where You Might Find Them
Azodicarbonamide	Cereal flour, breads
Acetone peroxide	Flour, breads & rolls
Benzoyl peroxide	
Hydrogen peroxide	
Calcium/potassium bromate	Breads
Sodium stearyl fumarate	Yeast-leavened breads, instant potatoes, processed cereals

Their Functions
Accelerate the aging process (oxidation) to develop the gluten characteristics of flour; improve baking qualities.

PURPOSE: To Aid in Processing or Preparation
CLASS: Anti-caking Agents

Some Additives	Where You Might Find Them
Calcium silicate	Table salt, baking powder, other powdered foods
Iron-ammonium citrate	Salt
Silicon dioxide	Table salt, baking powder, other powdered foods
Yellow prussiate of soda	Salt

Their Functions
Help keep salts and powders free-flowing; prevent caking, lumping, or clustering of a finely powdered or crystalline substance.

PURPOSE: To Affect Appeal Characteristics
CLASS: Flavor Enhancers

Some Additives	Where You Might Find Them
Disodium Guanylate	Canned vegetables
Disodium inosinate	Canned vegetables
Hydrolyzed vegetable protein	Processed meats, gravy/sauce mixes, fabricated foods
MSG (monosodium glutamate)	Oriental foods, soups, foods with animal protein
Yeast-malt sprout extract	Gravies, sauces

Their Functions
Substances which supplement, magnify, or modify the original taste and/or aroma of a food—*without* imparting a characteristic taste or aroma of its own.

PURPOSE: To Affect Appeal Characteristics
CLASS: Flavors

Some Additives	Where you Might Find Them
Vanilla (natural)	Baked goods
Vanillin (synthetic)	Baked goods
Spices and other natural seasonings and flavorings, e.g., clove, cinnamon, ginger, paprika, turmeric, anise, sage, thyme, basil	No restrictions on usage in foods—Found in many products

Their Functions
Make foods taste better; improve natural flavor; restore flavors lost in processing.

PURPOSE: To Affect Appeal Characteristics
CLASS: Natural/Synthetic (N/S) Colors

Some Additives	Where You Might Find Them
N Annatto extract (yellow-red)	No restrictions
N Dehydrated beets/beet powder	No restrictions
S Ultramarine Blue	Animal feed only .5% by wt.
N/S Canthaxanthin (orange-red)	Limit = 30 mg/lb of food
N Caramel (brown)	No restrictions
N/S Beta-apo-8' carotenal (yellow-red)	Limit = 15 mg/lb of food
N/S Beta carotene (yellow)	No restrictions

Their Functions
Increase consumer appeal and product acceptance by giving a desired, appetizing, or characteristic color. Any material which imparts color when added to a food. Generally not restricted to certain foods or food classes. May *not* be used to cover up an unwholesome food, *or* used in excessive amounts.
Must be used in accordance with FDA Good Manufacturing Practice Regulations.

PURPOSE: To Affect Appeal Characteristics
CLASS: Sweeteners

Some Additives	Where You Might Find Them
Nutritive Sweeteners: Mannitol—sugar alcohol Sorbitol—sugar alcohol	Candies, gum, confections, baked goods
Dextrose Fructose	Cereals, baked goods, candies, processed foods, processed meats
Glucose Sucrose (table sugar) Corn syrup/corn syrup solids Invert sugar	Cereals, baked goods, candies, processed foods, processed meats
Non-nutritive sweeteners: Saccharin	Special dietary foods, beverages

Their Functions
Make the aroma or taste of a food more agreeable or pleasurable.

N Cochineal extract/carmine (red)	No restrictions
N Toasted partially defatted cottonseed flour (brown shades)	No restrictions
S Ferrous gluconate (turns black)	Ripe olives
N Grape skin extract (purple-red)	Beverages only
S Iron oxide (red-brown)	Pet foods only .25% or less by wt.
N Fruit juice/vegetable juice	No restrictions
N Dried algae meal (yellow)	Chicken feed only

N Tagetes (Aztec Marigold)	Chicken feed only
N Carrot oil (orange)	No restrictions
N Corn endosperm (red-brown)	Chicken feed only
N Paprika/paprika oleoresin (red-orange)	No restrictions
N/S Riboflavin (yellow)	No restrictions
N Saffron (orange)	No restrictions
S Titanium dioxide (white)	Limit =1% by wt.
N Turmeric/Turmeric oleoresins (yellow)	No restrictions
S FD&C Blue No. 1	No restrictions
S Citrus Red No. 2	Orange skins of mature, green, eating-oranges. Limit = 2 ppm.
S FD&C Red No. 3	No restrictions
S FD&C Red No. 40	No restrictions
S FD&C Yellow No. 5	No restrictions

Synthetic color additives subject to certification: inspected and tested for impurities.

Source: FDA Consumer (June 1979):4–5.

flavor foods since early times, and it is said the expeditions of Marco Polo and Columbus were motivated in part by the desire to find new spices for these uses. Today's additives, however, are more diverse and used more extensively, and efforts to improve and preserve foods have moved from worldwide exploration to laboratory research.

As the use of additives proliferated, concern about their effects and hazards also increased. In 1938, the Federal Food, Drug, and Cosmetic Act strengthened the 1906 Pure Food and Drug Act, authorizing potency tests for some substances and banning formaldehyde use; the act also gave the Food and Drug Administration authority to inspect processing plants. It wasn't until 1958, however, that the United States passed legislation regulating food additives. The Food Additive Amendment prohibited use of additives in amounts known to produce cancers, and required that substances be proved safe before put into public use. To prove a product safe, manufacturers must first subject the additive to a battery of chemical tests and then feed the additive in large doses over an extended period to at least two kinds of animals, usually rodents and dogs. Manufacturers must then submit the results of all these tests to the FDA, and if they indicate the additive is safe, the agency establishes regulations for how it can be used in food. A basic rule is a 100-fold margin of safety for anything added to food. This means that the manufacturer may use in a food product only 1/100th the maximum amount of an additive that has been found not to produce any harmful effects in test animals.[67]

Under the Food Additives Amendment two major categories of additives are exempt from the testing and approval process. The first is a group of some 700 substances "generally recognized as safe" (GRAS) by qualified experts. The idea behind what has come to be known as the GRAS List was to free FDA and manufacturers from being required to prove the safety of substances already considered harmless because of past extensive use with no known harmful effect. Their efforts, it was felt, would be better spent on new additives and on those compounds about which less is known.

Also exempt from testing were "prior sanctioned substances," those that had been approved before 1958 for use in food by either FDA or the U.S. Department of Agriculture. Some prior sanctioned substances also were included on the GRAS List.

These lists of exemptions are not, however, engraved in stone. As testing methods and scientific understanding of toxicology improve, new evidence and questions may arise about the safety of old standbys. To make sure these substances are judged by the latest scientific standards, FDA is reviewing all categories of food additives.[68]

In 1960, the Color Additive Amendments were passed, subjecting coloring agents used in foods, drugs, and cosmetics to rigorous premarket testing. Colors in use when the amendment was passed were placed on a provisional approval list pending further investigation or confirmation of their safety. Nearly 200 coloring agents have been on the provisional approval list at one time or another, but only 31 colors are currently fully approved for use in foods. Chemicals were dropped from the list because manufacturers were no longer interested in marketing them or because they were found to be unsafe. In 1976, for example, the FDA banned Red Dye No. 2, then the most widely used red coloring agent, because tests done on animals could not resolve whether the dye caused cancer.[69]

In 1974, another piece of food additive legislation was passed. The Consumer Food Act was designed to close existing legal loopholes in the approval system, strengthen monitoring procedures, and extend labeling requirements.

Adverse Effects

Additives share with all drugs the potential for precipitating allergic reactions in some individuals. Though inconclusive, recent evidence suggests a link between processed "convenience" foods (rich in additives) and hyperkinesis in children. Certain additives, including cyclamates, nitrates, nitrites, saccharin, and diethyl-pyrocarbonate (DEPC), have also been linked to an increased incidence of various cancers.[70] However, later studies showed that food colorings Red Dye No. 2 and Red Dye No. 4 cause carcinogenic tumors in laboratory animals.[71]

Still other additives appear to have adverse effects. Nitrates and nitrites have been shown to reduce oxygen transportation by the blood, and are implicated in stomach and gastrointestinal cancers. Monosodium glutamate can cause headaches, sweating, nausea, thirst, flushing, tightness in the face or chest, and abdominal pains from doses of two to twelve grams. It is not totally clear what effects food additives have on the fetus, but many of these substances have low molecular weights and this may allow them to cross the placental barrier.

Sugar is an additive that may harm consumers through its contribution to obesity. At least one third of our population is overweight, and this extra weight can cause a number of health hazards. Sugar can also play a role in tooth decay. Sugar substitutes, such as saccharin, may be a cause of cancer. Research on rats conducted in Canada and the United States indicates that rats develop bladder cancer after regular ingestion of saccharin. In March 1977, the FDA banned saccharin, but many feel that carcinogen tests on animals may not apply to humans and that the large doses given to test animals are too unrealistic.

NutraSweet, a low-cal sweetener, has been a boon not only to its creator, G. D. Searle and Company, but also to the makers of a growing number of consumer products. Strong demand for NutraSweet products comes from aging baby boomers who are concerned about their weight and health. Mothers like NutraSweet because it doesn't promote tooth decay.

NutraSweet, which is patented under the generic name aspartame, was first introduced in 1981 in Searle's tabletop sweetener Equal.[72] Now it is available in more than sixty products, including hot cocoa, pudding, chewing gum, tea, and coffee preparations. Besides General Foods, Searle's clients include Coca Cola, Pepsi Cola, Seven Up, Borden, Carnation, H. J. Heinz, and Procter and Gamble.

At the moment you cannot bake with NutraSweet because high heat removes its sweetness. But one day consumers may be able to buy cookies and cakes sweetened with the above-mentioned aspartame, which is 180 times sweeter than sugar and is made from protein products. Many soft-drink companies substitute with 100 percent NutraSweet because of increased sales from the use of NutraSweet.

SUMMARY

The use of placebos in medicine is highly controversial. Should placebos be prescribed for patients? The answer is still unclear. However, with proper administration, placebos do appear to be effective.

Antibiotics, the Wonder Drugs, have revolutionized our society's expectations about drugs. Penicillin, streptomycin, and tetracycline preparations have been extremely effective in fighting harmful bacteria. However, bacterial resistance to antiobiotics is on the increase because certain bacteria tend to build up immunity to the drugs.

Antidepressants, such as nitrous oxide and lithium, have been used to elevate the spirits of depressed patients. Nitrous oxide may produce a dreamlike, euphoric state, but it may also result in delirium, disorientation, bronchial irritation, nausea, and vomiting. Lithium has been used with manic-depressive patients. Because it is not metabolized, a doctor can easily monitor the amount of lithium in a patient's blood.

Laetrile is a drug that is the subject of tremendous controversy. Made from apricot kernels, it has been promoted as an anticancer agent. However, current research indicates that Laetrile does not cure cancer.

Dimethyl sulfoxide (DMSO) may be the greatest drug discovery since the discovery of aspirin. Arthritis sufferers and individuals with muscular ailments are apparently finding great relief through this drug, although it must still undergo further testing before being made available to the public.

Oral contraception has tremendous potential for population control. It can dispel the fear of pregnancy as well as enhance sexual fulfillment. However, pills currently available sometimes lead to health problems. A male oral contraceptive called gossypol is being researched by the Chinese.

Fertility pills such as clomiphene citrate and HMG have been a blessing for many childless couples. These drugs, which encourage ovulation, have helped many women to become pregnant. Administration of fertility pills must be carefully monitored. In some cases, multiple births result.

Food additives are another source of continuous controversy. Though they help foods look more appealing and add to shelf life, tests indicate that some additives may contribute to hyperkinesis, obesity, cancer, and other adverse effects.

NutraSweet, a low cal sweetener, is making its way in the market place in a big way. It offers the person the taste of sweetness without the increase in calories. In our weight watching society this is a real attractive alternative to sugar.

NOTES

[1]Frederick J. Evans, "The Power of the Sugar Pill," *Psychology Today* 9, no. 11 (April 1974). Reprinted with permission from *Psychology Today Magazine*. Copyright © 1974 American Psychological Association (APA).

[2]Penny Webb, "Man, Magic and the Modern Placebo," *Health Education Journal* 37, no. 2 (June 1978):1–53.

[3]Ibid., p. 23.

[4]Ibid., p. 24.

[5]Carol E. Gammer and Vernon L. Allen, "Note on the Use of Drugs in Psychological Research." *Psychological Reports* 18, no. 2 (January–JUne 1966):64.

[6]Alfred Goodman Gilman, Louis S. Goodman, and Alfred Gilman, *The Pharmaceutical Basic of Therapeutics*, 6th ed. (New York: Macmillan, 1980), p.47.

[7]White Rabbit, *Drug Information Center (DIC)*, (Eugene: University of Oregon, 1975), p. 20.

[8]Richard Locscher, "Antibiotics: Use and Misuse" (lecture presented at Sacred Heart General Hospital, Eugene, Oregon, January 23, 1974.)

[9]William Boyd, *An Introduction to the Study of Disease* (Philadelphia: Lea & Febiger, 1971), p. 555.

[10]Locscher, "Antibiotics."

[11]Ibid.

[12]John R. Holum, *Elements of General and Biological Chemistry*, 3rd ed. (New York: John Wiley, 1972), pp. 390–91. p. 391.

[13]Ibid., p. 390.

[14]Locscher, "Antibiotics."

[15]White Rabbit, *Drug Information Center (DIC)*, p. 20.

[16]Ibid., p. 21.

[17]Harold Himwich and Hilma S. Alpers, "Psychopharmacology," *Annual Review of Pharmacology* 10 (1970):320.

[18]"Clinical Aspects of Amphetamine Abuse," *Journal of the American Medical Association* 240, no. 21 (November 17, 1978).

[19]White Rabbit, *Drug Information Center (DIC)*, p. 22.

[20]Arthur K. Shapiro, "A Historical and Heuristic Definition of Placebo," *Psychiatry* 27, no. 1 (February 1964).

[21]Joel Kotkin, Robert M. Post, and Frederick K. Goodwin, "Drug Treatment of Depressed Patients Referred for Hospitalization," *American Journal of Psychiatry* 130, no. 10 (October 1973):1141.

[22] Robert Julien, *A Primer of Drug Action*, 3rd ed. (San Francisco: W. H. Freeman & Company 1981), pp. 75–76.

[23]White Rabbit, *Drug Information Center (DIC)*, p. .

[24]Don Mcloud et al., *Drug Information Primer* (Eugene: University of Oregon 1980), p. 12.

[25]White Rabbit, *Drug Information Center (DIC)*, p. 20.

[26]Ibid., p. 21.

[27]Ibid.

[28]T. H. Corbett, "Anesthetics as a Cause of Abortion," *Fertility and Sterility* 23, no. 11 (November 1972):868; T. H. Corbett, "Effects of Low Concentrations on Rat Pregnancy," *Anesthesiology* 39, no. 3 (September 1973):301.

[29]D. L. Bruce, "Cause of Death among Anesthesiologists: A 20 Year Survey," *Anesthesiology* 29, no. 3 (May–June 1968):565; E. B. Johnson, "Harmful Pollution by Anesthetic Gases?" *Lancet* 2 (October 1972):824.

[30]James W. Long, *Essential Guide to Prescription Drugs*, 4th ed. (New York: Harper & Row Pub., 1985), p. 451.

[31]Julien, *Primer of Drug Action*, pp. 75–76.

[32]Samuel Gershen and Baron Shopoin, eds., *Lithium: Its Role in Psychiatric Research and Treatment* (New York: Plenum, 1973), p. 1.

[33]Ibid.

[34]Long, *Essential Guide to Prescription Drugs*, p.452.

[35]Joseph Mendels and Steven K. Secunda, eds., *Lithium in Medicine* (New York: Gordon & Breach, 1972), p. 11.

[36]Barbara J. Culliton and Wallace K. Waterfall, "Apricot Pits and Cancer," *British Medical Journal* 1, no. 61661 (March 24, 1979):11.

[37]"A Pharmacological and Toxicological Study of Amygadalin," *Journal of the American Medical Association* 245, no. 6 (February 13, 1981):591.

[38]"Toxicity of Laetrile," *FDA Bulletin* (November–December 1977).

[39]White Rabbit, *Drug Information Center (DIC)*.

[40]S. W. Jacob, "Dimethyl Sulfoxide (DMSO): Current Concepts in Toxicology," *American Surgeon* 35, no. 8 (August 1969):565.

[41]Ibid.

[42]White Rabbit, *Drug Information Center (DIC)*.

[43]S. W. Jacob et al., *Dimethyl Sulfoxide: Basic Concepts of DMSO* (New York: Marcel Dekker, 1971), p. 565.

[44]S. W. Jacob and D. C. Wood, "Dimethyl Sulfoxide (DMSO):A Status Report," *Clinical Medicine* 78 (November 1971):21–31.

[45]Ibid., p. 21.

[46]Ibid., p. 22.

[47]Ibid.

[48]John P. Bennett, *Chemical Contraception* (New York: Columbia University Press, 1974), p. 29.

[49]Quoted in Barbara Seaman, "The New Pill Scare," *MS* 3, no. 12 (June 1975):100.

[50]Saltman, *The Pill*, p. 36.

[51]Ibid.

[52]Long, *Essential Guide to Prescription Drugs*, p. 334.

[53]Josef Vana and Gerald Murphy, "Primary Liver Tumors and Oral Contraceptives:Results

of a Survey," *Journal of the American Medical Association* 238, no. 20 (November 14, 1977):2154–58.

[54]Seaman, "The New Pill Scare," p. 62.

[55]Alice Lake, "The Pill," *McCalls* 102, no. 4 (January 1975):114.

[56]"Chinese 'Pill' for Men 99% Effective," *Register-Guard* (Eugene, Oregon), May 5, 1979, p. 10.

[57]Roger Field, "Six for the Price of One: Pregnancy Pill," *Science Digest* 76, no. 6 (December 1974):44. Reprinted by permission from *Science Digest.* Copyright © 1974 The Hearst Corporation. All rights reserved.

[58]Ibid., pp. 14–15.

[59]Robert W. Kistner, "Induction of Ovulation with Clomiphene Citrate," in *Progress in Infertility,* 2nd ed., ed. M. D. Behrman and Robert Kistner (Boston: Little, Brown, 1975), p. 528.

[60]K. D. Schulz et al., "Oestrogen-like and Antioestrogenic Potencies of Clomiphene Citrate: Biochemical Investigations," in *Fertility and Sterility,* ed. Hasegawe et al. (New York:American Elsevier, 1973), p. 524.

[61]White Rabbit, *Drug Information Center (DIC),* p. 23.

[62]Frederick H. Meyers, Ernest Javetz, and E. Goldfein, *Review of Medical Pharmacology* (Los Altos, Calif.: Lange Medical Publications, 1968), p. 365.

[63]Clinter Sotrel, Rao Ramaa, and Antonio Scommegna, "Heterotropic Pregnancy following Clomid Treatment," *Journal of Reproductive Medicine* 16, no. 2 (February 1976):79.

[64]Field, "Six for the Price of One," p. 16.

[65]Phyllis Lehmann, "More Than You Ever Thought You Would Know about Food Additives," *FDA Consumer* (April, 1979).

[66]Ibid.

[67]Ibid.

[68]Ibid.

[69]Ibid.

[70]Nancy Glick, "Bringing Home the (Nitrite-less) Bacon," *FDA Consumer* 13, no. 4 (May 1979):25–26.

[71]White Rabbit, *Drug Information Center (DIC),* p. 30.

[72]"NutraSweet: How Sweet Is It?"*Register Guard* (Eugene, Oregon), March 10, 1985, p. 6F.

THE CONSUMER AND DRUG LEGISLATION

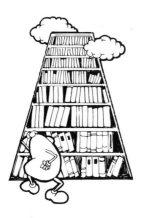

INTRODUCTION

How well the prescription-drug industry is regulated and functions directly affects the drug consumer. Both physicians and government regulatory agencies are involved in this supervision, as is the drug industry itself. Though all three groups are interested in safe and effective medians, they also work to protect their own interests. To understand the area of drug use and abuse, consumers must understand the roles physicians, business, and government play in that area.

THE PHYSICIAN'S ROLE

Though most doctors are well trained in their field of practice, most do not receive adequate training in the area of pharmacology. As doctors they are expected to prescribe drugs, but many may find it difficult to understand and apply correctly the constantly increasing barrage of pharmaceutical preparations:

1. The physician often lacks detailed information concerning several thousand pharmaceutical products. Most doctors rely on the *Physician's Desk Reference* (PDR) for this information. "But the PDR is as much an advertising catalogue as a reference tool because the information it contains has been supplied, edited, approved and paid for by the drug manufacturers."[1]
2. By contrast, the *Medical Letter on Drugs and Therapeutics,* an authoritative, non-profit, drug-evaluating service for physicians, is subscribed to by less than one fourth of the nation's practicing physicians.[2]
3. Surveys of physicians have indicated that drug salespersons or "detail people" and journal or direct-mail advertisements are their "most important sources of familiarization [with] new drugs."[3] Drug companies, whose incentives are to sell their particular product, exert a marked influence on the physician, so much so that the industry spends an estimated $5000 per year per physician on marketing and advertising.[4]
4. The American Medical Association has often called itself "the largest publisher of prescription drug advertisements in the world," with its weekly *Journal of the American Medical Association* and several specialty journals.[5]

What is the effect of most physicians' lack of understanding of pharmacology? They may prescribe drugs they know little about. To keep up with current pharmaceutical preparations, they must follow the advice of drug companies, not sound medical information. If physicians are misled, public health may be endangered. Already, for example, the indiscriminate use of antibiotics has had the following unfortunate consequences:

1. Many bacteria that were once susceptible to these drugs have mutated, becoming highly virulent strains resistant to available chemotherapy.[6]
2. Many thousands of Americans have died from adverse drug reactions.[7]
3. Physicians have been pressured by their patients into prescribing a medication that is not indicated, but is deemed psychologically necessary by the patient.

In addition to the problems of physicians, lack of training in pharmacology and the large-scale production and advertising of drugs, patients occasionally make mistakes with medications. Patients should carefully follow their doctor's instructions (some surveys show that a large percentage of patients receiving medication do not follow instructions) and be sure to ask for clarification of any points about the drug that are confusing or difficult to understand. On occasion it might even be a good idea to get instructions or special precautions in writing. Patients should promptly inform their doctors if they think they are experiencing side effects, adverse reactions, or overdose from a drug. Patients need to inquire if a particular drug from a physician can affect their driving behavior, or perhaps interfere or cause dangerous reactions if mixed with a second drug they are using. Finally, special precautions apply to use of medications by patients who are pregnant or nursing, and by elderly, who are more prone to side effects and adverse reactions because of their declining health as aging occurs.

THE DRUG INDUSTRY

Every year, approximately 1.5 billion prescriptions (or an average of 20 per family) are filled in this country. For these prescriptions, Americans pay $33 per year per person. In 1973, pharmaceutical companies made $5 billion; another $2 billion was garnered by middlemen such as distributors and pharmacists.[8] In 1978 the pharmaceutical industry made $10.5 billion, and an estimated $18 billion was spent in 1985.[9]

Profit and Production

The pharmaceutical industry is one of the most profitable of all industries. In 1973, its 9.1 percent return on sales was second only to mining among industrial groups.[10] Profitability is maintained even though drug prices haven't climbed as rapidly as other consumer prices. This continued profitability is attributed to a high degree of automation, the absence of price competition, and the inelastic demand for prescription drugs.

Marketing and Advertising

Many authorities believe that drug companies spend excessive amounts on marketing and advertising and too little on research and development. Most pharmaceutical houses do spend one out of every four dollars on advertising but only one quarter of that amount on research and development. In addition to the money they spend on salespeople, magazine and journal advertising, and other means of promotion, many pharmaceutical houses offer physicians and pharmacists prizes (freezers, color TV sets, camping equipment, all-expense-paid tours) and free samples of their products.[11]

Research and Development

Though the drug industry has spent up to $500 million a year on research and development, the return on research investments has shown a steady decline. A number of new drugs for treating hypertension, angina pectoris, and cardia arrythmias have recently been introduced on the market. In a Council of Economic Priorities Study, sixteen companies submitted 185 new-drug applications to the Federal Drug Administration. Nevertheless, only 33 drugs (18 percent) were found to be significant; the rest were simply new "packages" or minor chemical variations of existing drugs.[12] A 1969 study by an HEW task force on prescription drugs noted: "Since important chemical entities represent only a fraction—perhaps 10–20 percent—of all new products introduced each year, and the remainder consists merely of minor modifications or combination products, then much of the industry's research and development activities would appear only minor contributions to medical progress."[13] Though drug companies are spending more money, they are exhibiting less productivity.

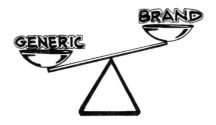

The High Cost of Prescription Drugs

To many observers, profits from the sale of drugs have depended too little on whether the drugs are beneficial and too much on whether they are successfully promoted.[14] This emphasis on promotion is part of the reason that prescription-drug costs are so high; buying brand names rather than generic medicines may cost the American consumer $1 billion per year.

Unfortunately, the consumer is not always given a choice. Though Henry Simmons, former director of the FDA's Bureau of Drugs, states that "we cannot conclude there is a significant difference in quality between the so-called generic and brand name products tested,"[15] many doctors continue to prescribe brand-name drugs. Efforts to correct this situation have been slow because the drug-industry lobby has been effective in blocking corrective legislation. Currently, however, a number of states have introduced generic legislation or "substitution" laws aimed at reducing the cost of prescription drugs. This trend appears to be spreading nationwide.

While the drug industry is often guilty of unrealistic drug prices and price fixing, the pharmaceutical lobby also shares in contributing to the high cost of prescription drugs. Avoiding price competition definitely maximizes profits for the manufacturer, especially when the consumer must buy a product with an inelastic demand.

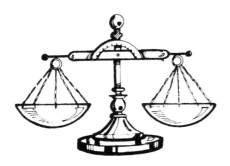

DRUG USE AND THE LAW

The effect of drug legislation is, paradoxically, sometimes both considerable and minimal. It has done little to dissuade illicit use: people use the chemical of their choice regardless of existing statutes. Drug legislation therefore becomes a number of hoops that people have to go through to achieve their goal and a list of the consequences of getting caught. Legislation of morality is the key issue. It seems that morality cannot be effectively legislated and that attempts to do so are always met with hazards to the individual greater than those posed by use of the drug.

Laws are sets of standards established by society for the regulation and preservation of its stability. Based on determined values (norms) of the society, their purpose is to prevent individuals from infringing upon the rights of others. It is important to keep in mind how these social values and norms are determined and assessed, and what the individual's legal rights are.

Societal norms are determined by examining the society's beliefs on a given issue.

> One of the amazing things is the almost magical belief many people have that the law and law enforcement are something separate from and independent of society. Failure to appreciate that the law is but one of the reflections of the culture is one of the points of contention in the drug scene today. Law enforcement works as a social control only when the society wants it to work, and that ocurs only when the law is in agreement with the major themes and beliefs of society.[16]

Throughout U.S. history, most Americans have believed that solutions to problems lay in the passing of restrictive laws. "The assumption of such legislation is that it will stop or deter the particular activity, e.g., drug use, and, if it fails to do so, will punish the individual and/or protect society from such antisocial behavior by imprisoning the offender."[17] Though many laws have been passed, they have failed to greatly reduce or restrict drug use. A look at narcotics legislation provides a clue as to why these laws often fail. "One reason for the failure . . . appears obvious. They [narcotics laws] were aimed at private transactions between willing sellers and willing, usually eager, buyers. Thus there were no [complainants]"[18]

Victimless Crimes

It is difficult to enforce crime legislation when the crime involved has no victim. Does society have the right to interfere with an individual's right to determine his or her own actions—in this case, to use drugs? Should drug use be a crime because society at large deems it to be? The answers to these questions remain uncertain, but the mere fact that the questions arise make it difficult to enforce legislation.

A further obstacle to narcotics-legislation enforcement is the inequitable treatment offenders often receive. Also, the types of drugs used in criminal acts are looked at in different lights. Finally, many penalties for drug use are not commensurate with the physical harm they may cause. With so many inequalities and concerns about drug-law enforcement, current regulations may be doing more harm than good.

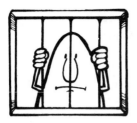

Drug Education

Publicizing a drug's effects can sometimes lure people to use it rather than deterring them. Certainly this was true for LSD in the 1960s, when passage of anti-LSD legislation led to an increase in LSD availability and demand. Also, after isolated instances of glue-sniffing among school-age children were widely reported in the nation's newspapers, that form of drug use increased. And when the nation was informed that "speed kills," methamphetamine use drastically increased too.

> Some speed users who inject almost suicidal doses of methamphetamine into their veins, without any regard for their safety and health, may actually be trying to test the truth of the youth slogan "Speed Kills." . . . To these individuals the slogan . . . may paradoxically carry more attraction than deterrent power—and thus may not serve the purpose for which it is being proposed.[19]

Publicizing false and misleading warnings about drugs can also have negative rather than positive effects. When LSD, marijuana, and heroin were grouped together in antidrug campaigns, many people believed that these drugs' effects and potency were similar. This is untrue, and "the fact that many of the warnings against marijuana were patently false . . . helped destroy the credibility of LSD warnings from the same sources."[20] Inappropriate drug education may not only fail to crack the "drug menace" but may in some instances help to make it even stronger.

A HISTORY OF MAJOR DRUG-RELATED LEGISLATION

Regulation of Opiates: 1865–1905

In the late nineteenth century, opiates were easy to obtain and could be purchased legally. They were known to be addictive yet were widely prescribed as pain-killers and tranquilizers and for menstrual and menopausal discomforts, diabetes, and countless other maladies. Since there were no laws governing the labeling of ingredients on patent medicines, many preparations contained morphine, cocaine, and heroin. Manufacturers of the time were remarkably effective in preventing any congressional action that would have required disclosure of dangerous drugs in commercial preparations.[21]

The Pure Food and Drug Act: 1906

"The medical consensus was that morphine had been overused by the physician, addiction was a substantial possibility, and addition of narcotics to patent medicines should be minimized or stopped."[22]

Also, feelings ran high that prolonged use of opiates led to criminal behavior and social decay. Lay reformers and Victorians began to take undaunted stands on the opiate issue. They looked to federal legislation as the most effective weapon against the sins of opiate use.

The first important federal legislation that regulated opiate use was the Pure Food and Drug Act of 1906. This act "prohibited interstate commerce of adulterated or misbranded food and drugs."

> In the section on misbranding, the act specifically referred to alcohol, morphine, opium, cocaine, heroin, Cannabis indica (marijuana), and several other agents. Each package was required to state how much (or what proportion) of these drugs was included in the preparation. This meant, for example, that the widely sold "cures" for morphine addiction had to indicate that they in fact contained another addicting drug.[23]

The act was a good beginning, but in 1911 a loophole was found. The law did not regulate claims of a medicine's curative powers or advertising of the preparation. Because few people read labels if accompanying advertising promises miracles, the Pure Food and Drug Act lost much of its clout.

The Shanghai International Conference: 1909

In 1906, in response to its growing opiate problem in the Philippines, the United States called for an international opium conference, the Shanghai Conference. But in asking for such a conference, the United States found itself in a difficult position: it had no exemplary opium laws of its own. The first attempt at such legislation grew out of the Shanghai Conference, but the bill met with defeat both at the conference and in the United States. The fight for opium legislation and international control continued. Two more international drug conferences were held—the Hague Conferences of 1911 and 1914—but since the United States still had no domestic legislation, there were no exemplary laws to pattern agreements after, and thus no concerted efforts to ratify the conventions.

The Harrison Narcotic Act: 1914

"In 1914, it was estimated that about 200,000 Americans—one in 400—were addicted to opium or its derivatives."[24] But when the Harrison Act was passed, the legal supply of opiates that led to that addiction was restricted. The Harrison Act allowed physicians to prescribe narcotics only "in the course of their professional practice," making possession of narcotics without a prescription a criminal offense. "Patent-medicine manufacturers [had to limit] themselves to preparations and remedies which do not contain more than 2 grains of opium, or more than one-fourth of a gram of morphine, or more than one-eighth of a grain of heroin . . . in one avoirdupois ounce."[25] The law focused not on prohibition but on regulation of the marketing and sale of opium, morphine, heroin, and other drugs and the prescribing of opiates by physicians.

Prohibition: 1920

Alcohol-prohibition legislation, sparked by the concerted efforts of such groups as the Anti-Saloon League and the Women's Temperance Union, became effective in 1920 with the enactment of the Volstead Act, which became the Eighteenth Amendment to the U.S. Constitution. The idea of national prohibition had been gaining ground for over twenty years prior to the bill's enactment. Many feel World War I was what finally put Prohibition over the top. "The United States had been at war since April 1917, and the hysteria that gripped the nation in its crusade against the Kaiser extended the firm belief that liquor sapped the nation's strength and willpower, and even depleted the cereal grains that could be used in bread for the troops and starving Europeans."[26]

Prohibition outlawed the manufacture, sale, and transportation (but not the possession) of domestic and foreign liquor within the United States. But this regulation only created a thriving alcohol black market, in which adulterated and contaminated "rotgut" was easy to obtain. Some of the ingredients in these bootleg beverages occasionally led to blindness, paralysis, and even death. In addition, "the disreputable saloon was replaced by the even less savory speakeasy."[27]

Prohibition not only resulted in impure alcoholic products sold illicitly, but initiated a shift from weak beers and wines to hard liquors. In addition, alcohol substitutes began to fill the void. Even before Prohibition, the states that had prohibition laws of their own found that morphine sales were rising rapidly. Marijuana, which was little used prior to Prohibition, also became popular during that time.

Despite Prohibition, alcohol remained an integral part of America's culture, as it had since the country's inception. The Eighteenth Amendment was unable to end either the use of alcohol or the problems that surrounded that use, and in 1933 Prohibition was repealed. But Prohibition wasn't ended because people decided that alcohol was a harmless drug. "On the contrary, the United States learned during prohibition, even more than in prior decades, the true horrors of the drug."[28] It also learned that making a drug illegal does not end its use, but can actually encourage more adverse drug situations.

Importation of Heroin Banned: 1924

Despite the passage of the Harrison Act, heroin use continued to rise. Law-enforcement officials made a further attempt to eradicate the drug's use by securing legislation banning the importation of heroin, even for medicinal use. "This legislation grew out of the widespread misapprehension that, because of deteriorating health, behavior and status of addicts from morphine to heroin, heroin must be a more damaging drug than opium or morphine."[29] This, of course, is not true: the two drugs' physiological effects are not drastically different. But no matter what the reasoning was behind it, "the 1924 ban on heroin did not deter the conversion of morphine addicts to heroin."[30]

Linder v. United States: 1925

In 1925, in the case of Linder v. United States, the Supreme Court decided that drug dependency was an illness. This decision allowed physicians to once again prescribe narcotics to help cure the addict, something the Harrison Act had made illegal.

Porter Narcotic Farms Bill: 1929

Though the Linder v. United States decision allowed doctors to consider drug dependents as patients and prescribe opiates for them as part of their treatment, many drug dependents were in prison for violating the Harrison Act. "This . . . abundance of narcotics prisoners led, at long last, to federal hospital care for addition."[31] Congress passed the Porter Narcotic Farms Bill in 1929, establishing "farms" in Lexington, Kentucky, and Fort Worth, Texas, for the treatment of drug dependents convicted of breaking federal law. Despite this seeming step forward in the treatment of drug abuse, the farms, operated by the Public Health Service until 1967 and from then on by the National Institute of Mental Health, maintained a consistently low cure rate.

Federal Bureau of Narcotics: 1930

In 1930 Congress reorganized the individuals responsible for opiate control into one separate body of enforcement within the Treasury Department. This bureau, the Federal Bureau of Narcotics (FBN), assumed all duties previously carried out by the Federal Narcotics Control Board. In April 1968 it became the Bureau of Narcotics and Dangerous Drugs in the Department of Justice. In 1972 President Nixon further reorganized the body and changed its name to the Drug Enforcement Agency.

The Marijuana Tax Act: 1937

Once the Federal Bureau of Narcotics was formed, it began to take a hard line on drug use, including marijuana use. FBN officials and others thought that marijuana was the cause of crime, violence, mental illness, sexual deviancy, and moral degeneration, and in 1937 the Marijuana Tax Act was passed to curtail these problems. Modeled after the Harrison Act, the Marijuana Tax Act did not actually ban the use of marijuana but merely taxed physicians, druggists, growers, manufacturers, and distributors for its prescription and distribution; only the nonmedicinal untaxed possession of marijuana was illegal.

And like the Harrison Act, the Marijuana Act was ineffective. As an editorial published in the *Journal of the American Medical Association* shortly after the act's passage stated,

> After more than twenty years of federal effort and the expenditure of millions of dollars, . . . opium and cocaine habits are still widespread. The best efforts of an efficient Bureau of Narcotics, supplemented by the efforts of an equally efficient Bureau of Customs, have failed to stop the unlawful flow of opium and coca leaves and their compounds and derivatives, on which the continuance and spread of narcotic addition depends. The best efforts of the Public Health Service to find means for prevention and cure of narcotic addiction cannot yet guarantee the cure of narcotic addiction. What reason is there, then, for believing that any better result can be obtained by direct federal efforts to suppress a habit arising out of the misuse of such a drug as cannabis? Certainly it is almost as easy to smuggle into the country and to distribute as are opium and coca leaves. Moreover, it can be cultivated in many parts of the United States and grows wild in field and forest along the highways in many places.[32]

The Food, Drug and Cosmetic Act: 1938

In the early 1930s President Roosevelt pushed for revision of the 1906 Pure Food and Drug Act, declaring it grossly inadequate. But Congress was unresponsive. It took until 1938 for major reform to be passed, and only then mainly because of a catastrophe. A product called Elixir of Sulfanilamide was marketed to meet a demand for sulfanilamide in liquid form. The drug, whose main ingredient was similar to radiator antifreeze, killed 108 persons, mostly small children. The product had been marketed without animal testing, a situation the resulting Food, Drug and Cosmetic Act of 1938 made illegal. The law closed the legal loophole of the original Food and Drug Act, gave the Federal Trade Commission (FTC) clear powers to regulate patent-medicine advertising, and, most importantly, required drugs to be found safe before distribution.

The Boggs Amendment: 1951

"Up until 1951, the control of narcotics was directed toward the medical profession and their dispensing of these drugs."[33] But at the end of World War II, illegal drug traffic spiraled. Continuing to align the evils of marijuana and heroin use, Congress responded to the increased drug traffic and to pressures from the FBN by passing the Boggs Amendment to the Harrison Act. This mandatory minimum-sentence law for opiate *and* marijuana offenders reflected the country's hard-line enforcement approach by imposing severe penalties and limiting suspension of sentence and probation or parole to first-time offenders. Penalties under this act were:

> first offense for possession: fine plus two- to five-year sentence, probation permitted

second offense for possession: fine plus five- to ten-year sentence, no probation or suspended sentence

third and subsequent offenses for possession: fine plus ten- to twenty-year sentence, no probation or suspended sentence

The Narcotic Drug Control Act: 1956

Though federal authorities expected a decrease in drug use after the passage of the Boggs Amendment, they saw none. Thoughts that "the laws must not be strict enough," that "drug usage is a Communist plot to demoralize and degenerate the American people" echoed throughout the land. In this emotion-laden environment, the Narcotic Drug Control Act was passed. This law increased the penalties of the Boggs bill at all levels. Fines were drastically increased, and third-time offenders were given mandatory ten- to forty-year sentences with no possibility of probation, suspension of sentence, or parole. Perhaps its most severe provision was that the death penalty could be imposed on anyone who sold, gave away, furnished, or conspired to sell heroin to a person under eighteen, even on the first conviction.

Kefauver-Harris Amendments: 1962

In 1960 a sleeping pill called Kevadon (thalidomide) was awaiting FDA approval. Though the drug had already been successfully marketed in Europe, and despite constant pressure from the manufacturers, the FDA was not satisfied with the new drug's application and insisted on proof of the product's safety. While this proof was being awaited, West Germany announced that the drug caused birth defects when taken by pregnant women. This tragic discovery gave impetus to a new drug-reform movement, and in 1962 the Kefauver-Harris Amendments to the Pure Food and Drug Act were passed. This legislation contained the following requirements:

1. All new drug applications had to be supported by substantial evidence of the product's effectiveness as well as its safety.
2. All drugs marketed between 1938 and 1962 were also to be subjected to the same efficacy demands as were new products.
3. Drug advertising and other printed media seen by the physician must state drug side effects as well as contraindicated uses.[34]

Robinson v. California: 1962

The 1925 Linder case affirmed that drug dependency is a medical condition that can be treated by physicians. This position was later supported by the decision handed down in *Robinson* v. *California*. In this case it was decided that to punish for opiate dependence was to impose cruel and unusual punishment, which is prohibited by the Bill of Rights. Since drug dependence was no longer illegal, it should not be punishable by imprisonment. Instead, states should have the right to compel drug-dependent people to undergo medical treatment.

The Community Mental Health Centers Act: 1963

"Although rival theories of deviance control were gaining credibility in the postwar period, the enforcement of narcotic laws did not become widely questioned and condemned until surveillance and penalties failed, even with mandatory minimum penalties and the death threat, to prevent a rapid rise in various forms of drug abuse in the 1960's."[35] At that time public officials and organizations slowly began to turn their ideas on drug abuse in the only direction afforded them—lessened penalties, medical treatment and rehabilitation, and possibly low-cost, legalized drug maintenance for drug-dependent individuals. Community mental-health centers, funded and supported by Congress, suggested that mandatory sentences and rigid controls on drug usage be modified.[36] In 1963 the Community Mental Health Centers Act was passed, emphasizing decentralized treatment, rehabilitation, and reintegration of mental patients (many of whom were drug dependents) back into society.

The Drug Abuse Control Amendments: 1965

It is ironic that at the same time rigid penalties for drug dependency began to soften, the desire for more stringent controls on nonnarcotic drug use began to grow. In 1965 the Drug Abuse Control Amendments to the 1938 Federal Food, Drug and Cosmetic Act were passed, classifying barbiturates, amphetamines, LSD, and other drugs with depressant, stimulant, or hallucinogenic effects as dangerous drugs. Penalties for possessing "dangerous drugs" were one year and/or a fine for a first offense and up to three years plus a fine for additional offenses. Penalties for selling these drugs to a minor were even greater. In 1968 a further amendment made simple possession a crime and increased maximum penalties but, ironically allowed for suspension of a first offender's sentence.

> The most important aspect of this [1965] law was its break with tradition in excluding possession for one's own use from the criminal penalties (as did the federal anti-alcohol laws) and instead concentrating on illegal manufacture and sale. The amendments, which came into effect in 1966, provide for more controls on distribution by manufacturers; limit physicians' prescription renewals of these drugs to five in any six-month period and, since 1967, bring LSD and related drugs under the same provision of control as the barbiturates and amphetamines. . . .[37]

Exempted from parts of this act was the Native American church, which was granted the right to use peyote in its religious ceremonies on the grounds that restriction of peyote would violate the Indians' freedom of religion.

The Narcotic Addict Rehabilitation Act: 1966

The concept of medical treatment and rehabilitation for drug users that started in the early 1960s became more widely accepted by the mid 1960s. The Narcotic Addict Rehabilitation Act of 1966 allotted federal monies to state and local communities and programs for the treatment of drug abusers. The act also changed the status of the two federal narcotics "farms" (in Lexington, Kentucky, and Fort Worth, Texas) from treatment centers to research centers.[38]

The Comprehensive Drug Abuse Prevention and Control Act (The Controlled Substances Act): 1970

When this bill was originally submitted to Congress, it was a liberal one, emphasizing research, education, and rehabilitation of drug users. As a result of the prevailing law-and-order sentiment of Congress, however, the bill that finally passed both houses was more enforcement-oriented. Still, the statute that passed was a major victory for those arguing for a reasonable drug law. It provided for the separation of law enforcement from the Department of Human Services, whose job was to scientifically evaluate which drugs to control. Other liberalizing changes from the strict 1951 and 1956 laws were the elimination of federal mandatory sentences for first-offense illegal possession, the reinstatement of the possibility of probation, and the complete erasure of conviction from public records relating to the case. "From a legal point of view, the individual is then restored to his prearrest status and can legally deny under oath that he was ever arrested on such a charge."[39]

The law's treatment of controlled drugs was divided into five dimensions called *schedules,* each carrying distinct penalties for manufacturing, distribution, and possession. A significant aspect of this law is that it focuses not on the user but on the distributor. More detailed information about the act follows.

THE CONTROLLED SUBSTANCES ACT

Procedures for Controlling Substances

The purpose of the Federal Controlled Substances Act (CSA) is to minimize the quantity of drugs of abuse which are available to persons who are prone to abuse drugs. Procedures for controlling a substance under the CSA are set forth in Section 201 of the Act. Proceedings may be initiated by the Department of Health, Education, and Welfare (HEW), by DEA, or by petition from any interested person. This may be a manufacturer, a medical society or association, a pharmacy association, a public interest group, a state or local government agency, or an individual citizen. When a petition is received by DEA, the agency begins its own investigation of the drug.

The Controlled Substances Act sets forth the findings which must be made to put a substance in any of the five schedules. These are as follows (Section 202(b)):

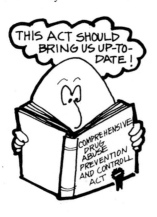

Schedule I

(A) The drug or other substance has a high potential for abuse.
(B) The drug or other substance has no currently accepted medical use in treatment in the United States.
(C) There is a lack of accepted safety for use of the drug or other substance under medical supervision.

Schedule II14-1

(A) The drug or other substance has a high potential for abuse.
(B) The drug or other substance has a currently accepted medical use in treatment in the United States or a currently accepted medical use with severe restrictions.
(C) Abuse of the drug or other substances may lead to severe psychological or physical dependence.

TABLE 14–1 Control Mechanisms of the CSA

Schedule	Registration	Recordkeeping	Manufacturing Quotas	Distribution Restrictions	Dispensing Limits
I	Required	Separate	Yes	Order forms	Research use only
II	Required	Separate	Yes	Order forms	Rx: written; no refills
III	Required	Readily retrievable	No *but* Some drugs limited by Schedule II quotas	DEA registration number	Rx:written or oral; with medical authorization, refills up to 5 times in 6 months
IV	Required	Readily retrievable	No *but* Some drugs limited by Schedule II quotas	DEA registration number	Rx: written or oral; with medical authorization, refills up to 5 times in 6 months
V	Required	Readily retrievable	No *but* Some drugs limited by Schedule II quotas	DEA registration number	OTC (Rx drugs limited to MD's order)

This chart summarizes the control mechanism in a format which permits comparison between the schedules in terms of the controls imposed.
Note that the distinction between Schedule III and Schedule IV is virtually nonexistent. Other than the penalties for criminal trafficking, the statute makes no distinction whatsoever. DEA, in imposing regulatory controls, has singled out narcotic drugs in Schedule III for coverage under the ARCOS system. By indirect means, some narcotics and non-narcotics in Schedule III are also under the quota system.
The differences between Schedule V and Schedules III and IV are also very small. The only practical distinction is that Schedule V drugs are generally over-the-counter, a differentiation imposed not by the CSA but by FDA.

Schedule III

(A) The drug or other substance has a potential for abuse less than the drugs or other substances in Schedules I and II.
(B) The drug or other substance has a currently accepted medical use in treatment in the United States.
(C) Abuse of the drug or other substance may lead to moderate or low physical dependence or high psychological dependence.

Schedule IV

(A) The drug or other substance has a low potential for abuse relative to the drugs or other substances in Schedule III.
(B) The drug or other substance has a currently accepted medical use in treatment in the United State.
(C) Abuse of the drug or other substance may lead to limited physical dependence or psychological dependence relative to the drugs or other substances in Schedule III.

Schedule V

(A) The drug or other substance has a low potential for abuse relative to the drugs or other substances in Schedule IV.
(B) The drug or other substance has a currently accepted medical use in treatment in the United States.
(C) Abuse of the drug or other substance may lead to limited physical dependence or psychological dependence relative to the drugs or other substances in Schedule IV.

In making these findings, DEA and HEW are directed to consider eight specific factors (Section 201(c)):

(1) Its actual or relative potential for abuse;
(2) Scientific evidence of its pharmacological effect, if known;
(3) The state of current scientific knowledge regarding the drug or other substance;
(4) Its history and current pattern of abuse;
(5) The scope, duration, and significance of abuse;
(6) What, if any, risk there is to the public health;
(7) Its psychic or physiological dependence liability;
(8) Whether the substance is an immediate precursor of a substance already controlled by this title.

A key criterion for controlling a substance, and the one which will be used most often, is the substance's potential for abuse. If the Attorney General through his designee the Administrator determines that the data gathered and the evaluations and recommendations of the Secretary of HEW constitute substantial evidence of potential for abuse, he may initiate control proceedings under this section. Final control by the Attorney General will also be based on the Administrator's findings as to the substance's potential for abuse.

Criminal Penalties for Trafficking

The most common and well-known control mechanism has not yet been mentioned: the criminal sanctions for illicit trafficking. Trafficking is defined as the unauthorized manufacture, the unauthorized distribution (i.e., delivery whether by sale, gift, or otherwise), or the possession for unauthorized manufacture or distribution of any controlled substance. The penalties for violation of this restriction are related to the schedules as well. For narcotics in Schedules I and II, a first offense is punishable by up to 15 years in prison and up to a $25,000 fine. For trafficking in a Schedule I and II non-narcotic drug or any Schedule III drug, the penalty is up to five years in prison and up to a $15,000 fine. Trafficking in a Schedule IV drug is punishable by a maximum of three years in jail and up to a $10,000 fine. And trafficking in a Schedule V substance is a misdemeanor punishable by up to one year in prison and up to a $5,000 fine. Second and subsequent offenses are punishable by up to twice the penalty imposed by the first offense.

It must be emphasized that possession for one's own use of any controlled substance is always a misdemeanor on the first offense, punishable by one year in jail and up to a $5,000 fine.[40]

The Black Market: 1971

"Most of the heroin that reaches the United States' black market has come (until recently) from Turkey. Farmers there have for years been required by law to sell their entire opium crop to the Turkish government, which resells it to legitimate pharmaceutical manufacturers. . . ." Despite this law, black-market operators have been able to secure all the Turkish opium they want; whatever portion of the crop they don't buy goes to the government and then to the legitimate pharmaceutical manufacturers.[41]

In 1971, the U.S. government announced it had persuaded Turkey to ban opium production altogether after 1972 in exchange for economic compensation. The bill laying out this agreement was hailed as a major victory for the United States' war on international opiate trade, but as it turned out the law only forced legitimate pharmaceutical companies as well as black-market entrepreneurs to seek available markets elsewhere in the world. Black-market operations found this availability in Southeast Asia, and opium from Asia as well as Mexico began to flood the country. It seems that as long as legal access to drugs is blocked for drug dependents, heroin and other illegal opiates will continue to enter the country through underground channels.

Consumer Issues and Legislation: 1973

How well the Food and Drug Administration implements drug-related laws has been the subject of much controversy for some time. In hearings before the Senate Health Subcommittee, Senator Edward Kennedy stated that

on one hand, timidity and bureaucratic delay are said to be holding up approval of valuable products that already are on sale and saving lives in foreign countries. On the other hand, FDA regulations are said to often cave in to industry pressure and release dangerous and ineffective products that haven't been adequately tested.[42]

Legislation designed to help consumers cope with this and other drug-related concerns was introduced in 1973. It strengthened consumer safeguards by:

TABLE 14–2 Controlled Substances: Uses and Effects

Drugs	Schedule*	Often Prescribed Brand Names	Medical Uses	Dependence Physical
Opium	II	Dover's Powder, Paregoric	Analgesic, antidiarrheal	High
Morphine	II	Morphine	Analgesic	High
Codeine	II, III, V	Codeine	Analgesic, antitussive	Moderate
Heroin	I	None	None	High
Meperidine (Pethidine)	II	Demerol, Pethadol	Analgesic	High
Methadone	II	Dolophine, Methadone, Methadose	Analgesic, heroin substitute	High
Other Narcotics	I, II, III, V	Dilaudid, Leritine, Numorphan, Percodan	Analgesic, antidiarrheal, antitussive	High
Chloral Hydrate	IV	Noctec, Somnos	Hypnotic	Moderate
Barbiturates	II, III, IV	Amytal, Butisol, Nembutal, Phenobarbital, Seconal, Tuinal	Anesthetic	High
Glutethimide	III	Doriden	Sedation, sleep	High
Methaqualone	II	Optimil, Parest, Quaalude, Somnafac, Sopor	Sedation, sleep	High
Tranquilizers	IV	Equanil, Librium, Miltown, Serax, Tranxene, Valium	Anti-anxiety, muscle relaxant, sedation	Moderate
Other Depressants	III, IV	Clonopin, Dalmane, Dormate, Noludar, Placydil,Valmid	Anti-anxiety, sedation, sleep	Possible
Cocaine†	II	Cocaine	Local anesthetic	Possible
Amphetamines	II, III	Benzedrine, Biphetamine, Desoxyn, Dexedrine	Hyperkinesis, narcolepsy, weight control	Possible
Phenmetrazine	II	Preludin	Weight control	Possible
Methylphenidate	II	Ritalin	Hyperkinesis	Possible
Other Stimulants	III, IV,	Bacarate, Cylert, Didrex, Ionamin, Plegine, Pondimin, Pre-Sate, Sanorex, Voranil	Weight control	Possible
LSD	I	None	None	None
Mescaline	I	None	None	None
Psilocybin Psilocyn	I	None	None	None
MDA	I	None	None	None
PCP‡	III	Sernylan	Veterinary anesthetic	None
Other Hallucinogens	I	None	None	None
Marijuana Hashish Hashish Oil	I	None	None	Degree unknown

*Scheduling classifications vary for individual drugs since controlled substances are often marketed in combination with other medicinal ingredients.
†Designated a narcotic under the Controlled Substances Act.
‡Designated a depressant under the Controlled Substances Act.

Potential		Duration of Effects (in hrs)	Usual Methods of Administration	Possible Effects	Effects of Overdose	Withdrawal Syndrome
High	Yes	3 to 6	Oral, smoked	Euphoria, drowsiness, respiratory depression, constricted pupils, nausea	Slow and shallow breathing, clammy skin, convulsions, coma, possible death	Watery eyes, runny nose, yawning, loss of appetite, irritability, tremors, panic, chills and sweating, cramps, nausea
High	Yes	3 to 6	Injected, smoked			
Moderate	Yes	3 to 6	Oral, injected			
High	Yes	3 to 6	Injected, sniffed			
High	Yes	3 to 6	Oral, injected			
High	Yes	12 to 24	Oral, injected			
High	Yes	3 to 6	Oral, injected			
Moderate	Probable	5 to 8	Oral	Slurred speech, disorientation, drunken behavior without odor of alcohol	Shallow respiration, cold and clammy skin, dilated pupils, weak and rapid pulse, coma, possible death	Anxiety, insomnia tremors, delirium, convulsions, possible death
High	Yes	1 to 16	Oral, injected			
High	Yes	4 to 8	Oral			
High	Yes	4 to 8	Oral			
Moderate	Yes	4 to 8	Oral			
Possible	Yes	4 to 8	Oral			
High	Yes	2	Injected, sniffed	Increased alertness, excitation, euphoria, dilated pupils, increased pulse rate and blood pressure, insomnia, loss of appetite	Agitation, increase in body temperature, hallucinations, convulsions, possible death	Apathy, long periods of sleep, irritability, depression, disorientation
High	Yes	2 to 4	Oral, injected			
High	Yes	2 to 4	Oral			
Possible	Yes	2 to 4	Oral			
Degree unknown	Yes	Variable	Oral	Illusions and hallucinations (with exception of MDA); poor perception of time and distance	Longer, more intense "trip" episodes, psychosis, possible death	Withdrawal syndrome not reported
Degree unknown	Yes	Variable	Oral, injected			
Degree unknown	Yes	Variable	Oral			
Degree unknown	yes	Variable	Oral, injected, sniffed			
Degree unknown	Yes	Variable	Oral, injected smoked			
Degree unknown	Yes	Variable	Oral, injected, sniffed			
Moderate	Yes	2 to 4	Oral, smoked	Euphoria, relaxed inhibitions, increased appetite, disoriented behavior	Fatigue, paranoia possible psychosis	Insomnia, hyperactivity, and decreased appetite reported in a limited number of individuals

1. establishing an independent federal drug-testing center, ending reliance on the FDA and drug manufacturers for drug analysis;[43]
2. requiring mandatory licensing of new drug patents at a "reasonable royalty," keeping new brand-name product prices down while still protecting company patents;[44]
3. requiring salespeople to pass a federally approved course in pharmacology;[45]
4. providing doctors and medical students with more training in pharmacology by offering government-subsidized courses through a National Center for Clinical Pharmacology.[46]

Though the public has generally shown little interest in food and drug legislation in the past, it is more concerned now and is becoming more involved with consumer protection.

DECRIMINALIZATION

Marijuana

Reasons for and against the decriminalization of marijuana have been presented by various parties for a number of years. In 1970, the Ledain Commission of the Canadian government urged decriminalization. After a thorough study of the nonmedical use of drugs, the commission issued the following conclusions in regard to marijuana:

1. The use of marijuana is increasing in popularity among all age groups of the population, and particularly among the young.
2. This increase indicates that the attempt to suppress, or even to control its use, is failing and will continue to fail—that people are not deterred by the criminal law prohibiting its use.
3. The present legislative policy has not been justified by clear and unequivocal evidence of short term or long term harm caused by cannabis.
4. The individual and social harm (including the incarceration of young people and growing disrespect for law) that caused the present use of criminal law to attempt to suppress cannabis far outweighs any potential for harm which cannabis could conceivably possess, having regard for the long history of its use and the present lack of evidence.
5. The illicit status of cannabis invites exploitation by criminal elements, and of the abuses such as adulteration; it also brings cannabis users into contact with other criminal elements and with other drugs as heroin, which they might not otherwise be induced to consider.[47]

The Oregon Law   One state in the United States seems to have agreed with the Ledain Commission's recommendation. Oregon became the first state to decriminalize marijuana. The Oregon law reduces the possession of one ounce (or "lid"), or enough to make twenty to thirty "joints," to a citation (misdemeanor) and a fine of no more than $100. However, stronger laws against possession of more than one ounce and transportation, sale, or cultivation of marijuana remain in effect.

A survey conducted for the Drug Abuse Council one year after Oregon decriminalized marijuana revealed no significant increase in the number of persons using marijuana in that state. In fact, a second study by the Oregon State Legislature concluded that decriminalization had not caused the major problems for the state which some had predicted. The state's successful legislation has now been used as a pattern for marijuana decriminalization in a number of other states. Currently, Alaska's decriminalization law, which legalized the growing of five marijuana plants for private use, is even more lenient than Oregon's, and in some states marijuana use has been approved for various medical illnesses, specifically glaucoma and cancer.

Recommendations for the Future   Judging from experience, there is little likelihood that continued reliance on legal penalties will solve this nation's marijuana problem. Legislators who look to law-enforcement techniques to eradicate marijuana use are failing to face the fact that despite every imaginable deterrent and social stigma, drug use is, and will continue to be, a part of our culture. Decriminalization may be one way to solve some of the problems marijuana use results in. The Oregon model has shown that at least decriminalization does not tend to increase marijuana use. More realistic attitudes toward marijuana use, as well as sound research on both short- and long-term effects, will also help resolve marijuana-related issues. Certainly, the current trend toward research and responsible drug education is a step in the right direction.

Opiates

Introduction   The issue of opiate decriminalization, specifically the legalization of heroin for known drug dependents, draws a negative reaction from most people. Yet proponents of heroin legalization claim that supplying morphine or heroin to users would in time reduce the size and influence of the black market, and possibly eliminate it.

For a nominal fee, users could buy their daily doses from clinic physicians, bypassing the black market and eventually causing it to collapse because it would be unable to compete with at-cost government pricing. Furthermore, by eliminating the need to prosecute users and other opiate-related police activities, significant amounts of time and monies would be saved. With no users to prosecute, court and jail congestion would quickly be reduced. The level of drug-related crime would also be likely to decline because users would no longer need to procure large amounts of money (through stealing or prostitution) to support their daily habit.

Decriminalization would help the user in another way. Clinically dispensed heroin would be pure and unadulterated, safely diluted in exact quantities in an appropriate vehicle. With proper doses, pure ingredients, and sterile packaging, needle-related diseases such as hepatitis and sepsis would be reduced, as well as the possibility of overdose.

Still, opponents argue that decriminalization of opiate use would be tantamount to government condonement. This, they feel, would encourage experimentation by individuals who otherwise would have remained untempted. Opponents also claim that recruitment of novice users would grow as heroin was illicitly diverted from the clinics to the streets. Psychologist Thomas Szasz feels otherwise:

> The fear that free trade in narcotics would result in vast masses of our population spending their days smoking opium or mainlining heroin, rather than working and taking care of their responsibilities, is a bugaboo that does not deserve to be taken seriously. Habits of work and idleness are deep-seated cultural patterns. . . .free trade in drugs [would not] convert [industrious people] to hippies.[48]

As with marijuana use, the law has failed to be an effective deterrent to opiate use; it is doubtful that it will be a significant deterrent in the future. It seems that people who wish to use opiates will do so regardless of the law. Alternatives to rigid legal penalties may need to be tried.

Opiate Maintenance   The 1970s saw a repeated call for the consideration of opiate-maintenance clinics. Perhaps the most concise and encompassing statement in this direction comes from Isador Chein, professor of psychology at New York University:

> There is obvious expedient for reducing the demand for black market narcotics— and that is to make a better quality of narcotics more cheaply available to addicts on a legal market. There are many advocates, the present [writer] included, of one variant or another of such a plan; and the numbers seem to be increasing. No one, of course, advocates putting narcotics on the open shelves of supermarkets. The basic idea is to make it completely discretionary with the medical profession whether or not to prescribe opiate drugs to addicts for reasons having to do only with the patient's addiction. . . .
> We think it is high time . . . to call a policy of forcing the addict from degradation, and all in the name of concern for his welfare, just what it is—vicious, sanctimonious, and hypocritical. . . . Every addict is entitled to assessment as an individual and to be offered the best available treatment in light of his condition, situation, and his needs. No legislator, no judge, no district attorney, no directors of a narcotics bureau, no police inspector and no narcotics agent is qualified to make such an assessment. If, as a result of such an assessment and continued experience in treating the individual addict, it should be decided that the best available treatment is to continue him on narcotics . . . then he is entitled to this treatment.[49]

A study of the British narcotics system may be useful in considering the idea of opiate-maintenance clinics. In 1924 the English government formed a medical commission, headed by a distinguished physician, Humphrey Rolliston, to formulate a national policy for their drug-dependence problem. In 1926 the Rolliston Commission decided that heroin could be issued to drug dependents under several circumstances: (1) if the client was undergoing gradual detoxification at the time and was subject to review as to any potential cure; (2) if it was found that prolonged attempts to cure were ill-advised because of the severity of the user's withdrawal symptoms following discontinuance of opiate administration; and (3) if the individual displayed the ability to lead a useful and relatively normal life style contingent upon his or her daily dose of opiates.[50]

The program went into effect, and British doctors were allowed to pre-

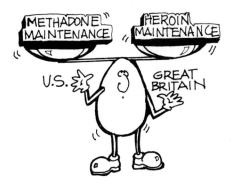

scribe heroin. Under the program, the number of known users in England remained insignificant, usually averaging under 500 a year.[51] This low rate continued until the early 1960s, when it became apparent that a small group of doctors were overprescribing the drugs. A committee was organized to review the problem and eventually a number of steps were taken. Administration of heroin was taken out of the hands of private physicians and delegated to specifically chosen doctors who were to operate in specific centers or clinics. Stricter controls on notification of users and duties of the doctors were also established.

By the spring of 1968, seventeen clinics had been authorized by the British government to dispense heroin. The clinics also offered various rehabilitation programs, and clients were consistently urged to consider detoxification and withdrawal as the final goal of their clinic experience.[52] The result of these clinics, according to one researcher, is that "in Britain, the supply of black market heroin has been almost completely eliminated—when the addict can obtain his supply for, at most, a few dollars a week, it is just not worth anyone's time to risk the penalties involved in smuggling or peddling the drug."[53] Another apparent result is that opiate-related crime is allegedly very low in England.

However, Avram Goldstein, professor of pharmacology at Stanford University and director of the Addiction Research Foundation in Palo Alto, California, feels that England's heroin black market has not substantially diminished:

> There will obviously have to be a ceiling on heroin dosage dispensed at a clinic. Then we can predict with fair confidence, on the basis of studies at the Lexington facility of the National Institute on Drug Abuse and elsewhere, that the addicts will escalate their dosage to that ceiling and will become tolerant to that dosage. . . . When their demands for more heroin are rejected, they are likely to look outside the clinic, and thus to sustain an illicit market after all. This has, indeed, happened in Britain. . . .[54]

Joseph L. Nellis, chief counsel for the House of Representatives' Select Committee on Narcotics Control, agrees:

> In Britain, approximately 300 doctors are licensed to supply heroin to certified addicts. Yet, there is a thriving black market in heroin. One reason is that certification is difficult to obtain. There are as many as five times the number of untreated addicts in England as those receiving heroin legally from doctors. Of the 10,000 heroin addicts in Britain, only 1,800 are "registered" for "treatment." The crime

rate continues to increase and the opportunities for fraud in the dispensing of heroin continue to be substantial. One section of Scotland Yard does nothing but look into abuse by doctors who are licensed to dispense heroin, and the violations are plentiful and continuous.[55]

The Future of Legalized Opiate Maintenance   From the inconclusive and varying opinions on Britain's opiate-maintenance program, it is impossible to know if that system is really working. It is also impossible to predict if such a system would work in this country. John Kaplan, of the Stanford University Law School, offers an opinion:

> I do not think that any system of heroin maintenance has yet been devised which can cope with the twin problems in that area: if the maintenance is convenient enough for the addicts . . . providing them with heroin outside secure clinics, the diversion problems, and hence the increase in use and addiction, will be substantial;. . . any method of securing clinics and checking on addicts to prevent diversion will be so inconvenient that most addicts will, in fact, prefer life on the street. . . .[56]

Kaplan states further that even if the British system is working, running a similar program in this country would be difficult because of the greater numbers of people who would be involved. Also, Great Britain's system of nationalized health care provides more economic support and assistance to opiate maintenance clinics than our own system of health care could provide. Finally, costs related to heroin maintenance in the United States would be substantially greater than in England. This alone could undermine any efforts to establish maintenance clinics.

Even if, despite their apparent drawbacks, maintenance clinics are given the go-ahead in this country, they will not solve the problems surrounding opiate dependency; even proponents of such clinics have never held their approach to be a curative one. Nonetheless, maintenance may be a necessary first step in the effort to reduce the personal consequences and the major social side effects of drug dependence.

SUMMARY

Historically, the United States has attempted to restrain drug consumption through legislation and judicial means. But because morality cannot be legislated and because extreme penalties often act as an incentive rather than a deterrent, drug use has continued and increased. Although a new, more realistic and sensitive approach to drug abuse is in the wind, it will be slow in reaching effectiveness. In the meantime, drug abuse continues.

Changes for the better in consumer laws have also been slow in coming. Only recently were consumers able to learn about and purchase generic drugs rather than brand-name drugs, an occurrence that often results in considerable monetary savings. Physicians, however, are still reluctant to prescribe anything but established brand-name drugs, and pharmacists compound the situation by being slow to effect generic substitutions. Because the drug industry has one of the most powerful lobbies in the country, as well as hard-hitting advertising campaigns, the slow changeover to generic drugs is not difficult to understand. Neither is the slow advance in legislation aimed at broadening and strengthening consumer rights.

While the number of new drugs on the market has grown, the physician's ability to understand and correctly prescribe many of the new drugs has not. Courses in pharmacology are sadly underemphasized in medical school, and busy physicians are rarely able to stay abreast of the numerous new pharmaceutical options that constantly flood their offices.

The FDA, too, has myriad problems with drug-related issues. It must determine which drugs are safe and effective, subjecting every present and potential product to a battery of tests. While this long and encumbered process often protects people from the distribution of harmful or ineffective drugs, it also frequently delays for years the availability of pharmacological agents with proven effectiveness.

MILESTONES IN ATTEMPTED DRUG REGULATION _____

1875   City of San Francisco adopts ordinance prohibiting the smoking of opium in smoking houses.

1882   New York State bans opium smoking.

1885   Federal law limits manufacture of opium for smoking.

1906   Pure Food and Drug Act passes, regulating labeling.

1909   Opium Exclusion Act prohibits importation of opium or its derivatives for nonmedicinal use.

1909   Shanghai International Opium Conference.

1911   Hague Conference.

1912   Townsend Act penalizes opiate use.

1914   Harrison Narcotic Act passes, making possession of narcotics without a prescription a legal offense.

1919   Volstead Act and Eighteenth Amendment (Prohibition).

1924   Importation of heroin banned.

1925   *Linder* v. *United States* establishes drug dependency as an illness.

1929   Porter Narcotic Farms Law passes, establishing federal treatment "farms" for jailed opiate dependents.

1930   Federal Bureau of Narcotics established.

1933   Twenty-first Amendment repeals Prohibition.

1937   Marijuana Tax Act passes, taxing physicians and marijuana distributors for marijuana prescription.

1938   Food, Drug and Cosmetic Act passes, requiring proof of product safety.

1942   Opium Exclusion Act requires domestic growers to register.

1956   Narcotic Drug Control Act.

1962   Kefauver-Harris Amendments to Pure Food and Drug Act passes, requiring proof of product safety and effectiveness.

1963   Community Mental Health Center Act passes, emphasizing rehabilitation of mental patients.

1965   Drug Abuse Control Amendments to the 1938 Food, Drug and Cosmetic Act pass, classifying depressant, stimulant, and hallucinogenic drugs as "dangerous drugs."

1966   National Addiction Rehabilitation Administration.

1968   Bureau of Narcotics and Dangerous Drugs established, replacing the Federal Bureau of Narcotics.

1968   1965 law further amended.

1970   Comprehensive Drug Abuse Prevention and Control Act passes, liberalizing penalties for drug-abuse offenders.

1972   Presidential Council on Marijuana and Drug Abuse recommends decriminalization.

1972   Drug Abuse Office and Treatment Act.

1973   Oregon becomes first state to decriminalize marijuana.

1974   Narcotic Addict Treatment Act.

1974   Alcohol and Drug Abuse Education Act.

1976   Amendments to National Security Act of 1947 prohibit CIA experimentation with drugs on unknowing or unwilling human subjects. PL 94-237 establishes the Office of Drug Abuse Policy within the executive office of the president.

1979   S-1075 revises FDA procedures and authority concerning new-drug introduction, testing, marketing, packaging, and recall and litigation powers.

NOTES

[1]"Drugged," *New Republic* 169, no. 22 (December 1, 1973):9. Reprinted by permission of *The New Republic,* © 1973 The New Republic, Inc.

[2]Ibid.

[3]Peter J. Ognibene, "RX: Inexpensive Pills with Costly Labels," *New Republic* 168, no. 22 (June 2, 1973):12. Reprinted by permission of *The New Republic,* © 1973 The New Republic, Inc.

[4]Ibid.

[5]James Goddard, "The Medical Business," *Scientific American* 229, no. 3 (September 1973):92A.

[6]"Clampdown on Drug Industry: Its Meaning," *U.S. News and World Report* 76, no. 25 (June 24, 1974):36.

[7]Ibid.

[8]"Drugged," p. 9.

[9]Gordon R. Trapnell, "What's the Estimated Cost of National Outpatient RX Program?" *Pharmacy Times* 46, no. 1 (January 1980):65.

[10]"Drugged," p. 9.

[11]"Clampdown on Drug Industry," p. 37.

[12]"Drugged," p. 10.

[13]Quoted in Ognibene, "RX," p. 12.

[14]Morton Mintz, *By Prescription Only* (Boston: Benson Press, 1967), p. 339.

[15]Ognibene, "RX", p. 12.

[16]Oakley S. Ray, *Drugs, Society and Human Behavior,* 2nd ed. (St. Louis: C.V. Mosby, 1978), pp. 431–32.

[17]Joel Forte, *The Pleasure Seekers: The Drug Crisis, Youth and Society* (New York: Grove Press 1970), p. 67. Reprinted with permission.

[18]Kenneth L. Jones, Louis W. Shainberg, and Curtis O. Beyer, *Drugs and Alcohol*, 2nd ed. (New York: Harper & Row 1973), p. 109.

[19]Edward M. Brecher et al., *Licit and Illicit Drugs* (Boston: Little, Brown, 1972), p. 292. Used with permission of the publisher.

[20]Ibid., p. 369.

[21]David F. Musto, *The American Disease: Origins of Narcotic Control* (New Haven: Yale University Press, 1973), p. 3.

[22]Jones, Shainberg, and Beyer, *Drugs and Alcohol*, p. 5.

[23]Ray, *Drugs, Society and Human Behavior*, p. 34.

[24]Ibid., p. 20.

[25]Brecher et al. *Licit and Illicit Drugs*, p. 49.

[26]Musto, *The American Disease*, p. 68.

[27]Brecher et al., *Licit and Illicit Drugs*, p. 265.

[28]Musto, *The American Disease*, p. 254.

[29]Brecher et al., *Licit and Illicit Drugs*, p. 51

[30]Ibid., p. 52.

[31]Musto, *The American Disease*, p. 184.

[32]Quoted in Brecher et al., *Licit and Illicit Drugs*, p. 417.

[33]Jones, Shainberg, and Beyer, *Drugs and Alcohol*, p. 62.

[34]Adapted from Mintz, *By Prescription Only*, pp. 93, 143.

[35]Musto, *The American Disease*, p. 235.

[36]Ibid.

[37]Forte, *The Pleasure Seekers*, pp. 75–76.

[38]Jones, Shainberg, and Beyer, *Drugs and Alcohol*, p. 103.

[39] Ray, *Drugs, Society and Human Behavior*, p. 42.

[40]*The Controlled Substances Act* (Washington, D.C.: Drug Enforcement Administration, 1980).

[41]Brecher et al., *Licit and Illicit Drugs*, p. 90.

[42]Quoted in Ognibene, "RX," p. 13.

[43]Ognibene, "RX," p. 13.

[44]"Clampdown on Drug Industry," p. 38.

[45]Ibid.

[46]"FDA's Policies and Practices for Clearing Drugs Are Criticized before Units," *Wall Street Journal* 184, no. 40 (August 26, 1974):10.

[47]Cited in Brecher, *Licit and Illicit Drugs, p. 466*.

[48]Thomas S. Szasz, "The Ethics of Addiction." in *Annual Editions Readings in Social Problems*, '73/'74 (Guilford, Conn.: Dushkin Publishing Group, 1973), p. 136.

[49]Quoted in Brecher, *Licit and Illicit Drugs*, p. 119.

[50]National Clearinghouse for Drug Abuse Information, *The British Narcotics System* (Washington, D.C., 1973), p. 2.

[51]Ibid.

[52]Ibid., p. 5.

[53]Phillip Whitter and Ian Robertson, in "A Way to Control Heroin Addiction," *Annual Editions Readings in Social Problems*, '73/'74 (Guilford, Conn.: Dushkin Publishing Group, 1973), p. 142.

[54]Avram Goldstein, "Heroin Maintenance: A Medical View," *Journal of Drug Issues* 9, no. 3 (Summer 1979):343.

[55]Joseph L. Nellis, "Controlling Heroin Addict Crime: Comments," *Journal of Drug Issues* 9, no. 3 (Summer 1979):318.

[56]John Kaplan, "Controlling Heroin Addict Crime: Comments," *Journal of Drug Issues* 9, no. 3 (Summer 1979):331.

ALTERNATIVES TO PSYCHOACTIVE DRUG ABUSE

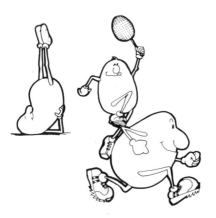

A NEW PHILOSOPHICAL PERSPECTIVE

Physician Andrew Weil reports on the system of drug education:

> I cannot help feeling that what we are now doing in the name of stopping the drug problem is the drug problem . . . . Society, either with or without drug education, will eventually learn about the effects of a given drug, but education may facilitate this learning process and increase knowledge of the risk/benefit ratio that accompanies the use of any drug. Such knowledge will ultimately be disseminated into the community, and as a society learns of a drug's risks and benefits, a level of drug use (and abuse) that will depend upon this knowledge will become established.[1]

The need to appropriately address drug use and abuse in this country is imperative. Between 9 and 12 million of our citizens suffer from alcohol dependency, at least 500,000 to 750,000 from opiate dependency, and several millions from barbiturate and tranquilizer use. But while these millions of citizens suffer, current laws and approaches to drug-abuse control seem too inadequate to help. Instead of more and more ineffective legislation, a new perspective on drug abuse seems necessary.

Drug Education in the Schools

One step toward a more realistic approach to the drug-abuse problem would be more realistic and up-to-date drug education. According to preliminary studies conducted jointly by the Center for Disease Control and the Office of Disease Prevention and Health Promotion, it appears that school health education is clearly effective in improving the health of our nation's youth. Those school districts willing to implement a comprehensive K–12 health program can take a major step toward reducing the drug problem. Further evidence of success is in the area of smoking-education programs, which are finally gaining some positive results in smoking cessation.

Other drug-education programs offer some hope in curtailing drug abuse. First Lady Nancy Reagan, has been instrumental in the National Federation of Parents for Drug Free Youth, which involves parents as key prevention groups. Numerous other groups throughout the country have been instrumental in reaching various groups and offering them support. It is imperative that these groups work in concert and not waste energy duplicating their efforts.

Updating information and looking at drug use in a new light could do much to reach young drug users or potential users. This process would entail in-depth study of the most current information and presentation of the facts in a value-free, nonjudgmental manner. With personal values and fervent emotions put aside, students could receive information and use it to make their own decisions. Though such an approach might not eliminate drug use, it would certainly help drug consumers become more informed and more aware of safety precautions. Responsible drug education might reasonably teach responsible drug use, especially if it emphasized nondestructive and responsible behavior.

Accepting Potential Drug Benefits

Along with more realistic drug education, a new attitude toward drug use seems needed. Though drug-free lifestyles may be morally and medically more desirable than lifestyles that include drug use, it seems probable that some people will always look to drugs to experience periodic states of altered consciousness—to look for a condition that is more preferable to actual life situations. Tolerance of this fact, and perhaps even belief that drug use under proper administration can be beneficial in understanding expressions of the unconscious mind, may help to ease the current drug-abuse problem and effect positive attitude changes among drug users. Andrew Weil suggests that if we are to begin to change things, we must start to look for the positive potential under (seemingly) negative experiences. As long as we continue to ridicule the possibility that drugs can help us, we have no chance of making them less harmful to us.[2]

To begin this shift toward a more positive way of looking at drug use, one might take two positive actions: (1) encourage people who use drugs to do so intelligently and for their own benefit, without harming society, and (2) encourage people to progress to better methods of altering consciousness, without drugs. The use of fear and repression have contributed to the current state of affairs; they have also been relatively ineffective in curbing drug abuse. Tolerance is the key trait. Much of our behavior is a composition of recurring themes and traits that are universal and therefore a fundamental link of humanity. The need to experience altered states may be one of these themes whose expression has many forms. People choose what they perceive to be best for them at any given time. The country-club, scotch-drinking businessperson is not totally unlike the university student who smokes marijuana.

People experience many of the same needs, desires, and pleasures, even though they may not be congruous for all people at one time. The key is viewing each other in the same light, subject to the same emotional and environmental pressures. If we can look at each other knowing that "I've been there before," perhaps tolerance will be more than a fleeting attitude.

This positive shift can "only be done by offering more desirable alternative involvement—activities, lifestyles and satisfactions which are more rewarding than drug experiences and incompatible with dependence on chemicals."[3]

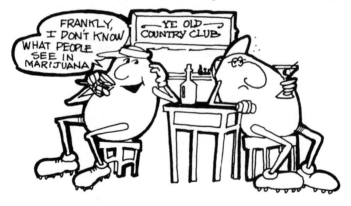

ALTERNATIVES

When looking for appropriate alternatives to drug use, we must look for activities that fill the same needs as drugs do. As this book has shown, people take drugs for a variety of reasons:

1. to feel better
2. to obtain pleasure and reward
3. to relieve discomfort
4. to pursue an altered state of consciousness
5. to test one's maturity
6. to feel part of a group

Alternatives to drug use must therefore afford these same experiences. Though virtually any activity may be considered an alternative, some realistic alternatives are exercise, wilderness experiences, work, social-political activism, religion, biofeedback, and meditation.

One of the goals of selecting alternatives is to substitute for a negative dependency a (series of) positive dependencies. Positive "addictions" usually meet the following six criteria:

1. It is something noncompetitive, you choose to do it, and you can devote approximately one hour a day to it.
2. It is possible to *do it easily:* you do not need a great deal of mental effort to do it well.
3. You can *do it alone,* or rarely with others, but you do not have to depend on others in order to do it.
4. You believe that it *has some value* (physical, mental, or spiritual) for you.
5. You believe that if you persist at it *you will improve,* but this is completely subjective.
6. You can do it *without criticizing yourself.* If you can't accept yourself during this time, the activity will not be addicting.[4]

Exercise

Preliminary research findings indicate that exercise seems likely to improve health. Depending on the intensity, exercise may aid in the decomposition of excess arterial cholesterol deposits that inhibit blood flow, increase cardiac effeciency by increasing blood output per beat, reduce blood pressure, aid in digestion by stimulating gastrointestinal secretion, improve respiration efficiency, stimulate production of biogenic amines (neurotransmitters that facilitate brain message sending), and stimulate production of testosterone and estrogen. Furthermore, exercise can improve muscle tone and muscle development, convert fat into caloric energy, and may aid in gradual weight reduction.

Despite all these potential physical benefits, the most important benefit exercise can result in may be psychological. Exercise can be an efficient way to reduce stress, develop or enhance a positive self-image, and increase personal awareness. Through intense physical movement, many people are better able to deal with daily pressure and obtain a sense of personal pride and accomplishment. Exercise's ability to produce this strong sense of self, coupled with its ability to improve strength and health, may make it a valued alternative to drug abuse.

Many people, in their efforts to survive the technocracy of our time, have forgotten, lost, or repressed the ability or desire to perceive subtle body cues, sensitive messages that tell us what's going on internally. Many people are physically out of touch. The so-called primitive people are in tune with their physiology because they have to be: it is their tool for survival. In the twentieth century, "civilized" people have placed greater emphasis on cognitive functioning, on the use of their minds, to the exclusion of body awareness. The body and its functions are an intergral contributor to the understanding of the complete person.

Exercise can help a person understand his or her movement characteristics, capabilities, and limitations. Increased self-awareness enhances self-appreciation and sensitivity and therefore increases the possibility of understanding one's environment and fellow human beings. Accomplishment, insight and awareness, a degree of meaning, and identification of the stimulation of emotion by motion— these are some of the issues addressed by physical movement.

Jogging Though exercise can include mountain climbing, calisthenics, walking, bicycling, canoeing, swimming, yoga, T'ai Chi, skiing, dancing, and many other forms of physical movement, jogging has become one of the more popular and more successful ways to feel good and stay in shape. After initial skepticism and hesitation, millions of Americans are finding jogging to be a real source of benefit and pleasure. Joggers are also discovering that running provides "therapeutic effects for the scars caused by the stresses of modern society— including depression, nervousness, inability to sleep, inability to cope with their environment, even in some cases, schizophrenia." Jogging results in "very measurable changes in depression levels . . . stimulates the unconscious . . . , [reduces] muscular electrical activity . . . [and] nerve electrical activity . . . ,[5] affects mental functioning in a positive way.

Jogging may work its effects by helping people to burn off the tension and frustration they encounter each day. Or, it may help to reduce tension and other adverse reactions by simply providing the opportunity to physically escape the causes of those reactions.

The term *timing out,* employed by behavioral psychologists, refers to the removal of an individual from his or her immediate environment to a neutral site of seclusion. It refers to taking a break from one's present involvement. Its application to jogging is quite simple. Jogging provides a break in the pattern of mounting daily tension that people often feel on stressful days. Says one writer on the subject:

> Any measurable psychological benefits from running may come not from the act itself, but from the opportunity that act gives the runner to get away from the stresses and pressures of modern civilization. You cannot answer a jangling telephone or pay bills while circling the running track, and long runs in the woods or on back country roads may permit otherwise harassed business executives or housewives to let their minds "spin free," engage in the form of conscious daydreaming and relaxation.[6]

As early as the 1940s, Veterans' Administration hospitals used running to help their clients relax. But later, as Carlyle H. Folkins, of the University of California at Davis, notes, "we went backwards . . . along came tranquilizers and other forms of drugs. All the psychiatrists got out their chemistry sets and forgot about the potential benefits of exercise. It was like the old Dupont slogan: 'Better things from chemistry.' "[7] Today, however, running may be an effective alternative to chemistry.

Robert Brown of the University of Virginia is exploring natural body chemistry as it relates to exercise. Working in conjuction with Fred Goodwin at the

National Institute of Mental Health, he is measuring neurotransmitter metabolite levels in response to physical exercise. Blood and urine specimens are taken from subjects before exercise and at one-, two-, and three-hour intervals following exercise to determine chemical fluctuations in the body. Brown reports that people suffering from depression obtain an antidepressant factor about two hours after exercise.

Wilderness Experiences

A wilderness environment offers a new perspective through which one may view his or her life. In such places, with positive counseling, drug users may be able to see their habits in new, more objective ways.[8] Eventually they may be able to reduce their drug consumption and perhaps eliminate it.

Though wilderness experiences may be obtained on one's own, various organizations offer opportunities to join in "risk sports" or "risk recreation." Bridge Over Troubled Waters, Inc., a drug-addiction treatment center headquartered in Berkeley, California, offers such out-of-the-ordinary experiences as river running, parachuting, skin diving, rock climbing, and skiing, and believes that participating in such adventures can address the need for risk taking that many heroin users have. The goal of the program is to show users alternative lifestyles and different ways of getting high, and to use success in an outdoor challenge as a step toward building confidence. Says one participant in the program:

> I thought it was going to be a complete bore. But then I got on that raft, and all the way down the river I felt light; I was singing, hollering. [River running] provided me with natural highs and challenges to supplant those I had been getting from involvement with heroin . . . when we finished that run I was eager to get off on more adventures. I had enjoyed the challenge of the river more than that of running the streets looking for a fix. . . . [9]

Confidence gained from a successful experience can spread to other areas of an individual's life. Believers in the wilderness-experience approach feel that outdoor living will help drug users develop fortitude and the drive to leave the street life. Proponents also believe that increased self-confidence will encourage increased self-esteem. A more positive self-concept, they feel, may reduce the drug dependent's desire to escape "reality."

To bring on all these positive changes, however, wilderness experiences, like all other drug alternatives, must make the participant feel good. As one Bridge Over Troubled Waters consultant says,

> dope makes you feel good, and unless you give drug addicts an alternative [that does the same], it's all a lot of talk. For them there's no feeling good without dope. It is a meaningless abstraction until we make the abstraction real. We are saying to them, "Hey, come do this with us. Get away from the whoring and the pimping and the buying of dope, come with us and feel good, come and get high on the 'natch.' "[10]

Work

Many people define themselves in terms of the function they perform in society—their work. People who like what they do usually feel content and consequently treat themselves with respect. People who are out of work or have a low-paying or dissatisfying job that leaves them with no sense of worth or personal accomplishment usually are not content, and may be driven to drink, take pills, or smoke to escape their unhappy state.

Meaningful work—work that is of genuine value to others and contributes to the production of quality goods or services—can do much to elevate feelings of self-worth and happiness. Such work can be fulfilling, occupy time, fill gaps, and be enjoyable and satisfying. Work can also cause fatigue, but this may actually provide an opportunity for relaxation. Finally, employment can result in paychecks, providing symbolic reinforcement of worth to society as well as purchasing power.

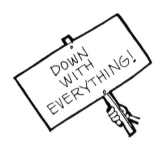

Social-Political Activism

Just as work in the form of gainful employment may serve as an alternative to drug dependency, so may work in the form of political or social involvement. People can gain satisfaction by identifying with a new value system or new political ideology, especially those organizations or theories that inspire and provide hope. Working for ideological change can help drug abusers fill empty time as well as address their need for self-worth.

A case in point is the People's Republic of China. For hundreds of years, this country had great problems with opium addiction. By 1920, 25 percent of the population were believed to be using the drug. But then something happened. By 1930, the total opium-dependent population had shrunk to 10 million, and as of the late 1960s the user population was virtually nonexistent.

What caused these opium users to turn away from their drug of choice? It was ideological change. The Communist takeover in 1949 was a chance for both the nation and its youth to redefine their worth and role:

> An American who lived in a Chinese village during and after liberation explained it in terms of a meaning of a new word, "Fenshen, . . . to turn the body or to turn over." To China's hundreds of millions of landless and land-poor peasants it meant to stand up to throw off the landlord yoke, to gain land, stock, implements, and houses. But, it meant much more than this. It meant to throw off superstition and

study science, to abolish "word blindness" and learn to read, to cease considering women as chattels and establish equality between the sexes, to do away with appointed village magistrates and replace them with elected councils. It meant to enter a new world.[11]

It also meant to help the millions of opium dependents move back into the mainstream of Chinese society. This process was effected nationwide through small street communities that offered political and cultural leadership as well as medical care. These small groups campaigned against opium use and were also responsible for detecting and censuring those who continued to use opium. Successes and failures were reported to higher authorities, and difficult cases were referred to rehabilitation centers. A disciplined Communist party of six million members supported the national campaign.[12]

> Meetings about addiction . . . were part of the national action program in which all people spent an hour a day discussing political and health topics of national importance. The testimony of former addicts was important to all levels of this reformation including newspaper stories, small community groups and rehabilitation centers. Mass meetings, slogans and flags used the words of the ex-addicts. Addiction was denounced as anti-social and unhealthy because it was an imperialist and capitalist activity.[13]

In this way, current and potential drug users were separated from drug involvement by involvement with the building of a new social order—one that decried the use of opiates. Although this example shows an extreme and undesired way to achieve alternative involvement, it does show that involvement can bring about change. Campaigning to elect officials can give people the enjoyable sense of being on the inside, of being useful and successful. Pushing for social reform can instill a sense of self-worth and pride, as well as result in a better world. Political and social activism may not work for everyone, but for many people it can provide the highs and rewards of drug use.

Religion

Religion can offer the same sense of involvement and exposure to new values that political and social activism can. Adopting ideas and beliefs that others also espouse can develop a sense of belonging and a better understanding of self. The "Jesus freak" movement that began in the mid 1960s is a good example of how involvement in religion can cause change. During the late 1960s and early 1970s, hundreds of thousands of young people, many of them drug dependents, became overwhelmed by their nonestablishment lifestyle and by prolonged drug use. They turned to religion, and in this straightforward and structured world found a new alternative. They found help in the form of strict adherence to religious philosophy, which was reinforced by group demands on baehavior. Specific rules and regulations gave participants a very clear and defined picture of their place in the world.

But though religion can be beneficial, extreme adherence to doctrine may discourage objective questioning and the consideration of new or different ideas. Religion, therefore, may be a successful alternative to drug abuse only if it is a temporary replacement. It may offer respite from a negative lifestyle and then spark the desire for a more positive one.

Biofeedback

Within the last ten years, biofeedback, the "immediate ongoing presentation of information to a person concerning his own physiologic processes,"[14] has emerged as a viable means of treating drug abuse, particularly alcoholism. This alternative to drug abuse, also known as alpha training, is simple to use and capable of producing numerous benefits, including personal control of physiological functions, golbular personality changes, (increased ability to relax under stress, diminished overreaction to problems, reduced frustration responses) feelings of well-being, new views toward one's individuality, and transcendental insights. Biofeedback encompasses a number of varied body-control techniques, the most publicized of which is the increased production of specific brain wavelengths known as alpha waves, which assist in reducing tension.

In 1924, while working with people with congenital brain openings, German psychiatrist Hans Berger first noted and recorded the electrical activity of the brain. Berger noticed that tiny cerebral voltages were being rhythmically emitted from the brain and that these waves were most visible when patients were in an alert but relaxed state. Berger continued to study the alpha waves, but little attention was paid to his discovery for many years.

In 1910 Swiss psychiatrist Johannes Schultz developed the forerunner to biofeedback—*autogenic* training, which centered on the control of blood flow. Somewhat likened to yoga and self-hypnosis, autogenic training affects even subtle processes such as blood sugar and white-blood-cell counts, and it has eventually become a major factor in European medicine and psychotherapy. It has been shown to be clinically effective in many patients suffering from migraine headache circulation in peripheral parts of the body.[15]

Encouraged by efforts in Europe, researchers started to experiment in the United States during the late 1960s. During this time conclusive evidence documenting the ability of individuals to control autonomic processes unfolded. (Previously, the autonomic nervous system, controlling visceral or internal body organs and processes, was thought to be involuntary, or out of the realm of "voluntary," conscious control.) Research, beginning with lower-phylogenic

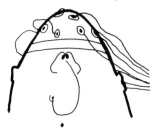

species, has shown that animals can learn conscious control over many involuntary metabolic functions.

By the mid 1960s, interest in alpha waves and their effects had grown. Joe Kamiya, at the University of Chicago, began training students to differentiate between alpha and nonalpha brain waves, and to maintain or turn off alpha-state production. He found that using a feedback device (in this case an audio tone) greatly aided skill acquisition and improved subsequent performance levels, and that the process, which is difficult to describe because of its sensory nature, helped students to detect the status of their visceral processes.[16]

Once students have learned body control through biofeedback, many report that the minor stresses in their daily lives seem to affect them less strongly. Though no explanation for this has been universally accepted to date, a number of theories have been postulated. Researcher Elmer Green has advanced his Psychophysiological Principle: "Every change in the physiological state is accompanied by an appropriate change in the mental-emotional state, conscious or unconscious . . . and conversely, every change in the mental-emotional state, conscious or unconscious, is accompanied by an appropriate change in the physiological state."[17] In other words, high levels of muscular activity cause high levels of mental anxiety and nervousness; reduced levels of muscular activity result in more relaxed mental states. Through biofeedback, a person may take note of his or her physiological state and then maintain or change that state with appropriate mental signals.

Many drug dependents will be able to use biofeedback in that way. The technique can teach these people to control the many processes that precipitate tension and stress and help them to see that they are not helpless victims of uncontrollable impulses and compulsions.

> By the time an alcoholic learns to . . . reduce his muscle tension levels to near zero, and increase his percentage of alpha rhythm, he will know, not just hope, or believe, that some processes are under his control. When that happens, he has essentially initiated a restabilization of maladjusted homeostatic processes . . . associated with total relaxation and . . . self-awareness. . . . [18]

He may then continue to choose biofeedback, instead of drugs, as a way to cope with tension and stress.

We are reminded that it is not life that "kills," but rather our reaction to the stress of everyday existence. We are the victims of our reactions to its frantic pace.[19] People choose and use various coping skills according to their behavioral repertoire, experience, and knowledge. The majority of people choose to use drugs to cope with the trepidations of everyday living. If the stress and strain become too great (or are perceived as such), drug use may become abuse. Biofeedback offers an alternative coping skill.

Meditation

Meditation is a psychological technique through which practitioners attempt to reach deep physiological relaxation. Developed several thousands of years ago by Indian philosophers and religious leaders, meditation works to exclude all thoughts from the mind through the repetition of sounds or words or through exercise or rhythmic breathing. Though there are a number of meditative techniques, transcendental meditation (TM) remains the most popular form in the United States.

TM was developed by Maharishi Mahesh Yogi, an Eastern philosopher who studied under Swami Brahamanda Saraswati. When using TM, followers repeat a specific phrase known only to themselves. The "objective of [this] mantra is to narrow the content of awareness to a fine point so that it may eventually break through to a higher, more intense plane [a more spiritual or higher state of consciousness]—as a narrow passageway might lead up toward an immense, lighted chamber."[20] The repetition of the words generates a rhythmic brain-wave pattern, which in turn generates a kind of sleep, or a turning down or quieting of the sympathetic nervous branch of the autonomic nervous system. During the relaxed state, the meditator remains conscious and aware of his or her surroundings. Analogous to a car resting in idle, the body is functioning but expending very little energy in its effort to recharge. Meditation is an energy-restoring "time out"—the continuous repetition of a brain-wave pattern. The brain tends to respond to rhythmic stimulation, especially if it is its own source. At this moment the brain begins producing alpha waves, bearing out sensory-deprivation researcher Donald Hebb's theory that an individual must experience *varying* stimuli in order to perceive normal awareness. At the moment the incoming stimuli become uniform, the mind begins to synchronize, anesthetize, and produce alpha waves, reducing autonomic nervous system functioning.

How does this relate to the average person on the street? We might define "stress" as excitement resulting in elevated body processes. Virtually all of us are subject to stress. Publication deadlines, luncheon dates, paper-processing time schedules, bills, unrequited love, economic insecurity, existential dilemma, stalled cars in an intersection, the boss who refused a raise and then increases the work load, the wife and/or husband who's "not in the mood"—these types of experiences generate stress. The cumulative effect of continuous subjection to stress is a state that psychologists identify as the "flight or fight" phenomenon, a series of biological processes that gear up an organism in preparation to meet a threat or crisis.

The sympathetic nervous system controls this diffuse arousal reaction by constricting the arteries in the digestive tract, dilating the skeletal-muscle arteries, and diverting increased amounts of blood to locomotor muscles. Heart-rate, blood pressure, respiration, and perspiration levels elevate. Norepinephrine is released at nerve synapses to further compound these reponses. With the influx of adrenalin an individual reacts in an accelerated fashion.

This system response is a defense reaction, mobilizing the body to accelerated states of readiness. It can become the basis of pathology when we fail to demobilize following a crisis. Some would further suggest that this 500,000 year-old machine, the human being, is in fact outmoded.

The issue is how people react to a perceived stress situation. Studies show that meditators have greater initial arousal levels and correspondingly faster recovery periods. Daniel Coleman writes:

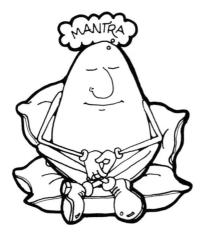

People who are chronically anxious or who have a psychosomatic disorder share a specific pattern of reaction to stress; their bodies mobilize to meet the challenge, then *fail to stop reacting* when the problem is over. The initial tensing up is essential for it allows them to marshal their energy and awareness to deal with a potential threat. But bodies stay aroused for danger when they should be relaxed, recouping spent energies and gathering resources for the next brush with stress.[21]

Anxious individuals overreact, perceiving normal events as crises. Each minor occurrence increases already existing levels of tension, in turn magnifying perception of stress concerning the forthcoming events. Because the anxious person's body stays mobilized after an event has passed, it has a lower threshold to the next. If the body is allowed to relax following a stress reaction, it is more likely to take the next *normal occurrence* in stride without becoming activated or alarmed. Those who have not learned to relax are exhausted at the end of the day. Relaxation comes in the form of four double scotches, two Valium, or a joint. Meditation can break the tension escalation of this threat–arousal–threat spiral by allowing relaxation to normalcy following a crisis. The "meditator relaxes after a challenge passes more often than the non-meditator. This makes him unlikely to see innocent occurrences as harmful. He perceives threat more accurately and reacts with arousal only when necessary. Once aroused, his rapid recovery makes him less likely than the anxious person to see the next deadline as a threat."[22]

Such a relaxed state of consciousness has been believed for centuries to cause neurophysiological and biochemical changes in its practitioners, mainly because meditators often become more physically and mentally healthy. Because of the diversity of meditative techniques, however, conclusive data on this theory has been virtually impossible to obtain until the last several years. Fortunately, TM's recent popularity has allowed in-depth research on this form of meditation, and literature resulting from this study is replete with conclusive data attesting to meditation's positive effects. The following list highlights some of the effects that occur during TM:

1. Oxygen consumption, respiration rate, and metabolic rate markedly decrease, indicating a deep state of rest.
2. Skin resistance increases significantly, indicating deep relaxation and a reduction of anxiety and emotional disturbances.
3. Cardiac output markedly decreases, reducing the heart's work load.
4. Concentration of blood lactate markedly decreases, indicating reduced blood pressure and lower anxiety level.
5. Brain waves alter, indicating a state of restful alertness.
6. Reaction time is speeded up, perceptual and auditory abilities are improved, and mind–body coordination is improved.
7. Spontaneous galvanic skin responses decrease, indicating more resistance to emotional stress, more efficiency in nervous system activities, and a greater ability to recover from stress. In addition, meditators perform better on recall tests and learn more quickly than nonmeditators, exhibit improved psychological traits, including reduced nervousness, reduced aggression, reduced depression, reduced self-criticism, and increased emotional stability, and become more accepting of themselves and others.[23]

Can drug abusers use TM or other forms of meditation to achieve these positive effects? The answer appears to be yes. TM apparently can help users to feel more in control of their lives,[24] and therefore less likely to use drugs for stress relief. Experiments conducted in the late 1960s indicated initial correlations between TM and lowered rates of drug use. Later, small, uncontrolled studies also gave evidence of significant drops in drug use following a period of TM practice.[25] Then, in 1972, a large study by Herbert Benson of the Harvard Medical School and Robert Wallace of UCLA's Department of Physiology was carried out. Benson and Wallace recruited 1950 subjects with documented drug-abuse backgrounds, trained them to meditate, and then had the group practice for three months or more prior to questioning. The results of the study indicated that

> in every drug category there was, with time, a significant increase in the number of non-users and decrease in the light, medium, and heavy users. The data on hard liquor use is especially pertinent to us. The study shows a 35 percent increase in non-users, a 25 percent decrease in light users, and a 13 percent decrease in moderate users. Twenty percent of the respondents sold drugs prior to TM and 71 percent of the sellers stopped selling after 0–3 months.[26]

Though some researchers feel that the procedures used in this study invalidate its conclusions, other studies have also presented data indicating that TM has a positive antidrug effect. In one study concerning TM and marijuana, researchers

> found that almost one-half of those who had practiced meditation for a period of 1–3 months decreased or stopped their use of marijuana. The longer a person had practiced meditation, the higher was the probability that he would discontinue his use. . . . Ninety-two percent of the meditators who had practiced TM for more

than two years had significantly decreased their use . . . and 72 percent had totally stopped.[27]

In yet another drug-use study concerning alcohol,

all of the meditation groups reported statistically significant decreases ranging from 25–33 percent in their use of wine and beer in the first three months of meditation compared to the 1–3 month pre-questionnaire period for control subjects . . . 6–20 percent of the subjects reported discontinuation during the first 3 months . . . 11–40 percent in the second 3 months . . . 60 percent had totally discontinued their use of beer and wine after 2 years. . . .[28]

Drug abusers, then, may use TM as an effective alternative to drugs. Through meditation, users can find stress relief as well as a means of achieving an altered state of consciousness—a nonchemical high. They can learn self-mastery and increase self-confidence.

SUMMARY

Uninformed as well as unrealistic attitudes toward drug consumption seem only to increase the drug problem. Rather than assuming that all reasons for drug use are unacceptable, or that legislation will end drug use, those involved with the problem might better use more up-to-date, unbiased drug education and a more understanding attitude to work on the problems. With a reasonable and calm approach, more responsible drug use can be taught and alternatives to drug use encouraged.

A variety of alternatives fill the same needs that drugs do. Exercise and wilderness experiences reduce stress, alter moods, and improve health. Work and social or political involvement help to build a sense of self-worth and social value. Religious involvement offers the opportunity to find a new and better set of values and beliefs. Meditation and biofeedback offer specific stress-reduction techniques as well as aid in the growth of self-confidence and self-mastery.

NOTES

[1]From *The Natural Mind* by Andrew Weil. Copyright © 1972 by Andrew Weil. Reprinted by permission of the publisher, Houghton-Mifflin Company.

[2]Ibid., pp. 195–96.

[3]Vista Hill Psychiatric Foundation, *Drug Abuse and Alcoholism Newsletter* 3, no. 3 (May 1974):1.

[4]William Glasser, *Positive Addiction* (New York: Harper & Row, Pub. 1976).

[5]Hal Higdon, "Running and the Mind: Can Running Cure Mental Illness?" *Runners World* 13, no. 1 (January 1978):36, 39.

[6]Ibid., p. 38.

[7]Quoted in ibid., p. 39.

[8]Marlene R. Ventura and Mike Durdon, "A Challenging Experience in Canoeing and Camp-

ing as a Tool in Approaching the Drug Problem," *Journal of Drug Education* 4, no. 1 (Spring 1974):124.

[9]John J. Fried, "High with a Little Help from a Friend," *Sports Illustrated* 40, no. 15 (April 15, 1974):88.

[10]Ibid, p. 91. Quote from a member of the group "Bridge Over Troubled Waters."

[11]Paul Lowinger, "How the People's Republic of China Solved the Drug Abuse Problem," *American Journal of Chinese Medicine* 1, no. 2 (1973):278.

[12]Ibid.

[13]Ibid., pp. 278–79.

[14]Elmer Green, Alyce Green, and Dale E. Walters, "Biofeedback Training for Anxiety Tension Reduction," *Annals of the New York Academy of Sciences* 233 (1974):157.

[15]Ibid., p. 157.

[16]Marilyn Ferguson, *The Brain Revolution: The Frontiers of Mind Research* (New York: Taplinger, 1973), p. 35.

[17]Quoted in Ibid., p. 38.

[18]Green, Green, and Walters, "Biofeedback Training,"pp. 158–59.

[19]Daniel Coleman, "Meditation Helps Break the Stress Spiral," *Psychology Today* 9, no. 9 (February 1976):82. Reprinted from *Psychology Today Magazine* Copyright © 1976 American Psychological Association (APA).

[20]Ibid., p. 10. Reprinted from *Psychology Today Magazine*. Copyright © 1976 American Psychological Association (APA).

[21]Ibid., p. 86. Reprinted from *Psychology Today Magazine*. Copyright © 1976 (American Psychological Association (APA).

[22]Maggie Scarf, "Turning Down with TM," *The New York Times Magazine,* February 9, 1979.

[23]*Scientific Research on Transcendental Meditation* (Los Angeles Maharishi International University Press, 1972), pp. 1–14.

[24]Coleman, "Meditation Helps Break the Stress Spiral," p. 84.

[25]Chester A. Swingyard, Chaube Shakauntala, and David B. Sutton, "Neurological and Behavioral Aspects of Transcendental Meditation Relevant to Alcoholism: A Review," *Annals of the New York Academy of Science* 233 (1974):167.

[26]Cited in ibid., p. 168.

[27]Mohammed Shafi, Richard Lavely, and Robert Jaffe, "Meditation and Marijuana," *American Journal of Psychiatry* 131 (January 1974):63.

[28]Mohammed Shafi, Richard Lavely, and Robert Jaffe, "Meditation and the Prevention of Alcohol Abuse," *American Journal of Psychiatry* 139 (1975):942–45. Copyright 1975, The American Psychiatric Association. Reprinted by permission.

INDEX

A, 243, 244, 245–46
Abdominal cramping, from nicotine, 101
Abdominal pain, 238, 275
Abortion, 109, 260
Abscesses, 256
Absences, from workplace by drug users, 42
Absorption
    of drugs, 52
    of oxygen, 107
Abstinence, 156, 171
Abstract thought, 64
Abuse of drugs, accidental, 45
Accidents, 158, 212
Acetaldehyde, 155, 161, 166
Acetaminophen, 235, 237, 238, 250
Acetate, 155
Acetic acid, 271
Acetic anhydride, 177

Acetone peroxide, 271
Acetylchloride, 234
Acetylcholine (ACH), 61, 65, 71
Acetylsalicylic acid, 40, 234
Acid, 202
Acid-base balance, 235
Acid head, 203
Acidic acid, 161
Acne, 245
Action potential, 59
Activism, social-political, 312–13
Acupuncture analgesia, 50
Addiction. See dependence
Addiction Research Foundation, 301
Addictive personality, 20
Adipic acid, 271
Adlerian theory of ego compensation,
    22

Administration
  improper, 257
  inhalation, 220, 263
  injection, 254, 256
  intramuscular, 263
  intravenous, 178, 263
  inunction, 52, 54–55
  oral, 263
Adolescents
  and deliriants, 141
  and smoking, 102
Adrenal glands, 102
Adrenaline, 65, 76, 105. *See also* epinephrine
Adrenergic, 61, 63
Adult drug scene, 39–41
Adulterants, in heroin, 181
Adults
  and alcohol, 147
  and marijuana, 216
Adverse effects
  of antidepressants, 259
  of fertility pills, 268
  of food additives, 275–76
  of lithium, 261
Adverse reactions, 140, 233
  to oral contraceptives, 265
  to over-the-counter drugs, 10
Advertising industry, 231, 232, 281, 282
  and alcohol, 148–49
  and recreational drugs, 11
  television, 10
  tobacco, 119
  and tranquilizers, 134
Aerosols, 30, 140
Age of Anxiety, 5
Aggression, and alcoholism, 164
Agitation, 260
AIDS, 84
Al-Anon, 170
Alaska, 299
Al-a-teen, 170
Al-a-tot, 170
Alcohol, 4, 5, 19, 216, 233, 319
  and adults, 147
  advertising of, 148–49
  and aspirin, 236
  with barbiturates, 132, 133
  and blood, 151–52
  and body temperature, 156
  and cancer, 156
  and central nervous system, 153–54
  and children, 30
  and circulatory system, 151–52
  in college, 32
  consumption in U.S., 146–47
  and crime, 159
  and digestive system, 155
  economic costs of, 157

effects on society, 157–59
  and elderly, 46–47
  and family, 159
  in high school, 30
  history of, 147–48
  information on, 68
  interaction with other drugs, 56,
    57
  and job-related problems, 158
  and kidneys, 155–56
  and liver, 154–55
  and marijuana, 221, 223
  and methaqualone, 133
  and minor tranquilizers, 135
  and motor-vehicle accidents, 158
  physiological effects of, 151–57
  reasons for consumption, 148–51
  as recreation, 11, 16
  and sex, 150–51
  study of use, 31
  and suicide, 159
  and testosterone levels, 157
  and tranquilizers, 140
  and Valium 136
  and women, 166–67
  in the workplace, 42
  and youth, 136–37
Alcoholdehydrogenase (ADH), 162
Alcoholics, 146, 149
  chronic and LSD, 207
Alcoholics Anonymous, 162, 168, 170
Alcoholism, 160–71, 314
  behavioral indicators of, 163–65
  causes of, 166
  chronic, 153
  and rehabilitation services, 167
  stages in, 163
  treatment approaches to, 169–71
Alertness, through amphetamines, 75
Algae meal, dried, 273
Alienation, 19
Alkaloid, 81
Allergic reactions, 242
  to barbiturates, 132
  to drugs, 55
Allergic shock reactions, 235
Allergies, 238, 245
  and smoking, 118
Alpert, Richard, 19
Alpha waves, 315
Alterations in the host, 257
Altered moods, from barbiturates, 132
Altered states, 18–19
Aluminum hydroxide, 240
Alveoli, 110
Amblyopia, 112
American Bar Association, 160
American Cancer Society, 107, 115

American Conference of Government Industrial Hygienists, 122
American Council on Science and Health, 103
American Heart Association, 115
American Hospitals Association, 168
American Indian, 207
American Lung Association, 115, 121, 123
American Medical Association, 74, 160, 178, 220, 281
American Rheumatic Association, 236
American Tobacco Company, 125
Ammonia, from side-stream smoke, 121
Ammonia poisoning, from free-base, 85
Ammonium alginate, 270
Amnesia, 152, 260
Amniotic fluid, nicotine in, 109
Amobarbital, 131
Amotivational syndrome, and marijuana, 225
Amphetamines, 73–78, 291, 296
    in adult drug scene, 41
    in college, 32
    counteraction by barbiturates, 132
    interaction with other drugs, 57, 58
    medical use of, 75–76
    misuse and abuse, 76
    physical effects of, 74–75
    in professional sports, 37
    psychological effects of, 74–75
    psychomimetic, 95
    psychosis from, 77
    as street drug, 3
    study of use, 31
Amputees, 207
Amyl alcohol, 146
Anabolic steroids, 35, 36
Analgesia, 146
Analgesics, 35, 218, 227, 231
    interaction with other drugs, 56–57
    properties of, 263
Anaphylactic shock, 257
Anastas, Robert, 172
Anatomy, 61–71
Androgen, 266
Anemia, 140, 245, 248
    iron-deficiency, 237
    pernicious, 246
Anesthetics, 140, 210, 227, 260
    cocaine as local, 86
    local, 242
Angel dust, 210
Angina pectoris, 122, 208
Animal crackers, 205
Animals, and antibiotics, 257
Annatto extract, 273
Anomalies, and smoking, 110
Anorexia, 133, 188, 191, 227
Anovulation, 267
Antabuse, 169

Antacid, interaction with other drugs, 58
Anthraquinones, 240
Antianxiety agent
    barbiturates as, 132
    Librium as, 138
Antibiotics, 256–58, 276
    effects of, 256–57
    interaction with other drugs, 58
    misuse of, 257–58
    resistance to, 257
Anticancer agent, 223, 261
Anticoagulants, 238
Anticonvulsants, 242
Antidepressants, 258–60, 276
    interaction with other drugs, 56, 57
    psychophysiological effects of, 259–60
Antidiabetics, and aspirin, 236
Antidiuretic action, of nicotine, 102
Antidiuretic hormones, 183
Antiepileptic effects, of Valium, 135
Antifreeze, 262
Antigens, 242
Antihistamines, 231, 242–43
    interaction with other drugs, 56, 57
    and tranquilizers, 140
Antiinflammatory agents, 35, 236
Antipsychotics. See tranquilizers, major
Antipyretic, 236
Anti-Saloon League, 287
Antispoilants, 269
Antitussives, 241–42
Anxiety, 133, 135, 139, 210, 212, 228, 249
    acute, 224
    cancer-caused, 228
    and minor tranquilizers, 134
    from nicotine withdrawal, 102
    reduction of, 227
    relief with methaqualone, 133
    relief with sedative-hypnotics, 131
    treatment with Valium, 135, 136
Anxiety reactions, 204, 219
Apathy, 135, 224
Aphrodisiac effects, 212
Appendix, 239
Appetite, 139
    increased, 268
    loss of, 183, 203, 246
    stimulated, 218, 227
Appetite control, with amphetamines, 41
Appetite reduction, 141
    and heroin, 180
    and tobacco, 108
Appetite suppressant, 249
Apricots, 243, 261
Arabia, 216
Arabians, 148
Army Chemical Corps Special Operations Division, 206

Arousal level, 63
Arteries
  plaque buildup in, 105
  in the uterus, 109
Arteriosclerosis, 105
Arthritis, rheumatoid, 234, 236
Ascending reticular activating system, 139
Aspartame, 276
Asphyxiation, 141
Aspirin, 234–38, 242, 250. *See also* salicylates
  in adult drug scene, 40
  in athletics, 35
  and heart attacks, 236–37
  interaction with other drugs, 56
  therapeutic effectiveness of, 236–37
  toxicology of, 237–38
Assaults, 159
Asthma, 55, 111, 238, 257
  bronchial, 237
AT&T, 115
Ataxia, 138
Atherosclerosis, 236, 245
Athletes, and drugs, 35–38
Atrophy, of brain, 154
Autistic children, 207
Autogenic training, 314
Autonomic functions, 63
Axon, 59
Azodicarbonamide, 271
Aztec Indians, 209

B_1, 245, 246
B_6, 243, 244, 245, 246
B_{12}, 111, 243, 244, 246
Bacteria, 242
  drug resistant, 257
  soil, 256
Bactericidal, 256
Bacteriostatic, 256
Bad breath, from nicotine, 110
Baden, Michael, 181
Baking powder, 271
Baking soda, 269, 271
Barbital, 131
Barbiturates, 131–33, 142, 187, 291, 296
  abuse of, 132–33
  in adult drug scene, 39
  classification of, 131
  in college, 32
  history of, 131
  information on, 67
  interaction with other drugs, 56, 57, 58
  medical use of, 132
  physical effects of, 132
  in professional sports, 37
  in senior citizens, 44
Barbituric acid, 131, 134

Bar mitzvahs, 20
Bayer, 234
Baylor College of Medicine, 120
Beans, 246, 247, 248
Beer, 146, 259
Bee stings, 242
Behavioral dependencies, 61
Behavioral-oral substitution, 108
Behavior modification, for hyperactivity, 80
Belladonna, 233
Benjamin Rush Hospital, 82
Benson, Herbert, 318
Benzedrine, 73, 74, 77
Benzodiazepines, 134, 135
Benzopyrene
  in cigarette tars, 100
  from side-stream smoke, 121
Benzoyl peroxide, 271
Berger, Hans, 314
Beriberi, 246
Berkeley Center for Drug Studies, 195
Beta endorphine, 25, 26
BHA (butylated hydoxyanisole), 269
BHT (butylated hydroxytoluene), 269
Biochemical theory, of dependency, 23
Biochemistry, of alcohol, 161
Biofeedback, 80, 314–15
Biotin, 244, 248
Biotransformation, 53
Bi-Phetamine T, 133
Birth control pills, 3
Birth defects, 140, 207
  and caffeine, 93
  and Pill, 266–67
Births, multiple, 268–69
Black market, 287, 295
Blackout, 152, 164
Bladder, 135, 140
Bleeding, 237, 243
  of gums, 247
  tendency toward, 237–38
Blindness, 287
Blood, and alcohol, 151–52
Blood abnormalities, 136
Blood alcohol content, 152
Blood-brain barrier, 53, 141, 209
Blood cells, development of red, 246
Blood chemistry, changes in, 105
Blood chloride levels, and alcoholism, 166
Blood clotting
  hindering of, 236
  time required for, 111
Blood coagulability, decrease in, 235
Blood-lipid values, and smoking, 108
Blood poisoning, 178
Blood pressure, 52, 61, 139, 140, 210, 218,
    228, 249, 265
  arterial and Valium, 136

and clove oil, 120
effect of nicotine on, 102
high, 152
increased, 212, 260
increase due to nicotine, 105
increase from smoking, 105
low, 135
reduction of, 227, 309
rise in, 169, 203, 221
and snuff, 120
Blood protein, 151
Bloodstream
increase in fatty acids in, 102
nicotine absorption into, 101
Blood sugar levels, 183, 203, 218
Blood vessels
constriction of, 106, 110
dilation of, 218, 235
permeability, 242
Blotter, 205
Blue, Vida, 38
Body functions, effects of marijuana on, 219
Body mass, 52
Body temperature, 140, 210
and alcohol, 156
basal, 267
reduction of, 218
rise in, 203
Body tissues, transport of oxygen to, 103
Body weight, and drug activity, 53
Boeing Aircraft, 115
Boggs Amendment, 1951, 289–90
Bolivia, 82
Bone deformities, 247
Bone formation, 246, 247
Bone marrow, 141, 246
Bone marrow depression, 236, 257
Borden, 276
Boredom, 17, 216
Boston Collaborative Drug Surveillance, 92,
    236
Brain, 183, 256
atrophy of, 154
chemicals found in, 135
damaging effects on, 153
effects of marijuana on, 223–24
effects of nicotine on, 102
and nicotine, 101
and opiates, 24
Brain damage, 154
and marijuana, 223–24
prevention of, 132
Brain stem, 63, 139
and morphine, 178
Brain tumor, 246
Brain waves, 318
Bran, 240
Breads, 246

Breast examination, 266
Breast feeding, and transfer of nicotine, 101
Breast soreness, 265, 268
Breathing capacity, after quitting smoking, 116
Breath odor, 263
Brecher, Edward, 180
Brewer's yeast, 243
Bridge Over Troubled Waters, 311
British Royal College of General Practitioners,
    266
Broccoli, 246
Bronchi, 106
Bronchial drainage, 242
Bronchial tubes, 100, 110
Bronchioles, 103
Bronchitis, 111, 219
chronic, 118
cigarette-induced, 40
Brown, Robert, 310
Brown & Williamson Tobacco, 124
Browner, Ross, 38
Bruises, 262
Bruising, 243, 247
Bruxism, 77
Buccal absorption, 100, 114
Buckwheat, 243
Buddhism, 19
Buerger's disease, 105
Bureau of Drugs, 283
Bureau of Narcotics and Dangerous Drugs,
    288
Burnout, 226
Burns, 227
Butabarbital, 131
Butler, 109
Butyrophenones, 139

C, 111, 236, 243, 244, 245, 246
Cabbage, 247
Cactus, 207
Cadium, 121
Caffeine, 5, 35, 87–94, 216, 233
addiction, 91–94
in adult drug scene, 40
and fibrocystic breast disease, 94
history of, 89–91
and hyperactivity, 80
physical effects of, 91
and PPA, 249
psychological dependence on, 88
as recreational drug, 11
as stimulant, 6
use with children, 93
and young people, 30
Caffeinism, 91–94
Calcification, 247
Calcium, 240, 244, 247, 269

Calcium alginate, 270
Calcium bromate, 271
Calcium lactate, 271
Calcium silicate, 272
Califano, Joseph, 101, 115
California, 7, 186, 205, 216, 227
California Rehabilitation Center, 186
Caloric utilization, increased, 108
Camp, 94
Campbell Soup, 115
Canadian Addiction Research Foundation, 219
Cancer, 220, 226, 245, 275, 276, 299
    and alcohol, 156–57
    bladder, 107, 117
    breast, 107
    from cigarette tars, 100
    and contraceptives, 266
    deaths from smoking, 107
    esophagus, 107, 117
    and exposure to chemicals, 11
    larynx, 107, 117
    of lip, 119
    lung, 107
    and marijuana, 227
    mouth, 107
    and non-inhaled smoke, 119
    of pancreas, 117
    from smoking, 102, 107
Cancer patients, 206, 207
    and heroin, 182
Cannabinoids, 227
Cannabis, 18, 215, 218, 223, 224. See also
        marijuana
Cannon, Walter, 65
Carbohydrates, 112, 248
Carbon dioxide, 161
Carbon monoxide
    absorbed by non-smoker, 122
    in cigarette smoke, 103
    and circulation, 105
    in environment from smoking, 122
    from side-stream smoke, 121
    from smoke, 100
Carboxyhemoglobin level, in nonsmokers, 122
Carcinogen, 11, 219
    in cigarettes, 100
Cardiac efficiency, 309, 318
Cardiac stimulation, 249
Cardiac tone, 208
Cardiomyopathy, 152
Cardiovascular disease
    marijuana and, 220–21
    from smoking, 102, 104–6
Carnation, 276
Carotene, 246
Carrageenan, 270
Carrot oil, 274
Castell, W. P., 152

Cauliflower, 247
Cell growth, new, 245
Cellular immunity, 108
Cellulose derivatives, 270
Center for Disease Control, 307
Center of Alcohol Studies, 168
Central nervous system, 61–65
    and alcohol, 146, 153–54
    and antidepressants, 259
    and clove oil, 120
    depression by sedative-hypnotics, 130
    effect of caffeine on, 92
    and marijuana, 7
    and nitrous oxides, 260
    and opiates, 24
    and psilocybin, 209
    stimulation of, 249
    and tranquilizers, 139
Central nervous system depressant methadone
        as, 183
Cereals, 246, 247
Cerebellum, 153, 154
Cerebral cortex, 64–65, 211
Cerebral palsy, and Valium, 135, 136
Cerebrovascular disease, 221
    and smoking, 106
Cerebrum, 153
Chandler, Asa G., 82
Chappel, John, 194
Chaw, 119
Cheese, 259
Chein, Isadore, 300
Chemical adulterants, 262
Chemical dependencies, 61
Chemical imbalances, 260
Chemicals, 11, 242
Chemotherapeutic agent, 223, 226
Chemotherapy, 195, 217, 227, 228
Chewing tobacco, and nicotine, 100
Chicken livers, 259
Chicken pox, 237
Childbirth, 227
Children
    and caffeine, 93
    and smoking, 102
Chills, 135, 259
Chippers, 7
Chloral hydrate, 296
Chloride ions, 59, 60
Chloroform, 141
Chlorpromazine, 78
Chocolate, 30
    and caffeine, 40, 87
    history of, 91
Cholesterol, 36
Cholesterol deposits, 105, 151, 309
Cholesterol levels, 245
Choline, 243

Cholinergic, 61, 63
Chromosome alterations, 202, 206, 223
Chronic bronchitis, from smoking, 106
Chronic obstructive pulmonary disease, 106
Churches, and morality of smoking, 123
CIA, 206
Ciapoline, 108
Cigarette companies, 114
Cigarettes
    clove, 120–21
    decrease in production of, 100
    effects on cardiovascular system, 104–6
    filtered, 114
    in high school, 30
    introduction, 99
    low tar and nicotine, 102
    smoke from, 100
Cigarette smoke, gases in, 103
Cigarette smokers, 220
Cigars, introduction of, 99
Cigar smokers, mortality rate of, 102
Cigar smoking, 116, 119
Cilia, 100, 103, 106
Cincinnati Bengals, 38
Circulation
    changes in, 221
    after quitting smoking, 116
Circulatory system, and alcohol, 151–52
Cirrhosis, 154
Citric acid, 269, 271
Citrus fruits, 246
Civil commitment, 186
Cleaning compounds, 141
Cleft lip, 110
Cleft palate, 110, 136
Clomid, 267
Clomiphene, 268
Clot, formation of, 106
Clotting
    blood, 247, 264
    prevented by aspirin, 237
Clotting time, 238
Clove, cigarettes, 120–21
Clove oil, 120
Co-alcoholics, 171
Coca, history of, 90–91
Coca-Cola, 82, 276
Cocaine, 81–87, 211, 233, 285, 296
    in college, 32
    history of, 82–83
    information on, 66
    medical use of, 86–87
    pharmacological effects of, 83–85
    physiological effects of, 83–85
    in professional sports, 37
    psychological effects of, 86
    as recreational drug, 6
    sociological effects of, 86

    in the workplace, 42
    and young people, 30
Coca plant, 12, 81
Co-carcinogenics, in cigarettes, 100
Cochineal extract/carmine, 273
Cocktail party, 16
Cocoa, 30
Codeine, 46, 177, 182–83, 240, 242, 296
Coffee, 30, 240
    and caffeine, 40, 87
    decaffeinated, 94
    history of, 89
    physical effects of, 91
Coffee intake, and nicotine, 111
Cohen, Maiman, 206
Cohen, Sidney, 220
CO intake, 110
Coke, 83
Cola drinks, 30, 40, 87
Cold, 245, 256, 263
Cold medications, 231
Cold sweat, from nicotine, 101
Coleman, Daniel, 316–17
Collapse, 238
College of Medicine, 94
College
    and drugs, 35
    and smokeless tobacco, 119
Colombia, 217
Colon, 240
Color Additive Amendment, 275
Colors, 255
Columbia University School of Public Health,
    193
Columbus, 274
Coma, 137, 178, 211, 261
Comfrey root, 243
Commercial drugs, 11
Committee on the Institute on Medicine, 221
Communist party, 313
Community Mental Health Centers Act, 291
Compassionate Pain Relief Act, 182
Compazine, 227
Comprehensive Drug Abuse Prevention and
    Control Act, 217, 292
Compulsive behavior, 77
Compulsive use, of alcohol, 160–61
Concentrate, inability to, 242
Confusion, 136, 141, 142, 191, 224, 243, 245,
    259
Congenital dependency, and barbiturates, 132
Congenital malformation, 110
Congestion, 242
Congestive heart failure, 151
Congress, 104, 217, 218, 288, 289, 291, 292
Conjunctival irritation, 122, 136
Constipation, 136, 183, 191, 239, 242
    understanding, 239–40

Constitution, 287
Consumer Food Act, 275
Consumer laws, 302
Consumer safety, and drugs, 51–59
Consumers Union Report, 193
Convenience foods, 275
Convulsions, 135, 138, 188
    prevention of, 227
Coordination, 141, 212, 248
Copper, 244
Corfman, Philip, 265
Corn, 246
Corn endosperm, 274
Corns, 227
Corn syrup, 269, 273
Coronary arteries, blockage of, 106
Coronary-artery blood flow, increase after
    smoking, 105
Coronary-artery spasms, 84
Coronary artherosclerosis, 221
Coronary bypass operations, and smoking, 105
Coronary deaths, and smoking, 105
Coronary heart disease, 151
    and carbon monoxide, 122
    and pipes or cigars, 119
    and smoking, 102, 118
Corpus collosum, 64
Correction fluid, 140
Cortex, 63
Cortisone, 234
Cosmetics, 11
Cost, 255
Costa Rica, 219
Cotton seed, 266
Cough, 227, 241
Cough medications, 182, 231. See also antitus-
    sives
Cough relievers, 250
Council of Economic Priorities Study, 282
Cowboy image, 115
Cramps, 135, 138, 248
Crime
    and alcohol, 159
    and methadone, 193
Crisis intervention, 185
    and alcoholism, 170–71
Crown Zellerbach, 262
Crystal, 76
Culbro, Inc., 125
Currants, 246
Current, 59
Cyanide, 261
Cyclamates, 275
Cyclazocine, 196

D, 243, 244, 245, 247
Dairy products, 256

Dallas Cowboys, 37
Dalmane, 19
Dangerous drugs, 204, 291
Darvon, 184, 194, 198
Dass, Ram, 19
Datril, 238
Daytop, 189
Death, 84, 135, 137, 141, 178, 210, 211, 235,
    238, 287
    from smoking, 102
    heroin-related, 180–81
    premature from cigarettes, 100
Death in the West, 115
Debakey, Lois, 232
Decongestants, 242, 249
Decriminalization, of drugs, 298–302
Delaney Amendment, 11
Deliriants, 140–42
    classification of, 140–41
    history of, 141
    physical effects of, 141–42
Delirium, 243, 260
    from clove oil, 120
Dendrites, 59
Dental problems, 120
Deodorants, 141
Department of Agriculture, 216
Department of Health and Human Services,
    217, 265
Department of Health, Education and Wel-
    fare, 115, 156, 222
Department of Human Services, 292
Department of Justice, 185, 288
Department of Psychiatry, 185
Dependence. See also specific drugs
    methadone, 183
    nonphysical, 180
    on opiates, 178
Dependence, physical
    and barbiturates, 132
    on Librium, 139
Dependence, physiological, on methaqualone,
    134
Dependence, potential for, 55
Dependence, psychological
    on Darvon, 184
    on minor tranquilizers, 135
    on sedative-hypnotics, 131
    on Valium, 137–38
Dependency states
    biological, 23–26
    psychological, 20–22
    sociological, 22–23
Depersonalization, 224
Dephenylmetanes, 134
Depressant, 151, 211, 296
Depression, 139, 210, 212, 248, 258, 265, 268
    from amphetamines, 75

and drugs, 19
and enkephalins, 50
from nicotine withdrawal, 102
Dermatitis, 263, 268
Dessicant, 218
DEPC (diethyl-pyrocarbonate), 275
Detoxification, 169, 187–88
Dexedrine, 73, 76, 77
Dextromethorphan, 242
Dextrose, 273
Diagnostic tests, and smoking, 111
Diaphragm, 102
Diarrhea, 133, 140, 188, 238, 247, 257
from nicotine, 102
Diet, improper, 240
Dietary supplement, 243
Diet pills, 249–50
Digestion, 246, 309
Digestive system, and alcohol, 155
Diglycerides, 269, 270
Dioctyl sodium sulfosuccinate, 270
Disaster Assistance and Mental Health Section, 159
Disodium guanylate, 272
Disodium inosinate, 272
Disorderly conduct, 159
Disorientation, 135, 235
Distance runners, 35
Distribution, of drug, 52–53
District of Columbia, 227
Diuretic actions, 93
Diuretics, 227, 236
Distillation, 148
Distilled spirits, 146
Dizziness, 133, 141, 169, 183, 184, 212, 235, 242, 246, 249
from LSD, 203
DMSO (dimethyl sulfoxide), 262–64, 276
physical effects of, 263–64
DNA, decreased syntheses of lymphocytes, 102
DNA metabolism, 223
Dr. Jekyll and Mr. Hyde, 82
Dogs, trained to find drugs, 43
Dole, Vincent P., 190
Domestic violence, 159
Dopamine, 18, 61, 161, 162
Dosage, 52–54
improper, 257
Dose-response curve, 53, 135
Doses, 245
Dose-time curve, 53
Double vision, 136
Dougherty, Ronald, 82
Doyle, Sir Arthur Conan, 82
Drew, John, 38
Drinking, responsible, 173
Drooling, 212

Drowsiness, 131, 136, 138, 178, 183, 238, 242, 259
Drug abuse, 4, 314
accidental, 45
alternatives to, 306–19
senior citizen, 43–47
Drug Abuse Control Amendments, 204, 291
Drug Abuse Council, 298
Drug Abuse Treatment and Referral System, 195
Drug Abuse Warning Network, 136
Drug activity
and body weight, 53
and sex, 53
Drug benefits, 307–8
Drug companies, 281
Drug dependency, among elderly, 46–47
Drug education, 285, 307
Drug Enforcement Agency, 288
Drug industry, 282–83
Drug interactions, 9
Drug regulation, milestones in, 303–4
Drugs
allergic reaction to, 55
and alteration of transmitters, 61
alternatives to, 308–19
and athletics, 35–38
on campus, 32
and consumer safety, 51–59
definition, 51
individual reaction to, 2
ingestion of, 52, 54
inhalation of, 52, 54
injection of, 52, 54
interaction of, 55, 56–59
interaction with food, 58–89
inunction of, 52, 54–55
legislation of, 285–98
look-alike, 95
in the military, 33–34
prescription, 87
psychoactive, 60
over-the-counter, 10–11, 87
Drug scene
adult, 39–43
youth, 29–38
Drug technology, 8–9
Drug treatment, for alcoholism, 169
Drug use, 4
and law, 283–85
Drug withdrawal, use of Librium in, 138
Drunk driving, movement against, 171–72
Drunkenness, 138
Dulles, Allen, 206
Dumas, Alexander, 18
DuPont, Robert, 83
Dust, 242
Dysfunction, alcoholism as, 160
Dysphoria, and drugs, 19

E, 243, 244, 247
Earaches, 227
Ecker, Tom, 35
Economic costs, of alcohol, 157
Edema, 105, 238, 246
Education, and hyperactive child, 80–81
EEG activity, 209
Effects, damaging on brain, 153
Eggs, 246, 247, 248
Ego compensation, 22
Egyptians, 148
Eighteenth Amendment, 287
Ejaculation, delayed, 191
Elderly, 220, 281
  and alcohol, 147
Electrochemical threshold, 59
Electroconvulsive therapy, 258
Elixir of Sulfanilamide, 289
Emotion, 64, 203
Emotional dysfunction, 210
Emotionally battered, 211
Emotionally disturbed children, and Librium,
  138
Emotional reactions, 136
Emphysema, 106–7, 219
  cigarette-induced, 40, 106
  pulmonary, 118
Employee assistance programs, 42, 43
Emulsifiers, 269
EN-1639, 196
Endocarditis, 78, 178
Endocrine functioning, effect of marijuana on,
  221–22
Endorphin, 50
Energy, loss of, 216
England, 218, 232
Enkephalins, 25, 26, 50
Environment, social and physical, 4
Environmental Protection Agency, 11
Enzymes, 242
Epilepsy
  and Ritalin, 78
  and Valium, 136
Epileptics, 64
Epinephrine, 76
  increase in, 111
  release due to nicotine, 102
Equal, 276
Equanil, 134
Ergogenic drugs, 35
Erickson, Kallen, and Westerholm, 110
Erythroxylon, 81
Esophagus, 241
Estrogen, 264, 309
Ether, 141
Ethical drugs. See prescription drugs
Ethyl alcohol, 146
Ethylene, 269

Euphoria, 141, 210, 224, 228
  through drugs, 19
Europe, 216, 263
Excitement, 131, 138, 243
Exercise, 309–11
  and smoking, 110
Existentialists, 21
Eye, 256
  bulging, 212
  reddened, 218
Eye disorder, 245

Fad drugs, 31
Fainting, 135, 238
Faintness, 259
Fair Oaks Hospital, 86
Fallopian tubes, 264
Family, and alcohol, 159
Family counseling, 185
Family life, 37
Family therapy, for alcoholics, 171
Fatigue, 136, 138, 235, 248, 268
Fat reservoir, 53
Fats, 248
Fatty acids
  increase in, 102
  release of, 107
Fatty tissue, 219
FDA (Federal Food and Drug Administra-
  tion), 2–3, 44, 76, 231, 233, 237, 239,
  243, 249, 261, 262, 263, 274, 275, 276,
  282, 290, 295, 302
  and caffeine, 93
  definition of drug use, 4
  and over-the-counter drugs, 10
  and tranquilizers, 36
  and Valium, 138
FD&C Blue No. 1, 274
FD&C Red No. 40, 274
FD&C Yellow No. 5, 274
Fears, 135
Feces, 219
Federal Bureau of Narcotics, 288
Federal Food, Drug, and Cosmetics Act, 274,
  291
Federal Narcotics Control Board, 288
Federal Register, 245
Federal Trade Commission, 104, 289
Federation of American Societies for Experi-
  mental Biology, 91
Feingold, Benjamin, 81
Felony, 217
Fermentation, 146
Ferrous gluconate, 273
Fertility, 246
Fertility pills, 267–69, 277
Fetal abnormalities, 202, 258

Fetal alcohol syndrome, 156
Fetal nutrition, and smoking, 109–10
Fever, 131, 135, 140, 235, 257
  reduction of, 234, 236, 238
Fibrocystic breast disease, and caffeine,
  94
Fibrosis, 218, 219, 241
Fifth World Congress of Psychiatry, 222
Fight or flight hypothesis, 65, 316
Filter tips, and cancer, 117
Firestone Tire and Rubber Company, 42
Firmers, 269
First Report of the National Commission on
  Marijuana and Drug Abuse, 218
Fish, 246, 247
Flashback, 204, 226
Flavorings, 255
Fleming, Alexander, 256
Floating sensation, 141
Florida, 227
Flour, 270
Flu, 237, 256
Fluid intake, insufficient, 240
Fluids, retention of, 265
Fluoride, 244
Fluoride rinses, 234
Flushing, 212, 275
Folic acid, 243, 244, 245, 248
Folkins, Carlyle H., 310
Folklore, 233
Food Additive Amendment, 274
Food additives, 11, 269–76, 277
  adverse effects of, 275–76
  reduction of for hyperactivity, 80
Food and Drug Act, 233
Food, Drug and Cosmetic Act, 289
Food starch, 270
Football players, 37
Ford Foundation, 137
Formaldehyde, 161
Fort Detrich, 206
Framington Heart Study, 105, 151, 152
Frank, Jerome, 188
Fraternal-club initiations, 20
Fraternity initiations, 20
Frederick, Calvin, 159
Frederickson, Donald T., 220
Free-base cocaine, 84–85
Freedom from Smoking, 115
Free Radical Assay Technique, 34
FRESHSTART, 115
Freud, Sigmund, 18, 82
Freudians, 21
Fright, 142
Frigidity, 206
Fructose, 273
Fruit juice, 273
Fruits, 247

Fumaric acid, 271
Furcelleran, 270

Galen, 177
Ganja, 18, 226
Gas chromatography, 36
Gases, from cigarettes, 103
Gasoline, as inhalant, 8, 140
Gastric hemorrhage, 237
Gastric upset, 93, 131, 235
Gastrointestinal bleeding, 235, 237
Gastrointestinal distress, 154, 257, 259
  and smoke, 108
Gastrointestinal hyperactivity, from nicotine,
  100, 102
G. D. Searle and Company, 276
Gelatin chips, 205
General Foods, 276
General hospitals, for alcoholism, 168
Genetic damage, and marijuana, 223–24
Genetic factors, and alcoholism, 166
Geriatric patients, and Librium, 138
Germany, 234, 290
Giddiness, from nicotine, 100, 261
Gilman, Alfred, 40
Gin, 148
Gitlow, Stanley, 162
Glaucoma, 217, 226–27, 228, 299
Glucose, 93, 273
Glue, 8, 19, 30
Glue sniffing, 285
Glutethimide, 296
Glycerine, 269, 271
Glycerol monostearate, 271
Glycogen release, 108
Gold, Mark, 86
Goldstein, Avram, 24, 301
Gonadotropin, 268
Goodman, Louis, 40
Goodwin, Frederick, 87, 310
Gooseflesh, 188
Gossypol, 266
Gout, 238
Grains, 247
Grape skin extract, 273
Grateful Dead, 83
Great Britain, 182
Greece, 219, 222
Greeks, 148
Green, David, 38
Green, Elmer, 315
Green pepper, 246
Group acceptance, 29
Group therapy, of alcoholics, 171
Growth, 246, 247, 257
Guatemala, 209
Gum, nicotine, 114

Gums, damage to, 111
Guru, 203

Hague Conference, 286
Haight-Ashbury Clinic, 138
Hair loss, 268
Hair sprays, 141
Halfway houses, for alcoholism, 168
Hallucinations, 77, 83, 141, 188, 191, 210, 249
  from clove oil, 120
  in college, 32
  information on, 69
  and rebellion, 19
Hallucinogens, 7, 218, 296
Halpern, Milton, 181
Halsted, William, 82
Hangover, 131, 133
Hapten, 108
Harkey, 108
Harrison Act, 82, 185, 186, 286
Harvard Medical School, 318
Hashish, 216, 218, 296
Hash oil, 218, 296
Hawaii, 216
Hazards, of PCP, 212
Headache, 131, 133, 135, 136, 139, 141, 184, 234, 235, 242, 248, 249, 250, 263, 268, 275
  from LSD, 203
  LSD for, 202
  migraine, 227
Health factors, and smoking, 111
Hearing loss, 257
Heart, 71
  changes in, 221
  effects of caffeine on, 92
Heart attacks, 250, 265
  cigarette-induced, 40
Heart beat, rapid, 212
Heartburn, 108
Heart convulsions, 260
Heart palpitations, 261
Heart rate, 169, 221
  drop in, 221
  effect of nicotine on, 102
  rise in, 203
  and snuff, 120
Hebb, Donald, 316
Hebrews, 148
Helms, Richard, 206
Hemoglobin, and carbon monoxide, 103
Hemoglobin-binding sites, 103
Hemorrhage, 247
Hemorrhoids, 227
Henderson, Thomas "Hollywood", 37
Hendrix, Jimi, 181

Henry, George, 197
Hepatic protein enzymes, 161
Hepatitis, 178, 236, 299
Hepperidin, 243
Herbal chemicals, 12, 215
Herbicide, 217
Heroin, 7–8, 177, 178–82, 285, 296
  importation banned, 287–88
  legalization of, 299
  medical uses of, 182
  in Vietnam, 33
  and young people, 30
Heroin dependent
  and barbiturates, 132
  and Valium, 136
Heroin Movement, 182
Herring, 259
Herschler, Jacob, 262
Herschler, Robert, 262
Hexachlorophene, 234
Hickey, 111
High-density lipoproteins, 36
High school
  alcohol in, 147
  drug use in, 30
  and marijuana, 216
  and smokeless tobacco, 119
Hilarity, 141
Hindu religious rites, 18
Hippocampus, 154
Hippocrates, 177
Histamine, 242
H. J. Heinz, 276
Hoffman, Albert, 202
Holmes, Sherlock, 82
Homeostasis, 61
Hormones, 61, 242
Hospices, 182
Hostility, 136
Hot flashes, 188
Household chemicals, 11
House Select Committee on Crime, 186
House Select Committee on Narcotics, Abuse, 216
Howe, Steve, 38
Hucker, 264
Hughes, John, 25
Huichol Indians, 18
Hunger, 61, 226
  suppression by amphetamines, 75
Hydraulic fluid, 262
Hydrocarbon solvents, 140
Hydrocortisone, 57, 263
Hydrogen cyanide, 261
  in cigarette smoke, 103
  and respiratory diseases, 106
  from smoke, 100
Hydrogen peroxide, 271

Hydrolyzed vegetable protein, 272
Hydrophillic compounds, 240
Hyperactivity, 142
  and education, 80–81
  and Ritalin, 79–81
Hyperkinesis, 275
Hyperphasias, focal modular, 266
Hypersensitivity reactions, to salicylates, 238
Hypertension, 136, 221, 247, 249
Hyperthemia, 260
Hyperventilating, 235
Hypodermic, 177, 178
Hypoglycemia, 93
Hyposensitivity, 55
Hypothalamus, 61, 156, 235, 267
Hypothermia, 156
Hypoxanthine, 135

Idaho, 216
Illegal drugs, 12
Illinois, 227
Illusions, 224
Immunological system
  effect of marijuana on, 221
  and smoking, 108
Immunosuppressant, 221
Impotence, 183, 245
Impulse, 59
Incestuous relationships, 211
Indian Health Service, 159
Indian remedies, 233
Indians, and cocaine, 82
Industrial chemicals, 11
Infants, transfer of nicotine to, 101
Infection, upper respiratory, 84
Infections, 245
Inflammation, 250, 262, 263
Ingestion, of drugs, 52, 54
Ingredients, listing of, 245
Inhalants, as drugs for children, 30
Inhalation, 220, 263
  of drugs, 52, 54
  of heroin, 7
  of pipe and cigar smoke, 119
Initiation rites, 20
Injection, 254, 256
  of drugs, 52, 54
Innervation, 65
Inorganic wastes, 11
Inosine, 135
Insomnia, 135, 136, 139, 184, 191, 249, 250
  reduction of, 227
  treatment with barbiturates, 132
  and Valium, 136
Institute of Medicine of National Academy of
  Sciences, 219
Instructions, doctor's, 281

Insulin, 93
  and aspirin, 236
Insurance premiums, 115
  increased by smokers, 104
  after quitting smoking, 116
Interaction
  adverse drug, 233
  of drugs, 55, 56–69
  between food and drugs, 58–59
Intercourse, timing of, 267
Interstitial cystitis, 263
Intestinal tract, 235
Intestines, 219, 246, 250
Intoxication, 141, 210, 235, 260
  legal, 152
Intramuscular administration, 263
Intraocular pressure, 226
Intravenous administration, 263, 178
Inunction, of drugs, 52, 54–55
Invert sugar, 273
Investigational New Drug, 263
Iodine, 244
I Quit Kit, 115
Iron, 244
Iron-ammonium citrate, 272
Iron oxide, 273
Irradiation, 263
Irregularity. See constipation
Irritability, 136, 247
  from nicotine withdrawal, 102
Itching, 242
IUD, 265

Jacob, Stanley, 262
Jamaica, 219, 226
Jaundice, 192
Jenever, 148
Job placement, 185
Job-related problems, and alcohol, 158
Jogging, 310–11
Johns Hopkins School of Medicine, 24, 82,
  188, 192
Johns-Manville, 115
Johnson, Pete, 38
Joint cough, 220
Joplin, Janis, 181
Journal of the American Medical Association,
  281, 289
Junior high, and alcohol, 30

K, 243, 244, 247
Kalbe and Lauteman, 234
Kale, 246, 247
Kamiya, Joe, 315
Kansas City Royals, 38
Kaplan, John, 302

Kardong, Don, 35
Kasterlitz, Hans W., 25
Kefauver-Harris Amendments, 290
Kelp, 243
Kennedy, Edward, 295
Kesey, Ken, 19
Kidney, 140, 183, 247, 264
  and alcohol, 155–56
  changes in, 141
  and excretion of nicotine, 101
  and morphine, 178
Kidney damage, 236
Kidney functions, impaired, 259
Kidney stones, 245
Klinefelter's syndrome, 110
Kolansky, Harold, 224
Koller, Karl, 82
Korsicoff's syndrome, 163

Lacrimation, 187
Lactation, 246
Lactic acid, 271
Lactose, 85
Laetrile, 261–62, 276
Language, 64
Lassitude, 247
Laws
  and drug use, 283–85
  about smoking, 123
Laxatives, 231, 239–41, 250
  types of, 240–41
  use of, 241
Leary, Timothy, 19, 204
Lecithin, 243, 270
Ledain Commission, 298
Lee, Samuel, 233
Legal intervention, 185
Legislation, and consumer issues, 295, 298
  on drug abuse, 184–87
  drug-related, 285–98
Lemmon Company, 6, 133
Lethargy, 136
Lettuce, 247
Leukoplakia, 120
Lewin, Lewis, 207
Lexington facility, 185
Liberty Park, 189
Libido
  changes in, 136
  weakened, 259
Librium, 6, 131, 134, 138–39
  current use of, 139–40
  physical effects of, 138
Licensing tests, 20
Life expectancy, shortened by smoking, 117
Liggett Group, 124
Lighter fluid, 140

Lightner, Candy, 171–72
Lilly, John, 17
Limbic/endocrinal system, 61
Linder v. United States, 288
Lipids, metabolism of, 112
Lipid-soluble, 52
Lipoproteins, 151
Liquiprin, 238
Lithium, 260–61, 276
  and alcoholism, 169
Little, Ralph B., 21
Liver, 140, 183, 245, 246, 247, 248, 250
  and alcohol, 154–55, 161
  changes in, 141
  disorders from amphetamines, 75
  and drugs, 53, 55
  effects of caffeine on, 93
  and glycogen release, 108
  impairment of, 265
  and metabolism of nicotine, 101
  and morphine, 178
Liver damage, 238, 247, 259
Liver tumors, 266
Livingston, Louisiana, 42
Loftus, Elizabeth, 154
Lorillard, 125
Los Angeles Dodgers, 38
Louisiana, 227
Love drug, 133
LSD, 7, 94, 202–7, 212, 285, 291, 296
  and medical research, 206–7
  psychological effects of, 203–4
  psychophysiological effects of, 208–9
  and society, 204–6
Lucas, John, 38
Lundy, Bob, 37
Lung cancer
  cigarette-induced, 40, 117
  and nicotine, 114
  and women, 102
Lung damage, 218
Lung diseases
  and pipe or cigar smoke, 119
  from smoking, 102
Lung function, 219
Lungs, 183, 219
  and morphine, 178
Lymphatic system, 103
Lymphocytes
  decreased synthesis of, 102
  decrease in, 108

Macrophages, 103
MADD, 171–72
Maddox and Desmond, 180
Magnesium, 244
Maharishi Mahesh Yogi, 316

Maimonides Medical Center, 93
Mainlining, 7
Maletzky and Klotter, 138
Malic hydroazide, 269
Malt extract, 243
Manganese, 244
Manic-depressive illness, 260
Mannitol, 85
Manufacturers, cigarette, 101
Marathoners, 35
March of Dimes, 93
Marco Polo, 274
Margarine, 247
Marijuana, 3, 7, 19, 285, 287, 296
    in adult drug scene, 41
    and alcohol, 221
    and brain damage, 223–24
    and cardiovascular complications, 220–21
    in college, 32
    decriminalization of, 298–99
    effect on immunology system, 221
    endocrine functioning and, 221–22
    and genetic damage, 223–24
    information on, 70
    medical uses of, 226–28
    pharmocological classification of, 218
    physiological effects of, 218–24
    psychological effects of, 224–26
    and psychomotor impairment, 222–23
    and rebellion, 19
    and society, 225–26
    study of use of, 31
    use in the U.S., 216–17
    use in the world, 215–16
    in Vietnam, 33
    in the workplace, 42
Marijuana and Health, 219, 222
Marijuana Tax Act, 217, 288–89
Marlboro Man, 115
Massachusetts, and snuff, 120
Mass spectrometry, 36
Maxwell Report, 100
Mayo Clinic diet, 107
MDA (methylene dioxyamphetamine), 94–95, 296
Measles, 256
Meats, 247, 248
Medial forebrain bundle, 63
Medical cost, cigarette-induced, 103
Medical Letter on Drugs and Therapeutics, 281
Medical research, and LSD, 206–7
Medical uses,
    of heroin, 182
    of lithium, 261
Medication effectiveness, and smoking, 111
Medications, 315–19
Medulla, 63, 153
Medullary center, depressing, 241

Melges, 225
Membrane, of nerve, 59
Membrane permeability, increase in, 105
Memorial University, 169
Memory
    disturbances in, 212
    impairment of short-term, 224
    improvement with enkephalin, 50
    and Valium, 136
Menadione, 247
Menopausal stress, 264
Menopause, 268
Menstrual cycle, 264
Menstrual disturbance, 133, 135, 136, 264
Menstrual flow, changes in, 265
Menstruation, 167, 268
Mental confusion, 235
Mental derangement, acute temporary, 249
Mental disorders, 247
Mental illness, 206, 245, 258
Mental retardation, 212
    from FAS, 156
Meperidine, 296
Meprobamate, 134
Merrel Dow Pharmaceuticals, 114
Mescaline, 7, 12, 18, 207–9, 210, 212, 296
Metabolic rate, 318
Metabolism, 139, 248
    of an alcoholic, 161
    carbohydrate, 246
    of DMSO, 263–64
    and smoking, 107–8
    sugar, 93
Metabolites, 53, 219
Methadone, 8, 183–84, 187, 198, 296
    as detoxification for opiates, 183
    maintenance, 190–95
    physical effects of, 183
    side effects of, 191–92
Methadone maintenance
    rate of success of, 193–94
    social implications of, 194–95
Methamphetamine, 31, 73, 76–78, 285
    adverse effects of, 78
    intravenous use of, 6
    treatment of, 78
Methapyrilene, 234
Methaqualone, 6, 19, 31, 133–34, 142,
    effects of, 133–34
    history of, 133
Methylene chloride, 94
Methylphenidate, 296
Metzger, Ralph, 206
Mexico, 217, 295
Miami Dolphins, 37, 38
Michigan, 7

Microbial contamination, 262
Microdots, 205
Microorganisms, 256
Middle age, 197
Military, drug use in, 33–34
Milk, 246, 247, 248, 256
Miltown, 134
Mind control, 206
Minerals, 243–49
Minimum-sentence law, 289
Minnesota Lipid Research Clinic, 108
Minton, John, 94
Miscarriages, and smoking, 109
Misuse of drugs, by senior citizens, 45
MKULTRA, 206
Model glue, 140, 141
Molasses, 243
Molds, 256
Monetary benefits, of quitting smoking, 116
Monoamine oxidase, 61
Monoglycerides, 269, 270
Monosodium glutamate, 275
Mood swings, 208
Moore, William, 224
Moral norms, 32
Morpheus, 177
Morphine, 177, 178, 233, 285, 287, 296
Morris, Mercury, 37–38
Morrison, Jim, 181
Motion sickness medicine, 242
Motor coordination, 222
Motor vehicle accidents, and alcohol, 158
Mouth ulcers, 141
MSG, 272
Mucosa, and absorption of nicotine, 100
Multiple sclerosis, 245
Mumps, 256
Muncie, Chuck, 38
Muscle activity, skeletal, 102
Muscle contractions, 246
Muscle cramps, 188
Muscle impulses, 203
Muscle relaxant, Librium as, 138
Muscle rigidity, 212, 261
Muscle spasms, and Valium, 135, 136
Muscle tone, 140, 309
    reduction in, 102
Muscular dysfunction, 212
Musculoskeletal injuries, 263
Mushroom poisoning, 210
Mushrooms, 12, 209
    hallucinogenic, 7
Mustard, 269
Mustard greens, 246
Myocardial infarction, 84, 105, 111, 236
Myocardium, 105
Myopia, 262
Mystical experiences, 203

Nabilone, 228
Naditch, 225
Naloxone, 24, 196
Narcolepsy, 41, 74, 76
    and amphetamines, 75
Narcotic Addict Rehabilitation Act, 291–92
Narcotic antagonists, 195–96
Narcotic Drug Control Act, 290
Narcotics. See opiates
National Addiction Rehabilitation Administration, 184, 198
National Basketball Association, 38
National Cancer Institute, 11
National Center for Drugs and Biologics, 88
National Center for Health Statistics, 40
National Clearinghouse for Drug Abuse Information, 39, 41
National Committee for the Treatment of Intractable Pain, 182
National Conference on Uniform State Laws, 217
National Council on Alcoholism, 156, 168
National Federation of Parents for Drug Free Youth, 307
National Heart, Lung, and Blood Institute, 151
National Institute on Alcohol Abuse and Alcoholism, 156, 160, 167
National Institute on Drug Abuse, 30, 83, 136
National Institute of Mental Health, 17, 87, 136, 159, 185, 186, 258, 288, 311
    study on Jamaica, 219
National Interagency Council on Smoking and Health, 123
National Transportation Safety Board, 42–43
National Youth and Polydrug Study, 31
Native American church, 18, 208, 212, 291
Native Americans, 159
Nausea, 133, 135, 136, 139, 140, 141, 169, 183, 188, 191, 207, 221, 228, 235, 238, 242, 243, 246, 247, 248, 257, 260, 261, 263, 268, 275
    from giddiness, 101
    from LSD, 203
    relief of, 227
    from sedative-hypnotics, 131
n-butyl alcohol, 146
Needle contamination, 78
Nellis, Joseph L., 301
Nerve fibers, effect of nicotine on, 102
Nerve-impulse transmitters, 260
Nerve synapses, 259
Nerve tissue, 246
Nervous disturbances, 246
Nervousness, 249
Nervous system, 235, 246. See also central nervous system
    blocked impulse transmission of, 241

and drugs, 59–61
  effect of nicotine on, 102
  parasympathetic, 65
  peripheral, 65–71
  sympathetic, 316
Netsworth, John, 79
Neuromuscular irritability, 260
Neuronal-function depression, 102
Neuron membrane, 60
Neurons, 59
Neurosis, 206
Neurotransmitters, 60, 203, 259
  endogenous, 25
  systems of, 24
New Mexico, 227
New York, 7, 206
New York Medical College, 191
New York Metropolitan Hospital Center, 192
New York, State Health Department, 266
New York University, 220, 300
Niacin, 243, 244, 247
Nicorette, 114
Nicotine, 5–6, 216
  in adult drug scene, 40
  in amniotic fluid, 109
  antigenicity of, 108
  in cigarettes, 100–101
  and coffee intake, 111
  and constriction of blood vessels, 106
  effects on cardiovascular system, 105
  and filtered cigarettes, 114
  in mother's milk, 109
  and oral contraceptives, 111
  physiological effects of, 102
  in pill form, 114
  as recreational drug, 11
  and respiratory diseases, 106
  from side-stream smoke, 121
  from smoke, 100
  and teeth discoloration, 110
Nicotine alkaloid, 100
Nicotine substitute, 114
Night blindness, 246
Nitrates, 275
Nitrites, 275
Nitrous oxide, 141, 260, 276
  in cigarette smoke, 103
  and respiratory diseases, 106
  from smoke, 100
Nixon, 288
Noncompliance, by senior citizens, 45
Nonprescription drugs, 243
Nonsmokers, death rate of, 102
  level of COHb, 103
  paying costs of smoking, 104
  rights of, 122–23
  and tobacco, 121–23
Nonsmoking sections, 123

Norepinephrine, 18, 61, 65, 83, 259, 260
  increases in, 111
North America, 216
North Carolina Council of Churches, 123
Nosebleeds, 133
Novocaine, 35, 86
Nuclei, 64
Numbness, 191, 212
  facial, 131
NutraSweet, 276, 277
Nutritional deficiencies, and alcoholism, 166
Nuts, 246, 248
Nyswander, Marie, 190

Obesity, 275
  and methamphetamine, 76
Odyssey House, 189
Office of Disease Prevention and Health Promotion, 307
Office of Drug Abuse Policy, 218
Ohio, 7
Ohio State University, 94
Olson, Frank, 206
Olympics
  drug use in, 35–37
  1984 Summer, 36
One Flew Over the Cuckoo's Nest, 19
Ontario Prenatal Mortality Study, 109
Operant conditioning, and alcoholism, 162
Ophthalmologists, and cocaine, 87
Opiate-receptor mechanism, 24
Opiate maintenance, 300–302
  future of legalized, 302
Opiates, 7–8, 198, 233, 296
  in adult drug scene, 41
  decriminalization of, 299–302
  information on, 69
  nonsynthetic, 177–83
  regulation of, 285
  synthetic, 183–84
  and tranquilizers, 140
  in Vietnam, 33
Opium, 177, 198, 295, 296
Opium addiction, 312
Optimal, 133
Oral administration, 263
Oral contraceptives, 264–67, 277
  and nicotine, 111
Oral dose, 256
Oranges, 248
Oregon, 7, 216, 217
Oregon Law, 298–99
Organic compounds, 243
O'Shaughnessy, 216
Osteoporosis, 245
Ovarian cysts, 268
Ovarian enlargement, 268

Ovaries, 267
Overdosage, 233
Overdose, 235, 238, 261
    of methadone, 183, 191
    of methaqualone, 133, 134
Overexcitement, 136
Overprescribing, 134
Oversedation, 191
Over-the-counter drugs, 231. *See also* specific medications
    development of in the U.S., 232–33
    reform of use of, 233–34
Ovulation, prevention of, 264
Owens-Illinois, 43
Oxford, 256
Oxygen consumption, 318
Oxygen debt, 169
Oxygen transportation, 103
Oxyhemoglobin bond, 103

Pain, 133, 188, 236, 265
    decreasing, 238
    indifference to, 212
    intractable, 182
    joint, 257
    muscle, 191, 248
    reduction by enkephalins, 50
    relieving during surgery, 216
Pain killers, 35, 111
Pain relief, 234, 235
    with amphetamines, 37
Paleospinothalmic pain pathway, 24–25
Pancreas, effect of caffeine on, 93
Pantothenic acid, 243, 244, 247–48
Paprika, 274
Pap smears, 266
Paralysis, 287
Paranoia, 77, 203, 210, 228
    transient mild, 225
Paraquat, 217–18
Parasympathetic nervous system, 65
Parest, 133
Parkinson's disease, 76
Patent medicines, 232, 233
Patients, and drug responsibility, 9
PCP, 19, 31, 210–12, 213
    effects of society on, 210
    information on, 70
    psychophysiological effects of, 211–12
Peanuts, 248
Pearson, Manuel M., 21
Peas, 246, 247
Pectin, 270
Peer acceptance, and alcohol, 149–50
Peer pressure, 20
Peers, 216
Pellagra, 247

Pellets, 205
Penalties, marijuana, 217
Penicillins, 256, 276
    and aspirin, 236
    interaction with other drugs, 58
Pentazocine, 111
Pentobarbital, 131, 189
People's Republic of China, 312
Pepper, 269
Pepsi Cola, 276
Peptic ulcers, 237
    activation of, 235–36
    and smoking, 108, 118
Perception, distortions in, 203
Pergonal, 267, 268
Peridontal disease, and smoking, 111
Periventricular system, 63
Personality, 64
Perspiration, 136, 187, 191
Pert, Candice B., 24
Peru, 82
Peyote. *See* mescaline
Pharmaceutical companies, 3, 134
Pharmacist, 3, 302
    and drug use by elderly, 44
Pharmacological classification of marijuana, 218
Pharmacology, 280, 303
    altered by smoking, 118
Phenmetrazine, 296
Phenobarbital, 131
Phenols, in cigarette tars, 100
Phenothiazines, 19, 139
Philadelphia Veteran's Administration Drug Dependence Treatment and Research Center, 136
Philip Morris Inc., 124
Philippines, 286
Phlegm, 106
pH level, 60, 235
Phoenix House, 189
Phosphates, 271
Phosphoric acid, 271
Phosphorus, 244, 247
Physical effects
    of amphetamines, 74–75
    of barbiturates, 132
    of Darvon, 184
    of deliriants, 141–42
    of DMSO, 263–64
    from FAS, 156
    of Librium, 138–39
    of major tranquilizers, 140
    of minor tranquilizers, 135
    of methadone, 183
    of salicylates, 235
    of sedative-hypnotics, 131
    of Valium, 136–37

Physicans, 302
and drug responsibility, 8–9
and drug use of elderly, 44
role of, 280–81
and tranquilizers, 134
and Valium, 138
Physician's Desk Reference, 8, 281
Physiological effects
of marijuana, 218–24
of methaqualone, 133–34
Physiology, 61–71
Pill, the, 264
and birth defects, 266–67
for males, 266–67
and smoking, 265–66
Pipe smokers, mortality rate of, 102
Pipe smoking, 99, 116, 119
Pittle, Stephen, 195
Pituitary gland, 25, 61, 267
Placebos, 253–55, 276
Placental barrier, 140, 183, 222, 258, 259, 275
Plant accidents, 42
Plants, and chemicals, 12
Plasma proteins, 53
Platelet aggregation, decrease in, 236
Platelet production, 250
Platelets
effect of smoking on, 105
increased adhesiveness of, 102
Pleasure center, 63
Plug, 119
Pneumonia patients, 208
Poisoning, by over-the-counter drugs, 10
Pollen, 242
Polypharmacy, 9
Polysaccharides, 240
Polysorbate 60, 270
Pork, 246
Porter Narcotic Farms Bill, 288
Post, Robert, 87
Postuse depression, from nicotine, 102
Potassium, 244
Potassium alginate, 270
Potassium bromate, 271
Potassium depletion, 235
Potassium ions, 59, 60, 71
Potatoes, 246, 247
PPA (phenylpropanolamine), 249, 250
Preaddiction state, 21
Pregnancy, 222, 240, 245
and barbiturates, 132
and methadone, 191
and smoking, 109–10
and Valium, 136
Pregnant women, 238
and antibiotics, 258
and heroin, 179
Prehistoric brain, 61

Prescription drugs, cost of, 283
Preservative, 247
Pressure, increased inside skull, 246
Price, Frank, 43
Procaine, 86
Procter and Gamble, 276
Productivity, loss through drugs, 42
Professional sports, 37–38
Progesterone, 264
Progestin, 264
Prohibition, 287
Prolixin, 19
Proof, 146
Propellants, 140
Proprietary drugs. *See* over-the-counter drugs
Propylene glycol, 270, 271
Proteins, 248
metabolism, 112
utilization of, 246
Pseudoaphrodisiac, 95
Psilocin, 12
Psilocybin 7, 12, 209–10, 212, 296
psychophysiological effects of, 209–10
Psychedelic drugs, 7
Psychiatry, experimental, 209
Psychoactive substances, 12
nicotine as, 102
reasons for use of, 15–16
Psychodrama, 171
Psychological benefit, 309
Psychological considerations, of narcotic antagonists, 196
Psychological disorders, 142
Psychological effects, 216
of alcohol, 151–57
of deliriants, 142
of LSD, 203–4
of marijuana, 224–26
of methaqualone, 133–34
of smoking, 148
Psychology, of drug users, 15–16
Psychomotor impairment
by marijuana, 222–23
by smoking, 122
Psychopathology, 197
of marijuana, 224–25
Psychophysiological effects
of antidepressants, 259–60
of LSD, 208–9
of PCP, 211–12
of psilocybin, 209–10
Psychosis, 139, 142
Psychotherapists, 207
Psychotherapy, 185
Psychotic episodes, 211, 249
Psychotic reactions, 202
Psyllium, 240
Public Health Service, 109

Public Welfare programs, 104
Pulmonary effects, of marijuana, 219–20
Pulmonary embolism, 265
Pulse, 178
Pulse rate, 139, 140, 210
Pupil dilation, 188, 203, 209
Pupils, 178
    constriction of, 183
    dilation of, 210
    pinpoint, 178
Pure Food and Drug Act, 274, 286, 289, 290
Pure Food and Drug Law, 82
Purgative oils, 240
Purification ritual, 215–16

Quaalude, 31, 133
    information on, 67
Quarterly Journal of Studies on Alcohol, 168
Quitting, 102
    behavioral programs for, 115
    benefits of, 115–16, 117–18
    company programs for, 115

Randall v. FDA, 227
Rape, 159
Raphae nuclei, 63–64
Rashes, 131, 135, 136, 139, 184, 238, 257
Rauwolfia alkaloids, 139
Ray, Oakley, 40
Reaction, adverse, 52
    of individual to drugs, 2
Reaction time, 222, 318
Reagan, Nancy, 307
Reagent, 262
Rebellion, 19
Receptor mechanisms, 51–52
Receptor, 61
Receptor site, 59, 60
Recreational drugs, 11–12
    and children, 30
Red blood cells, 110
    manufacture of, 248
    size of, 111
Red Dye No. 2, 275
Red Dye No. 4, 275
Red meats, 246
Reed, John, 4
Referral, 185
Reform, of over-the-counter drug use, 233–34
Rehabilitation services
    for alcoholics, 167–68
    for Vietnam veterans, 34
Relaxation, 227
Religion, 313–14
Religious factors, and drug use, 18
Remorse, and alcoholism, 165

REM sleep
    and barbiturates, 132
    and methaqualone, 133
Rerlman, 109
Research and development, 282
Resistance-transferring system, 257
Respiration, 178, 235
    reduced, 183
    suspension of, 139
Respiration efficiency, 309
Respiration rate, 318
Respiratory depression, 141
    from Valium, 136
Respiratory diseases, and smoking, 106–7
Respiratory infection, 245
Respiratory stimulation, from nicotine, 100
Respiratory tract, 220
    and absorption of nicotine, 100
Restlessness, 133
    from nicotine withdrawal, 102
Restorative drugs, 35
Reticular formation, 63, 139
Retina, 226
Retinal thrombosis, 265
Reye's Syndrome, 237
Rhinitis, 84
Rhinorrhea, 187
Riboflavin, 243, 244, 274
Richardson, Michael Ray, 38
Richmond, Julius, 101
Rickets, 247
Ritalin, 76, 78–81
    and hyperkinesis, 79–81
    psychological effects of, 79
    physical effects of, 79
R. J. Reynolds Tobacco Co., 124
Robinson v. California, 290
Roche Laboratories, 135
Rolliston, Humphrey, 300
Rolliston Commission, 300
Romans, 148
Roosevelt, 289
Rose hips powder, 243
Russia, 262
Rutgers University, 168

Saccharin, 273, 275, 276
Saffron, 274
Saint Elizabeth's Hospital, 211
Saint Louis Cardinals, 38
Salicylates, 81, 234–38
    physical effects of, 235
    poisoning, 40
    side effects of, 235–36
Salicylic acid, 234, 238
Salicylism, 235
Saliva, production of, 102

Salts, 240, 260, 269
Samples, free, 282
San Francisco, 206, 210
 and smoking regulations, 123
Santa Clara County Methadone Program, 193
Save a SweetHEART, 115
Schedule I, 217, 293
Schedule II, 80, 217, 293
Schedule III, 293, 294
Schedule IV, 293, 294
Schedule V, 293, 294
Schedules, 292
Schirren, Carl, 110
Schizophrenia, 207
 and enkephalins, 50
 and tranquilizers, 139
Schnacker, Robert, 80
School dances, 30
Schredorf and Ivy, 108
Schultz, Johannes, 314
Scurvy, 247
Secobarbital, 131
Seconal, 19
Sedation, 140, 141, 184
Sedative-hypnotics, 130–34, 231
 in drug scene, 39
 information on, 67
 physical effects of, 131
Sedatives, 6, 218, 227, 240
 smoking as, 113
Seizures, 211
 from clove oil, 120
 grand mal, 137
 lowering of threshold, 259
Select Committee on Narcotics Control, 301
Selective cultivation, 216
Self-awareness, disturbed, 224
Self-fulfillment, 32
Self-help programs, for alcoholics, 170
Self-medication, 231, 233
 by elderly, 45
Semipermeable, 60
Senate Health Subcommittee, 295
Senate hearings, 74
Senility, 76, 139
Sensation seeking, 16–18
Sense of smell, 120
Sense of taste, 120
Senses, 153
Sensitivity, increased, 259
Sensory deprivation research, 17
Sensory distraction, 224
Sensory information, regulation of, 203
Sensory perception, 208
Sepsis, 299
Serotonin, 18, 61, 63, 203
Serum cholesterol levels, 108
Serum hepatitis, 78

Serum triglycerides, rise in, 108
Set, 3
Seven Up, 276
Sex
 and alcohol, 150–51
 and drug activity, 53
Sex drive, 139
Sex roles, and alcohol, 150
Sexual activity, and smoking, 110
Sexual behavior, 61
Sexual deviancy, treatment of, 206
Sexual drugs, 86
Shaffer Commission, 219
Shakespeare, 150
Shanghai International Conference, 286
Shapiro, Harvey, 132
Shellfish, 246
Shell Oil Company, 43
Shen-Nung, 215
Shilgin, Alexander, 16
Side effects, 52, 210
 of antibiotics, 257
 of antihistamines, 242
 of codeine, 183
 of deliriants, 141
 of DMSO, 263
 of fertility pills, 268
 of heroin, 182
 of methadone, 191–92
 of minor tranquilizers, 135
 of nitrous oxide, 260
 of oral contraceptives, 265–66
 of over-the-counter drugs, 10
 of PPA, 249
 of salicylates, 235–36
 of sedative-hypnotics, 131
 of tobacco, 107–12
 of Valium, 136
Silicon dioxide, 272
Silver, Walter, 93
Silvette, 108
Simmons, Henry, 283
Sineoff, 249
Sinequan, 19
Skeletal muscles, and caffeine, 93
Skin, and absorption of nicotine, 100
Skin rash, 55
Skin responses, galvanic, 318
Skin tumors, 119
Sleep, 178
 light, 64
 promotion with methaqualone, 133
Sleep disturbances, 135
Sleeping aids, 234
Sleeping pills, 37
Sleeplessness, 248
Sleep-walking cycle, 61
Sloan-Kettering Cancer Center, 182

Slurred speech, 136
Small-group support, 188–89
Small intestine, 240
Smith, David E., 138
Smith, Lonnie, 38
Smith, Robert, 79
Smith, Kline, and French, 74
Smoke
    absorbed into body, 101
    cigarette, 100
    and gastrointestinal disturbances, 108
    mainstream, 121
    not inhaled, 119
    side-stream, 121
Smokeless tobacco, harmful effects of, 120
Smokers
    types of, 113
    women, 112
Smoker's cough, 100, 106
Smoking
    addictive, 113
    alternatives to, 114
    of cannabis, 215
    cigar, 116, 119
    as habit, 112
    harmful effects of, 101–2
    and metabolism, 107–8
    pipe, 116, 119
    quitting, 115–21
    reasons for and against, 112–13
    as sedative, 113
    as stimulant, 113
    and taking Pill, 265–66
Sneezing, 242
Snell Laboratories, 114
Snuff, and nicotine, 100
Snuff dipping, 119–20
Snyder, Solomon H., 24, 25, 26
Social environment, and alcoholism, 166
Social facilitation, 16
Social forces, and smoking, 112
Social-political activism, 312–13
Society
    effects of alcohol on, 157–59
    effects of PCP on, 210–11
    and LSD, 204–6
    and marijuana, 225–26
Sociological factors, and drug use, 20
Sociology, of drug users, 15–16
Sodium acetate, 271
Sodium alginate, 270
Sodium citrate, 271
Sodium ions, 59, 60
Sodium propionate, 269
Sodium, salicylate, 234, 238
Sodium stearyl fumarate, 271
Soft drinks, and caffeine, 87
Softron, 134

Solvent, 262, 263
Soma, 59, 134
Sometimes a Great Notion, 19
Somnafac, 133
Sopor, 133
Sorbitan monostearate, 270
Sorbitol, 271
Sorority initiations, 20
South Africa, 227
Southeast Asia, 295
Soybeans, 246
Spatial images, 65
Speech, impaired, 212
Speed, 31
    use in junior high, 30
Speed freak, 77
Speed increase, through amphetamines, 37
Sperm counts, 266
    low, 222
Sperm motility, disturbance of, 110
Sperm production, impaired, 266
Spices, 272
Spinach, 247
Spinal cord
    degeneration of, 246
    effect of nicotine on, 102
    upper, 235
Spleen, 183
Sports idols, and smokeless tobacco, 119
Sprains, 262
Spray cans, 141
Squires, 120
Stabilizers, 269
Stammering, 136
Stanford University, 301
Stanford University Law School, 302
Stanford University School of Medicine, 24
Staphylococci, 256, 257
State University of New York at Buffalo,
    206
Steiner, Claude, 160
Sternbach, Leo, 135
Steroids, 35, 36
Stevenson, Robert Louis, 82
Stewart, 180
Stillbirth, and smoking, 109, 118
Stimulant, 100, 218, 296
    information on, 66
    smoking as, 113
    use of, 6
Stimuli, sorting of, 139
Stomach, 235, 237
Strauss, M. E., 192
Strawberries, 246
Street acid market, 205
Street drugs, 3
Street market, and methadone, 194
Streptomycins, 256, 258, 276

Stress, 5
  coping with, 216
Stress clinics, 133
Strokes, 236, 265
  after smoking, 106
Students Against Driving Drunk (SADD), 172
Stupor, 141, 178
Suavitil, 134
Subarachnoid hemorrhage, 111
Subcutaneous administration, 263
Sucrose, 273
Sudden infant death syndrome (SIDS), 109
Sugar, 269, 275
  in cocaine, 85
Sugar cubes, 205
Suicidal tendencies, 258
Suicide, 258
  and alcohol, 159
Superinfections, 257
Supreme Court, 186, 288
Surgeon General's Report
  1964, 100, 220
  1979, 101–2, 111
  1983, 105
  1984, 107
Swami Brahamanda Saraswati, 316
Sweating, 135, 138, 183, 212, 238, 259, 260, 275
Sweden, 126
Sweeteners, nutritive, 273
Sydney Farber Cancer Institute, 227
Sympathetic nervous system, 65, 203
  hyperactivity of, 105
Sympathomimetics, 73
Synapses, 59, 60
Synar, Mike, 120
Synergism, 181, 249
  of Valium, 136–37
Synergistic effect, of alcohol and barbiturates, 132
Snyergistic response, 55
Synesthesia, 203, 208
Szasz, Thomas, 300

Tachycardia, 228, 249
Tagetes, 274
Tarahumara Indians, 18
Tardive dyskinesia, 140
Tars
  and respiratory diseases, 106
  from side-stream smoke, 121
  from smoke, 100
Tartaric acid, 271
Tartrates, 271
Tashkin, Donald P., 220
Taste, unpleasant, 255
Taste-bud sensitivity, 108

Taylor, Norman, 178
Tea, 240
  and caffeine, 87
  history of, 90
Teenager-parent contract, 172
Temperature, body, 61
Temperature, of skin, 102
Tendon reflex, deep, 210
Terenius, Lars, 25
Terminals, 59, 60
Testes, 266
Testosterone, 35, 309
  and alcohol, 150, 157
  impaired production of, 110
Tetanus, 227
Tetracyclines, 256, 276
  interaction with other drugs, 58
Tetrahydraisoquardrelone, 161
Texas Lutheran College, 120
Tetrahydrocannabinol, 210, 218, 219, 222, 225, 226, 227
Thalidomide, 3, 290
Theobroma tree, 90
Theophylline, 111
Therapeutic approaches, to drug problems, 188–90
Therapeutic communities, 189–90
Therapeutic effectiveness, of aspirin, 236–37
Therapy, aid to, 206
Thiamine, 243, 244
Thickeners, 269
Thiopental, 131, 132
Thioxanthines, 139
Thirst, 61, 136, 275
Thompson, David, 38
Thrombophlebitis, 78, 265
Thrombosis, 245
Tingling sensations, 210
Tinnitus, 235
Tiredness, 261
Tissue bleeding, 235
Tissue repair, 246
Titanium dioxide, 274
Toasted cottonseed flour, 273
Tobacco, 5–6
  and alcohol, 156
  and appetite reduction, 108
  and cancer, 107
  chemistry of, 100–101
  chewing, 99
  and chronic disease, 103–7
  and exercise, 110
  and health factors, 111
  and medication effectiveness, 111
  and nonsmoker, 121–23
  and peridontal disease, 111
  physiological effects of, 102–3
  and pregnancy, 109–10

Tobacco (*cont.*)
  psychological effects of, 112–13
  and respiratory diseases, 106–7
  and sexual activity, 110
  side effects of, 107–12
  smokeless, 119–20
  and strokes, 106
  and vitamins, 111–12
Tobacco companies, 112
  diversification of, 123–25
Tobacco industry
  advertising by, 119
  opposition to laws on smoking, 123
Tolerance
  to alcohol, 160, 163
  of amphetamines, 75
  and barbiturates, 132
  of cocaine, 85
  for heroin, 179
  to Librium, 139
  to marijuana, 224
  of methamphetamine, 76
  of methaqualone, 134
  of minor tranquilizers, 135
  to nicotine, 102
  of opiates, 178
  to PCP, 211
  potential for, 55
  and Valium, 138
Tomatoes, 246
Tongue
  changes in, 133
  swelling, 140
Topical administration, 263
Toxicity, 236, 261
  drug, 233
  of elements in smoke, 100
Toxicology, of aspirin, 237–38
Toxic reactions, to penicillin, 256
Toxic Substances Act, 11
Trachea, swelling of, 110
Tracks, 178
Trafficking, criminal penalties for, 294–95
Tranquilizers, 9, 142, 242, 260, 285, 296
  in adult drug scene, 39
  and alcoholism, 169
  animal, 210, 213
  information on, 68
  interaction with other drugs, 56, 57
  major, 139–40
  minor, 134–39
  as muscle relaxants, 35
Transcendental meditation (TM), 316, 317, 318
Transmitters, 61
Transport mechanisms, of drugs, 52
Treasury Department, 288
Treatment approaches
  to alcoholism, 169–71
  for opiates, 197–98

Treatment milieu, 159
Tremors, 138, 139, 188, 209, 259, 260, 261
  from LSD, 203
Trichloroethylene, 94
Trip, 203
Turkey, 295
Turmeric, 274
Turnip greens, 246
Twins, 166
Tylenol, 238
Typewriter correction fluid, 8

UCLA, 227, 318
Ulcers
  corneal, 245
  peptic, 108, 118, 235–36, 237
  stress, 245
Ultramarine Blue, 273
Ultraviolet rays, 247
Unconsciousness, 141, 260
Underleider, J. Thomas, 219
Uniform Narcotic Drug Act, 217
University of Aberdeen, 25
University of California at Davis, 310
University of California at Los Angeles, 36
University of Chicago, 315
University of Kentucky, 197
University of Oregon Health Science Center, 262
University of Pittsburgh, 103
University of Uppsala, 25
University of Virginia, 310
Upset stomach, 135
Urban ghetto, 22
Urinalysis, 186
Urinary retention, 259
Urinating, difficulty, 243
Urination, 191
  excessive, 247
  increased, 268
Urine, 219
  increase in, 155
  pH of, 101
  sample of, 192
Uterus, arteries in, 109
U. S. Army, 34, 226
U.S. Center for Population Research, 265
U. S. Public Health Service Hospital, 187, 197
U. S. Tobacco Company, 125

Vaccines and smoking, 111
Valium, 6, 19, 131, 134, 135–38
  dependence on, 137–38
  history of, 135–36
  physical effects of, 136–37
  in senior citizens, 44
  withdrawal from, 137–38

Vanilla, 272
Vasodilation, 242
Vasomotor collapse, from nicotine, 101
Vegetable colors, 269
Vegetable gums, 270
Vegetable juice, 273
Vegetable oils, 247
Vegetables, 247, 248
Vegetarians, 246
Vertigo, 257
Vesicles, 60
Vick's Day Care, 249
Victimless crime, 284
Vietnam, and drugs, 33–34
Violence, 261
Violent behavior, 211, 212
Viral infections, 256
Viruses, 242
Vision, 203, 268
  blurred, 131, 135, 212, 243, 259
Visual distortion, 208
Visual perception, 222
Vitamins, 29, 231, 243–49
  mega madness, 248–49
  misconceptions, 248
  and smoking, 111–12
  specific use of, 244–45
  vitamin A, 243, 244, 245–46
  vitamin B_1, 245, 246
  vitamin B_6, 243, 244, 245, 246
  vitamin B_{12}, 111, 243, 244, 246
  vitamin C, 111, 236, 243, 244, 245, 246
  vitamin D, 243, 244, 245, 247
  vitamin E, 243, 244, 247
  vitamin K, 243, 244, 247
Vocal cords, 141
Vocational training, 185
Volatile substances, 8, 142. *See also* deliriants
Volunteer-run organizations, 168
Vomiting, 131, 135, 139, 140, 141, 169, 183, 188, 191, 207, 221, 228, 235, 238, 243, 246, 257, 260, 261, 268
  from nicotine, 101
  relief of, 227

Wallace, Robert, 318
Walnut Creek study, 111
Warnings, on cigarette packages, 104
Warts, 227, 245
Washington, Claudell, 38
Washington, D. C., 211
Washington University National Alcohol Research Center, 150
Waxman Bill, 182
Wayland High School, 172
Weakness, 238, 242, 247
Weed control, 218

Weg, Ruth, 44
Weight gain, 107, 140, 191, 265, 268
Weight loss, 188, 246, 247
  through amphetamines, 37
Weil, Andrew, 1, 306, 307
Wernicky's disorder, 163
Wheat germ, 243
Whelan, Elizabeth, 103
White blood cells, 103, 111
Wilderness experiences, 311
Windowpanes, 205
Wine, 146, 259
Withdrawal, 55, 187
  from alcohol, 160
  from barbiturates, 132
  easing of, 227
  from methadone, 183
  from methaqualone, 134
  from sedative-hypnotics, 131
  from Valium, 137–38
Withdrawal symptoms, 26
  of heroin, 179
  of minor tranquilizers, 135
  from nicotine, 102–3
Withdrawal syndrome and amphetamines, 75
Women
  and alcohol, 150, 166–67
  and cocaine, 81
  and lung cancer, 102, 107
  pregnant, and barbiturates, 132
  and smoking, 112
  and Valium, 136
Women's Temperance Union, 287
Work, 312
Workplace, drugs, in, 41–43
World Health Organization, 219
World War I, and smoking, 112

Xanthines, 87, 92. *See also* caffeine
Xylocaine, 86

Yankelovich, Daniel, 32
Yawning, 187
Yeast, 270
Yeast infections, 265
Yeast-malt sprout extract, 272
Yellow prussiate of soda, 272
Yolles, Stanley, 186
Young, Rickey, 38
Young user, and narcotic antagonists, 196
Youth, and alcohol, 146–47

Zelson, Carl, 191
Zinc, 244
Zuckerman, Marvin, 17